LIST OF LOW CARB FOODS

Copyrights:

No part of the materials available through this book (except for personal use) may be copied, photocopied, reproduced, translated or reduced to any electronic medium or machine-readable form, in whole or in part, without prior written consent of the publisher.

Disclaimer

The information contained in this book should be used aa a reference only, and it is not intended to give any medical advice.

How to use this list

This is the extensive list of foods with their carb content.

The list is organized by alphabet, so yiu can use it as you use a normal dictionary to find out if a food is low, medium or high in carbs.

Every food that has a carb count **less than 50 g** per 100 g (1 serving) it is considered **low in carbs**.

Every food that has a carb count **between 51 g and 57 g** per 100 g (1 serving) it is considered **medium in carbs.**

Every food that has a carb count **greater than 57** g per 100 g (1 serving) it is considered **high in carbs**.

If you follow a low carb diet, then you should not consume more than 150 g of carbs per day

If you follow a keto diet, then you should not consume more than 57 g of carbs per day.

Left blank

Food name/ Category (100 g)	Status	Carbs content in g
Acerola juice, raw",	LOW	4.8
Alcoholic beverage, beer, light, BUD LIGHT",	LOW	1.3
Alcoholic beverage, beer, light, BUDWEISER SELECT",	LOW	0.87
Alcoholic beverage, beer, light, higher alcohol",	LOW	0.77
Alcoholic beverage, beer, light, low carb",	LOW	0.73
Alcoholic beverage, beer, light",	LOW	1.64
Alcoholic beverage, beer, regular, all",	LOW	3.55
Alcoholic beverage, beer, regular, BUDWEISER",	LOW	2.97
Alcoholic beverage, creme de menthe, 72 proof",	MEDIUM	41.6
Alcoholic beverage, daiquiri, canned",	LOW	15.7
Alcoholic beverage, daiquiri, prepared-from-recipe",	LOW	6.94
Alcoholic beverage, distilled, all (gin, rum, vodka, whiskey) 100 proof",	LOW	0
Alcoholic beverage, distilled, all (gin, rum, vodka, whiskey) 80 proof",	LOW	0
Alcoholic beverage, distilled, all (gin, rum, vodka, whiskey) 86 proof",	LOW	0.1
Alcoholic beverage, distilled, all (gin, rum, vodka, whiskey) 90 proof",	LOW	0
Alcoholic beverage, distilled, all (gin, rum, vodka, whiskey) 94 proof",	LOW	0
Alcoholic beverage, distilled, gin, 90 proof",	LOW	0
Alcoholic beverage, distilled, rum, 80 proof",	LOW	0
Alcoholic beverage, distilled, vodka, 80 proof",	LOW	0
Alcoholic beverage, distilled, whiskey, 86 proof",	LOW	0.1
Alcoholic beverage, liqueur, coffee with cream, 34 proof",	LOW	20.9
Alcoholic beverage, malt beer, hard lemonade",	LOW	10.07
Alcoholic beverage, pina colada, canned",	LOW	27.6
Alcoholic beverage, rice (sake)",	LOW	5
Alcoholic beverage, tequila sunrise, canned",	LOW	11.3
Alcoholic beverage, whiskey sour, canned",	LOW	13.4
Alcoholic beverage, whiskey sour, prepared from item 14028",	LOW	12.82
Alcoholic beverage, whiskey sour, prepared with water, whiskey and powder mix",	LOW	15.85

Food name/ Category (100 g)	Status	Carbs content in g
Alcoholic beverage, wine, cooking",	LOW	6.3
Alcoholic beverage, wine, table, all",	LOW	2.72
Alcoholic Beverage, wine, table, red, Merlot",	LOW	2.51
Alcoholic beverage, wine, table, red",	LOW	2.61
Alcoholic beverage, wine, table, white, Chardonnay",	LOW	2.16
Alcoholic beverage, wine, table, white",	LOW	2.6
Alcoholic beverages, beer, higher alcohol",	LOW	0.27
Alcoholic beverages, wine, rose",	LOW	3.8
Amaranth grain, uncooked",	HIGH	65.25
Amaranth leaves, cooked, boiled, drained, with salt",	LOW	4.11
ANDREA'S, Gluten Free Soft Dinner Roll",	MEDIUM	40.24
Apple juice, canned or bottled, unsweetened, with added ascorbic acid, calcium, and potassium",	LOW	11.49
Apple juice, canned or bottled, unsweetened, with added ascorbic acid",	LOW	11.3
Apple juice, canned or bottled, unsweetened, without added ascorbic acid",	LOW	11.3
APPLEBEE'S, 9 oz house sirloin steak",	LOW	0
APPLEBEE'S, chicken tenders platter",	LOW	17.98
APPLEBEE'S, chicken tenders, from kids' menu",	LOW	18.36
APPLEBEE'S, chili",	LOW	4.57
APPLEBEE'S, coleslaw",	LOW	13.17
APPLEBEE'S, crunchy onion rings",	MEDIUM	40.17
APPLEBEE'S, Double Crunch Shrimp",	LOW	25.96
APPLEBEE'S, fish, hand battered",	LOW	16.65
APPLEBEE'S, french fries",	LOW	39.5
APPLEBEE'S, KRAFT, Macaroni & Cheese, from kid's menu",	LOW	21.08
APPLEBEE'S, mozzarella sticks",	LOW	22.87
Apples, canned, sweetened, sliced, drained, heated",	LOW	16.84
Apples, canned, sweetened, sliced, drained, unheated",	LOW	16.7
Apples, dehydrated (low moisture), sulfured, uncooked",	HIGH	93.53
Apples, dried, sulfured, uncooked",	HIGH	65.89
Apples, frozen, unsweetened, heated",	LOW	12

Food name/ Category (100 g)	Status	Carbs content in g
Apples, frozen, unsweetened, unheated",	LOW	12.31
Apples, raw, fuji, with skin",	LOW	15.22
Apples, raw, gala, with skin",	LOW	13.68
Apples, raw, golden delicious, with skin",	LOW	13.6
Apples, raw, granny smith, with skin",	LOW	13.61
Apples, raw, red delicious, with skin",	LOW	14.06
Apples, raw, with skin",	LOW	13.81
Apples, raw, without skin, cooked, boiled",	LOW	13.64
Apples, raw, without skin, cooked, microwave",	LOW	14.41
Apples, raw, without skin",	LOW	12.76
Applesauce, canned, sweetened, without salt (includes USDA commodity)",	LOW	17.49
Applesauce, canned, unsweetened, with added ascorbic acid",	LOW	11.27
Applesauce, canned, unsweetened, without added ascorbic acid (includes USDA commodity)",	LOW	11.27
Apricot nectar, canned, with added ascorbic acid",	LOW	14.39
Apricot nectar, canned, without added ascorbic acid",	LOW	14.39
Apricots, canned, extra light syrup pack, with skin, solids and liquids",	LOW	12.5
Apricots, canned, heavy syrup pack, with skin, solids and liquids",	LOW	21.47
Apricots, canned, heavy syrup, drained",	LOW	21.31
Apricots, canned, juice pack, with skin, solids and liquids",	LOW	12.34
Apricots, canned, light syrup pack, with skin, solids and liquids",	LOW	16.49
Apricots, canned, water pack, with skin, solids and liquids",	LOW	6.39
Apricots, dehydrated (low-moisture), sulfured, stewed",	LOW	32.62
Apricots, dried, sulfured, stewed, with added sugar",	LOW	29.26
Apricots, dried, sulfured, stewed, without added sugar",	LOW	22.15
Apricots, frozen, sweetened",	LOW	25.1
Apricots, raw",	LOW	11.12
ARBY'S, roast beef sandwich, classic",	LOW	22.21
ARCHWAY Home Style Cookies, Chocolate Chip Ice Box",	HIGH	65.02
ARCHWAY Home Style Cookies, Coconut Macaroon",	HIGH	61.23

Food name/ Category (100 g)	Status	Carbs content in g
ARCHWAY Home Style Cookies, Date Filled Oatmeal",	HIGH	68.16
ARCHWAY Home Style Cookies, Dutch Cocoa",	HIGH	69.44
ARCHWAY Home Style Cookies, Frosty Lemon",	HIGH	64.78
ARCHWAY Home Style Cookies, Iced Molasses",	HIGH	69.12
ARCHWAY Home Style Cookies, Iced Oatmeal",	HIGH	66.76
ARCHWAY Home Style Cookies, Molasses",	HIGH	69.41
ARCHWAY Home Style Cookies, Oatmeal Raisin",	HIGH	69.27
ARCHWAY Home Style Cookies, Oatmeal",	HIGH	68.17
ARCHWAY Home Style Cookies, Old Fashioned Molasses",	HIGH	70.55
ARCHWAY Home Style Cookies, Old Fashioned Windmill Cookies",	HIGH	72.23
ARCHWAY Home Style Cookies, Peanut Butter",	HIGH	58.48
ARCHWAY Home Style Cookies, Raspberry Filled",	HIGH	65.92
ARCHWAY Home Style Cookies, Reduced Fat Ginger Snaps",	HIGH	76.23
ARCHWAY Home Style Cookies, Strawberry Filled",	HIGH	65.92
ARCHWAY Home Style Cookies, Sugar Free Oatmeal",	HIGH	67.2
Arrowhead, cooked, boiled, drained, with salt",	LOW	16.14
Arrowroot flour",	HIGH	88.15
Artichokes, (globe or french), cooked, boiled, drained, with salt",	LOW	11.39
Artichokes, (globe or french), cooked, boiled, drained, without salt",	LOW	11.95
Artichokes, (globe or french), frozen, cooked, boiled, drained, with salt",	LOW	9.18
Artichokes, (globe or french), frozen, cooked, boiled, drained, without salt",	LOW	9.18
Artichokes, (globe or french), frozen, unprepared",	LOW	7.75
Artichokes, (globe or french), raw",	LOW	10.51
Artificial Blueberry Muffin Mix, dry",	HIGH	77.45
Asparagus, canned, drained solids",	LOW	2.46
Asparagus, canned, regular pack, solids and liquids",	LOW	2.48
Asparagus, cooked, boiled, drained, with salt",	LOW	4.11
Asparagus, frozen, cooked, boiled, drained, with salt",	LOW	1.92
Asparagus, frozen, cooked, boiled, drained, without salt",	LOW	1.92
Asparagus, raw",	LOW	3.88
AUSTIN, Cheddar Cheese on Cheese Crackers, sandwich-type, reduced fat",	HIGH	68
AUSTIN, Cheddar Cheese on Cheese Crackers, sandwich-type",	HIGH	60
AUSTIN, Cheddar Cheese on Wafer Crackers, sandwich-type",	HIGH	62.6
AUSTIN, Cheddar Cheese on Wheat Crackers, sandwich-type",	HIGH	61.4
AUSTIN, Chocolatey Peanut Butter Crackers, sandwich-type",	HIGH	66.2
AUSTIN, Grilled Cheese on Wafer Crackers, sandwich-type",	HIGH	62
AUSTIN, PB & J Crackers, sandwich-type",	HIGH	65.7
AUSTIN, Peanut Butter on Cheese Crackers, sandwich-type, reduced fat",	HIGH	66.3
AUSTIN, Peanut Butter on Cheese Crackers, sandwich-type",	HIGH	59
AUSTIN, Peanut Butter on Toasty Crackers, sandwich-type, reduced fat",	HIGH	67.2
AUSTIN, Peanut Butter on Toasty Crackers, sandwich-type",	HIGH	60.2
Avocados, raw, Florida",	LOW	7.82

Food name/ Category (100 g)	Status	Carbs content in g
Babyfood, apple-banana juice",	LOW	12.3
Babyfood, apple-cranberry juice",	LOW	11.49
Babyfood, Baby MUM MUM Rice Biscuits",	HIGH	83.21
Babyfood, baked product, finger snacks cereal fortified",	HIGH	76.68
Babyfood, banana juice with low fat yogurt",	LOW	17.54
Babyfood, banana no tapioca, strained",	LOW	21.34
Babyfood, banana with mixed berries, strained",	LOW	21.31
Babyfood, carrots and beef, strained",	LOW	5.7
Babyfood, carrots, toddler",	LOW	5.23
Babyfood, cereal, barley, prepared with whole milk",	LOW	9.94
Babyfood, cereal, high protein, prepared with whole milk",	LOW	11.6
Babyfood, cereal, high protein, with apple and orange, dry",	HIGH	57.6
Babyfood, cereal, high protein, with apple and orange, prepared with whole milk",	LOW	13.4
Babyfood, cereal, mixed, dry fortified",	HIGH	73.4
Babyfood, cereal, mixed, prepared with whole milk",	LOW	12.3
Babyfood, cereal, mixed, with applesauce and bananas, junior, fortified",	LOW	18.4
Babyfood, cereal, mixed, with applesauce and bananas, strained",	LOW	18
Babyfood, cereal, mixed, with bananas, dry",	HIGH	77.1
Babyfood, cereal, mixed, with bananas, prepared with whole milk",	LOW	10
Babyfood, cereal, mixed, with honey, prepared with whole milk",	LOW	15.9
Babyfood, cereal, oatmeal, prepared with whole milk",	LOW	15.3
Babyfood, cereal, oatmeal, with applesauce and bananas, junior, fortified",	LOW	15.8
Babyfood, cereal, oatmeal, with applesauce and bananas, strained",	LOW	15.4
Babyfood, cereal, oatmeal, with bananas, prepared with whole milk",	LOW	10
Babyfood, cereal, oatmeal, with honey, dry",	HIGH	69.3
Babyfood, cereal, oatmeal, with honey, prepared with whole milk",	LOW	15.3
Babyfood, cereal, rice with pears and apple, dry, instant fortified",	HIGH	88.5
Babyfood, cereal, rice, prepared with whole milk",	LOW	10.31
Babyfood, cereal, rice, with applesauce and bananas, strained",	LOW	17.1
Babyfood, cereal, rice, with bananas, dry",	HIGH	79.9
Babyfood, cereal, rice, with bananas, prepared with whole milk",	LOW	10.49
Babyfood, cereal, rice, with honey, prepared with whole milk",	LOW	17.1

Food name/ Category (100 g)	Status	Carbs content in g
Babyfood, cereal, with eggs, strained",	LOW	8
Babyfood, cherry cobbler, junior",	LOW	19.2
Babyfood, cookies, arrowroot",	HIGH	75.4
Babyfood, cookies",	HIGH	67.1
Babyfood, crackers, vegetable",	HIGH	66.85
Babyfood, dessert, banana pudding, strained",	LOW	14.14
Babyfood, dessert, cherry vanilla pudding, junior",	LOW	18.4
Babyfood, dessert, cherry vanilla pudding, strained",	LOW	17.8
Babyfood, dessert, custard pudding, vanilla, strained",	LOW	16
Babyfood, dessert, dutch apple, junior",	LOW	19.18
Babyfood, dessert, dutch apple, strained",	LOW	19.74
Babyfood, dessert, fruit dessert, without ascorbic acid, junior",	LOW	17.2
Babyfood, dessert, fruit dessert, without ascorbic acid, strained",	LOW	16
Babyfood, dessert, fruit pudding, pineapple, strained",	LOW	20.3
Babyfood, dessert, peach cobbler, junior",	LOW	18.3
Babyfood, dinner, beef lasagna, toddler",	LOW	10
Babyfood, dinner, beef stew, toddler",	LOW	5.5
Babyfood, dinner, beef with vegetables",	LOW	6.36
Babyfood, dinner, chicken and noodle with vegetables, toddler",	LOW	8.89
Babyfood, dinner, chicken noodle, strained",	LOW	9.08
Babyfood, dinner, macaroni and cheese, junior",	LOW	8.2
Babyfood, dinner, macaroni and cheese, strained",	LOW	8.95
Babyfood, dinner, macaroni and tomato and beef, strained",	LOW	9.45
Babyfood, dinner, mixed vegetable, junior",	LOW	7.88
Babyfood, dinner, mixed vegetable, strained",	LOW	9.5
Babyfood, dinner, spaghetti and tomato and meat, toddler",	LOW	10.8
Babyfood, dinner, turkey, rice, and vegetables, toddler",	LOW	7.5
Babyfood, dinner, vegetables and dumplings and beef, junior",	LOW	8
Babyfood, dinner, vegetables and dumplings and beef, strained",	LOW	7.7

Food name/ Category (100 g)	Status	Carbs content in g
Babyfood, dinner, vegetables and turkey, junior",	LOW	7.55
Babyfood, fortified cereal bar, fruit filling",	HIGH	68.63
Babyfood, fruit and vegetable, apple and sweet potato",	LOW	15.3
Babyfood, fruit dessert, mango with tapioca",	LOW	19
Babyfood, fruit supreme dessert",	LOW	17.18
Babyfood, fruit, apple and blueberry, junior",	LOW	16.6
Babyfood, fruit, apple and blueberry, strained",	LOW	16.3
Babyfood, fruit, apple and raspberry, junior",	LOW	15.4
Babyfood, fruit, apple and raspberry, strained",	LOW	15.6
Babyfood, fruit, applesauce and apricots, junior",	LOW	12.4
Babyfood, fruit, applesauce and apricots, strained",	LOW	11.64
Babyfood, fruit, applesauce and cherries, junior",	LOW	14.1
Babyfood, fruit, applesauce and cherries, strained",	LOW	14.1
Babyfood, fruit, applesauce and pineapple, junior",	LOW	10.5
Babyfood, fruit, applesauce and pineapple, strained",	LOW	10.1
Babyfood, fruit, applesauce with banana, junior",	LOW	16.16
Babyfood, fruit, applesauce, junior",	LOW	10.3
Babyfood, fruit, applesauce, strained",	LOW	10.8
Babyfood, fruit, apricot with tapioca, junior",	LOW	17.3
Babyfood, fruit, apricot with tapioca, strained",	LOW	16.3
Babyfood, fruit, banana and strawberry, junior",	LOW	25.78
Babyfood, fruit, bananas and pineapple with tapioca, junior",	LOW	18.4
Babyfood, fruit, bananas and pineapple with tapioca, strained",	LOW	17.8
Babyfood, fruit, bananas with apples and pears, strained",	LOW	19.31
Babyfood, fruit, bananas with tapioca, junior",	LOW	17.8
Babyfood, fruit, bananas with tapioca, strained",	LOW	15.3
Babyfood, fruit, guava and papaya with tapioca, strained",	LOW	17
Babyfood, fruit, papaya and applesauce with tapioca, strained",	LOW	18.9

Food name/ Category (100 g)	Status	Carbs content in g
Babyfood, fruit, peaches, junior",	LOW	14.48
Babyfood, fruit, peaches, strained",	LOW	14.48
Babyfood, fruit, pears and pineapple, junior",	LOW	11.4
Babyfood, fruit, pears and pineapple, strained",	LOW	10.9
Babyfood, fruit, pears, junior",	LOW	11.6
Babyfood, fruit, pears, strained",	LOW	10.8
Babyfood, fruit, plums with tapioca, without ascorbic acid, junior",	LOW	20.5
Babyfood, fruit, plums with tapioca, without ascorbic acid, strained",	LOW	19.7
Babyfood, fruit, prunes with tapioca, without ascorbic acid, junior",	LOW	18.7
Babyfood, fruit, prunes with tapioca, without ascorbic acid, strained",	LOW	18.5
Babyfood, green beans, dices, toddler",	LOW	5.7
Babyfood, juice treats, fruit medley, toddler",	HIGH	86.68
Babyfood, juice, apple - cherry",	LOW	11.2
Babyfood, juice, apple and cherry",	LOW	9.9
Babyfood, juice, apple and grape",	LOW	11.34
Babyfood, juice, apple and peach",	LOW	10.5
Babyfood, juice, apple and plum",	LOW	12.3
Babyfood, juice, apple-sweet potato",	LOW	11.4
Babyfood, juice, apple, with calcium",	LOW	11.1
Babyfood, juice, fruit punch, with calcium",	LOW	12.7
Babyfood, juice, orange and apple and banana",	LOW	11.5
Babyfood, juice, orange and apple",	LOW	10.1
Babyfood, juice, orange and banana",	LOW	11.9
Babyfood, juice, orange and pineapple",	LOW	11.7
Babyfood, juice, orange",	LOW	10.2
Babyfood, juice, prune and orange",	LOW	16.8
Babyfood, macaroni and cheese, toddler",	LOW	11.2
Babyfood, mashed cheddar potatoes and broccoli, toddlers",	LOW	7.47

Food name/ Category (100 g)	Status	Carbs content in g
Babyfood, meat, beef, junior",	LOW	2.43
Babyfood, meat, beef, strained",	LOW	2.43
Babyfood, meat, chicken sticks, junior",	LOW	1.5
Babyfood, meat, chicken, junior",	LOW	0
Babyfood, meat, chicken, strained",	LOW	0.1
Babyfood, meat, lamb, junior",	LOW	0
Babyfood, meat, lamb, strained",	LOW	0.85
Babyfood, meat, meat sticks, junior",	LOW	1.1
Babyfood, meat, turkey sticks, junior",	LOW	1.4
Babyfood, meat, turkey, junior",	LOW	1.4
Babyfood, meat, turkey, strained",	LOW	1.4
Babyfood, meat, veal, strained",	LOW	1.51
Babyfood, mixed fruit juice with low fat yogurt",	LOW	14.68
Babyfood, oatmeal cereal with fruit, dry, instant, toddler fortified",	HIGH	74.1
Babyfood, peas, dices, toddler",	LOW	10.3
Babyfood, plums, bananas and rice, strained",	LOW	12.7
Babyfood, potatoes, toddler",	LOW	11.73
Babyfood, pretzels",	HIGH	82.2
Babyfood, prunes, without vitamin c, strained",	LOW	23.52
Babyfood, ravioli, cheese filled, with tomato sauce",	LOW	16.3
Babyfood, Snack, GERBER, GRADUATES, LIL CRUNCHIES, baked whole grain c	HIGH	61.59
Babyfood, snack, GERBER, GRADUATES, YOGURT MELTS",	HIGH	71.43
Babyfood, vegetable, butternut squash and corn",	LOW	9.26
Babyfood, vegetables, beets, strained",	LOW	7.7
Babyfood, vegetables, carrots, junior",	LOW	7.2
Babyfood, vegetables, carrots, strained",	LOW	6
Babyfood, vegetables, corn, creamed, junior",	LOW	16.25
Babyfood, vegetables, corn, creamed, strained",	LOW	14.1
Babyfood, vegetables, green beans, junior",	LOW	5.8
Babyfood, vegetables, mix vegetables junior",	LOW	8.2

Food name/ Category (100 g)	Status	Carbs content in g
Babyfood, vegetables, mix vegetables strained",	LOW	8.25
Babyfood, vegetables, peas, strained",	LOW	8.36
Babyfood, vegetables, spinach, creamed, strained",	LOW	5.7
Babyfood, vegetables, squash, junior",	LOW	5.73
Babyfood, vegetables, squash, strained",	LOW	5.73
Babyfood, water, bottled, GERBER, without added fluoride.",	LOW	0
Babyfood, yogurt, whole milk, with fruit, multigrain cereal and added DHA fortified",	LOW	13.22
Babyfood, yogurt, whole milk, with fruit, multigrain cereal and added iron fortified",	LOW	13
Bagels, cinnamon-raisin, toasted",	HIGH	59.3
Bagels, cinnamon-raisin",	MEDIUM	55.2
Bagels, egg",	MEDIUM	53
Bagels, multigrain",	MEDIUM	47.47
Bagels, oat bran",	MEDIUM	53.3
Bagels, plain, enriched, with calcium propionate (includes onion, poppy, sesame), t	HIGH	57.39
Bagels, plain, enriched, with calcium propionate (includes onion, poppy, sesame)",	MEDIUM	52.38
Bagels, plain, enriched, without calcium propionate (includes onion, poppy, sesame	MEDIUM	53.4
Bagels, plain, unenriched, with calcium propionate (includes onion, poppy, sesame)	MEDIUM	53.4
Bagels, plain, unenriched, without calcium propionate(includes onion, poppy, sesam	MEDIUM	53.4
Bagels, wheat",	MEDIUM	48.89
Bagels, whole grain white",	MEDIUM	54.52
Baking chocolate, MARS SNACKFOOD US, M&M's Milk Chocolate Mini Baking Bi	HIGH	68.4
Baking chocolate, MARS SNACKFOOD US, M&M's Semisweet Chocolate Mini Bal	HIGH	65.96
Baking chocolate, mexican, squares",	HIGH	77.41
Balsam-pear (bitter gourd), leafy tips, cooked, boiled, drained, with salt",	LOW	6.16
Balsam-pear (bitter gourd), pods, cooked, boiled, drained, with salt",	LOW	4.32
Balsam-pear (bitter gourd), pods, raw",	LOW	3.7
Bamboo shoots, cooked, boiled, drained, with salt",	LOW	1.52
Bamboo shoots, cooked, boiled, drained, without salt",	LOW	1.92
Bamboo shoots, raw",	LOW	5.2
Bananas, dehydrated, or banana powder",	HIGH	88.28
Bananas, raw",	LOW	22.84
BANQUET, Salisbury Steak With Gravy, family size, frozen, unprepared",	LOW	6.96
BARBARA DEE, Winter Mints Cookies",	HIGH	67.1
Barley flour or meal",	HIGH	74.52
Barley, pearled, cooked",	LOW	28.22
Basil, fresh",	LOW	2.65
Beans, adzuki, mature seed, cooked, boiled, with salt",	LOW	24.77

Food name/ Category (100 g)	Status	Carbs content in g
Beans, adzuki, mature seeds, canned, sweetened",	MEDIUM	55.01
Beans, adzuki, mature seeds, raw",	HIGH	62.9
Beans, baked, canned, no salt added",	LOW	20.49
Beans, baked, canned, plain or vegetarian",	LOW	21.14
Beans, baked, canned, with beef",	LOW	16.91
Beans, baked, canned, with franks",	LOW	15.39
Beans, baked, home prepared",	LOW	21.63
Beans, black turtle, mature seeds, canned",	LOW	16.55
Beans, black turtle, mature seeds, cooked, boiled, with salt",	LOW	24.35
Beans, black turtle, mature seeds, cooked, boiled, without salt",	LOW	24.35
Beans, black, mature seeds, canned, low sodium",	LOW	16.55
Beans, black, mature seeds, cooked, boiled, with salt",	LOW	23.71
Beans, black, mature seeds, cooked, boiled, without salt",	LOW	23.71
Beans, black, mature seeds, raw",	HIGH	62.36
Beans, chili, barbecue, ranch style, cooked",	LOW	16.9
Beans, cranberry (roman), mature seeds, canned",	LOW	15.12
Beans, cranberry (roman), mature seeds, cooked, boiled, with salt",	LOW	24.46
Beans, cranberry (roman), mature seeds, cooked, boiled, without salt",	LOW	24.46
Beans, french, mature seeds, cooked, boiled, with salt",	LOW	24.02
Beans, great northern, mature seeds, canned, low sodium",	LOW	21.02
Beans, great northern, mature seeds, canned",	LOW	21.02
Beans, great northern, mature seeds, cooked, boiled, with salt",	LOW	21.09
Beans, great northern, mature seeds, cooked, boiled, without salt",	LOW	21.09
Beans, kidney, all types, mature seeds, canned",	LOW	14.5
Beans, kidney, all types, mature seeds, cooked, boiled, with salt",	LOW	22.8
Beans, kidney, all types, mature seeds, cooked, boiled, without salt",	LOW	22.8
Beans, kidney, california red, mature seeds, cooked, boiled, with salt",	LOW	22.41
Beans, kidney, california red, mature seeds, cooked, boiled, without salt",	LOW	22.41
Beans, kidney, red, mature seeds, canned, drained solids, rinsed in tap water",	LOW	20.8

Food name/ Category (100 g)	Status	Carbs content in g
Beans, kidney, red, mature seeds, canned, drained solids",	LOW	21.49
Beans, kidney, red, mature seeds, canned, solids and liquid, low sodium",	LOW	14.83
Beans, kidney, red, mature seeds, canned, solids and liquids",	LOW	14.83
Beans, kidney, red, mature seeds, cooked, boiled, with salt",	LOW	22.8
Beans, kidney, red, mature seeds, cooked, boiled, without salt",	LOW	22.8
Beans, kidney, royal red, mature seeds, cooked, boiled with salt",	LOW	21.85
Beans, kidney, royal red, mature seeds, cooked, boiled, without salt",	LOW	21.85
Beans, liquid from stewed kidney beans",	LOW	2.8
Beans, mung, mature seeds, sprouted, canned, drained solids",	LOW	2.14
Beans, navy, mature seeds, canned",	LOW	20.45
Beans, navy, mature seeds, cooked, boiled, with salt",	LOW	26.05
Beans, navy, mature seeds, cooked, boiled, without salt",	LOW	26.05
Beans, navy, mature seeds, raw",	HIGH	60.75
Beans, pink, mature seeds, cooked, boiled, with salt",	LOW	27.91
Beans, pink, mature seeds, cooked, boiled, without salt",	LOW	27.91
Beans, pinto, canned, drained solids",	LOW	20.22
Beans, pinto, immature seeds, frozen, cooked, boiled, drained, with salt",	LOW	30.87
Beans, pinto, immature seeds, frozen, cooked, boiled, drained, without salt",	LOW	30.87
Beans, pinto, immature seeds, frozen, unprepared",	LOW	32.5
Beans, pinto, mature seeds, canned, drained solids, rinsed in tap water",	LOW	20.77
Beans, pinto, mature seeds, canned, solids and liquids, low sodium",	LOW	15.18
Beans, pinto, mature seeds, canned, solids and liquids",	LOW	15.18
Beans, pinto, mature seeds, cooked, boiled, with salt",	LOW	26.22
Beans, pinto, mature seeds, cooked, boiled, without salt",	LOW	26.22
Beans, shellie, canned, solids and liquids",	LOW	6.19
Beans, small white, mature seeds, cooked, boiled, with salt",	LOW	25.81
Beans, small white, mature seeds, cooked, boiled, without salt",	LOW	25.81
Beans, snap, canned, all styles, seasoned, solids and liquids",	LOW	3.49

Food name/ Category (100 g)	Status	Carbs content in g
Beans, snap, green, canned, no salt added, drained solids",	LOW	4.32
Beans, snap, green, canned, regular pack, drained solids",	LOW	4.32
Beans, snap, green, canned, regular pack, solids and liquids",	LOW	3.27
Beans, snap, green, cooked, boiled, drained, with salt",	LOW	7.88
Beans, snap, green, cooked, boiled, drained, without salt",	LOW	7.88
Beans, snap, green, frozen, all styles, microwaved",	LOW	6.98
Beans, snap, green, frozen, all styles, unprepared",	LOW	7.54
Beans, snap, green, frozen, cooked, boiled, drained without salt",	LOW	6.45
Beans, snap, green, frozen, cooked, boiled, drained, with salt",	LOW	6.45
Beans, snap, green, microwaved",	LOW	6.41
Beans, snap, yellow, canned, no salt added, drained solids",	LOW	4.5
Beans, snap, yellow, canned, regular pack, drained solids",	LOW	4.5
Beans, snap, yellow, canned, regular pack, solids and liquids",	LOW	3.5
Beans, snap, yellow, cooked, boiled, drained, with salt",	LOW	7.88
Beans, snap, yellow, cooked, boiled, drained, without salt",	LOW	7.88
Beans, snap, yellow, frozen, all styles, unprepared",	LOW	7.58
Beans, snap, yellow, frozen, cooked, boiled, drained, with salt",	LOW	6.45
Beans, white, mature seeds, canned",	LOW	21.2
Beans, white, mature seeds, cooked, boiled, with salt",	LOW	25.09
Beans, yellow, mature seeds, cooked, boiled, with salt",	LOW	25.28
Beans, yellow, mature seeds, cooked, boiled, without salt",	LOW	25.28
BEAR NAKED, Double Chocolate Cookies",	HIGH	66.9
BEAR NAKED, Fruit & Nut Cookies",	HIGH	61.6
Beef composite, separable lean only, trimmed to 1\/8\" fat, choice, cooked",	LOW	0
Beef macaroni with tomato sauce, frozen entree, reduced fat",	LOW	17.99
Beef Pot Pie, frozen entree, prepared",	LOW	22.05
Beef sausage, fresh, cooked",	LOW	0.35
Beef sausage, pre-cooked",	LOW	0.03
Beef stew, canned entree",	LOW	7.85

Food name/ Category (100 g)	Status	Carbs content in g
Beef, Australian, imported, grass-fed, external fat, raw",	LOW	0.39
Beef, Australian, imported, grass-fed, ground, 85% lean \/ 15% fat, raw",	LOW	0
Beef, Australian, imported, grass-fed, loin, tenderloin steak\/roast, boneless, separable lean and fat, raw",	LOW	0.01
Beef, Australian, imported, grass-fed, loin, tenderloin steak\/roast, boneless, separable lean only, raw",	LOW	0
Beef, Australian, imported, grass-fed, loin, top loin steak\/roast, boneless, separable lean and fat, raw",	LOW	0.11
Beef, Australian, imported, grass-fed, loin, top loin steak\/roast, boneless, separable lean only, raw",	LOW	0
Beef, Australian, imported, grass-fed, loin, top sirloin cap-off steak\/roast, boneless, separable lean and fat, raw",	LOW	0.01
Beef, Australian, imported, grass-fed, loin, top sirloin cap-off steak\/roast, boneless, separable lean only, raw",	LOW	0
Beef, Australian, imported, grass-fed, rib, ribeye steak\/roast lip-on, boneless, separable lean and fat, raw",	LOW	0.11
Beef, Australian, imported, grass-fed, rib, ribeye steak\/roast lip-on, boneless, separable lean only, raw",	LOW	0
Beef, Australian, imported, grass-fed, round, bottom round steak\/roast, boneless, separable lean and fat, raw",	LOW	0.01
Beef, Australian, imported, grass-fed, round, bottom round steak\/roast, boneless, separable lean only, raw",	LOW	0
Beef, Australian, imported, grass-fed, round, top round cap-off steak\/roast, boneless, separable lean and fat, raw",	LOW	0
Beef, Australian, imported, grass-fed, round, top round cap-off steak\/roast, boneless, separable lean only, raw",	LOW	0
Beef, Australian, imported, Wagyu, external fat, Aust. marble score 4\/5, raw",	LOW	0
Beef, Australian, imported, Wagyu, external fat, Aust. marble score 9, raw",	LOW	0.97
Beef, Australian, imported, Wagyu, loin, tenderloin steak\/roast, boneless, separable lean and fat, Aust. marble score 4\/5, raw",	LOW	0
Beef, Australian, imported, Wagyu, loin, tenderloin steak\/roast, boneless, separable lean and fat, Aust. marble score 9, raw",	LOW	0.58
Beef, Australian, imported, Wagyu, loin, tenderloin steak\/roast, boneless, separable lean only, Aust. marble score 4\/5, raw",	LOW	0
Beef, Australian, imported, Wagyu, loin, tenderloin steak\/roast, boneless, separable lean only, Aust. marble score 9, raw",	LOW	0.57
Beef, Australian, imported, Wagyu, loin, top loin steak\/roast, boneless, separable lean and fat, Aust. marble score 4\/5, raw",	LOW	0.17
Beef, Australian, imported, Wagyu, loin, top loin steak\/roast, boneless, separable lean only, Aust. marble score 4\/5, raw",	LOW	0.2
Beef, Australian, imported, Wagyu, loin, top loin steak\/roast, boneless, separable lean only, Aust. marble score 9, raw",	LOW	0.13
Beef, Australian, imported, Wagyu, loin, top loin steak\/roast, separable lean and fat, Aust. marble score 9, raw",	LOW	0.22
Beef, Australian, imported, Wagyu, rib, small end rib steak\/roast, boneless, separable lean and fat, Aust. marble score 4\/5, raw",	LOW	0
Beef, Australian, imported, Wagyu, rib, small end rib steak\/roast, boneless, separable lean and fat, Aust. marble score 9, raw",	LOW	0.42
Beef, Australian, imported, Wagyu, rib, small end rib steak\/roast, boneless, separable lean only, Aust. marble score 4\/5, raw",	LOW	0
Beef, Australian, imported, Wagyu, rib, small end rib steak\/roast, boneless, separable lean only, Aust. marble score 9, raw",	LOW	0.46

Food name/ Category (100 g)	Status	Carbs content in g
Beef, bologna, reduced sodium",	LOW	2
Beef, bottom sirloin, tri-tip roast, separable lean and fat, trimmed to 0\" fat, all grades, cooked, roasted",	LOW	0
Beef, bottom sirloin, tri-tip roast, separable lean and fat, trimmed to 0\" fat, all grades, raw",	LOW	0
Beef, bottom sirloin, tri-tip roast, separable lean and fat, trimmed to 0\" fat, choice, cooked, roasted",	LOW	0
Beef, bottom sirloin, tri-tip roast, separable lean and fat, trimmed to 0\" fat, choice, raw",	LOW	0
Beef, bottom sirloin, tri-tip roast, separable lean and fat, trimmed to 0\" fat, select, cooked, roasted",	LOW	0
Beef, bottom sirloin, tri-tip roast, separable lean and fat, trimmed to 0\" fat, select, raw",	LOW	0
Beef, bottom sirloin, tri-tip roast, separable lean only, trimmed to 0\" fat, all grades, raw",	LOW	0
Beef, bottom sirloin, tri-tip roast, separable lean only, trimmed to 0\" fat, choice, cooked, roasted",	LOW	0
Beef, bottom sirloin, tri-tip roast, separable lean only, trimmed to 0\" fat, choice, raw",	LOW	0
Beef, bottom sirloin, tri-tip roast, separable lean only, trimmed to 0\" fat, select, cooked, roasted",	LOW	0
Beef, bottom sirloin, tri-tip roast, separable lean only, trimmed to 0\" fat, select, raw",	LOW	0
Beef, brisket, flat half, boneless separable lean only, trimmed to 0\" fat, all grades, raw",	LOW	0
Beef, brisket, flat half, boneless, separable lean and fat, trimmed to 0\" fat, all grades, raw",	LOW	0
Beef, brisket, flat half, boneless, separable lean and fat, trimmed to 0\" fat, choice, raw",	LOW	0
Beef, brisket, flat half, boneless, separable lean and fat, trimmed to 0\" fat, select, raw",	LOW	0
Beef, brisket, flat half, boneless, separable lean only, trimmed to 0\" fat, choice, raw",	LOW	0
Beef, brisket, flat half, boneless, separable lean only, trimmed to 0\" fat, select, raw",	LOW	0
Beef, brisket, flat half, separable lean and fat, trimmed to 0\" fat, all grades, cooked, braised",	LOW	0
Beef, brisket, flat half, separable lean and fat, trimmed to 0\" fat, choice, cooked, braised",	LOW	0
Beef, brisket, flat half, separable lean and fat, trimmed to 0\" fat, select, cooked, braised",	LOW	0
Beef, brisket, flat half, separable lean and fat, trimmed to 1\/8\" fat, all grades, cooked, braised",	LOW	0
Beef, brisket, flat half, separable lean and fat, trimmed to 1\/8\" fat, all grades, raw",	LOW	0
Beef, brisket, flat half, separable lean and fat, trimmed to 1\/8\" fat, choice, cooked, braised",	LOW	0
Beef, brisket, flat half, separable lean and fat, trimmed to 1\/8\" fat, choice, raw",	LOW	0.12
Beef, brisket, flat half, separable lean and fat, trimmed to 1\/8\" fat, select, cooked, braised",	LOW	0
Beef, brisket, flat half, separable lean and fat, trimmed to 1\/8\" fat, select, raw",	LOW	0
Beef, brisket, flat half, separable lean only, trimmed to 0\" fat, all grades, cooked, braised",	LOW	0

Food name/ Category (100 g)	Status	Carbs content in g
Beef, brisket, flat half, separable lean only, trimmed to 0\" fat, choice, cooked, braised",	LOW	0
Beef, brisket, flat half, separable lean only, trimmed to 0\" fat, select, cooked, braised",	LOW	0
Beef, brisket, flat half, separable lean only, trimmed to 1\/8\" fat, all grades, cooked, braised",	LOW	0
Beef, brisket, flat half, separable lean only, trimmed to 1\/8\" fat, all grades, raw",	LOW	0
Beef, brisket, flat half, separable lean only, trimmed to 1\/8\" fat, choice, cooked, braised",	LOW	0
Beef, brisket, flat half, separable lean only, trimmed to 1\/8\" fat, choice, raw",	LOW	0
Beef, brisket, flat half, separable lean only, trimmed to 1\/8\" fat, select, cooked, braised",	LOW	0
Beef, brisket, flat half, separable lean only, trimmed to 1\/8\" fat, select, raw",	LOW	0
Beef, brisket, point half, separable lean and fat, trimmed to 0\" fat, all grades, cooked, braised",	LOW	0
Beef, brisket, point half, separable lean and fat, trimmed to 1\/8\" fat, all grades, cooked, braised",	LOW	0
Beef, brisket, point half, separable lean and fat, trimmed to 1\/8\" fat, all grades, raw",	LOW	0
Beef, brisket, point half, separable lean only, trimmed to 0\" fat, all grades, cooked, braised",	LOW	0
Beef, brisket, whole, separable lean and fat, trimmed to 0\" fat, all grades, cooked, braised",	LOW	0
Beef, brisket, whole, separable lean and fat, trimmed to 1\/8\" fat, all grades, cooked, braised",	LOW	0
Beef, brisket, whole, separable lean and fat, trimmed to 1\/8\" fat, all grades, raw",	LOW	0
Beef, brisket, whole, separable lean only, all grades, raw",	LOW	0
Beef, brisket, whole, separable lean only, trimmed to 0\" fat, all grades, cooked, braised",	LOW	0
Beef, carcass, separable lean and fat, choice, raw",	LOW	0
Beef, carcass, separable lean and fat, select, raw",	LOW	0
Beef, chuck eye Country-Style ribs, boneless, separable lean and fat, trimmed to 0\" fat, all grades, cooked, braised",	LOW	0
Beef, chuck eye Country-Style ribs, boneless, separable lean and fat, trimmed to 0\" fat, all grades, raw",	LOW	0
Beef, chuck eye Country-Style ribs, boneless, separable lean and fat, trimmed to 0\" fat, choice, cooked, braised",	LOW	0
Beef, chuck eye Country-Style ribs, boneless, separable lean and fat, trimmed to 0\" fat, choice, raw",	LOW	0
Beef, chuck eye Country-Style ribs, boneless, separable lean and fat, trimmed to 0\" fat, select, cooked, braised",	LOW	0
Beef, chuck eye Country-Style ribs, boneless, separable lean and fat, trimmed to 0\" fat, select, raw",	LOW	0
Beef, chuck eye Country-Style ribs, boneless, separable lean only, trimmed to 0\" fat, all grades, cooked, braised",	LOW	0
Beef, chuck eye Country-Style ribs, boneless, separable lean only, trimmed to 0\" fat, all grades, raw",	LOW	0
Beef, chuck eye Country-Style ribs, boneless, separable lean only, trimmed to 0\" fat, choice, cooked, braised",	LOW	0

Food name/ Category (100 g)	Status	Carbs content in g
Beef, chuck eye Country-Style ribs, boneless, separable lean only, trimmed to 0\" fat, choice, raw",	LOW	0
Beef, chuck eye Country-Style ribs, boneless, separable lean only, trimmed to 0\" fat, select, cooked, braised",	LOW	0
Beef, chuck eye Country-Style ribs, boneless, separable lean only, trimmed to 0\" fat, select, raw",	LOW	0
Beef, chuck eye roast, boneless, America's Beef Roast, separable lean and fat, trimmed to 0\" fat, all grades, cooked, roasted",	LOW	0
Beef, chuck eye roast, boneless, America's Beef Roast, separable lean and fat, trimmed to 0\" fat, all grades, raw",	LOW	0
Beef, chuck eye roast, boneless, America's Beef Roast, separable lean and fat, trimmed to 0\" fat, choice, cooked, roasted",	LOW	0
Beef, chuck eye roast, boneless, America's Beef Roast, separable lean and fat, trimmed to 0\" fat, choice, raw",	LOW	0
Beef, chuck eye roast, boneless, America's Beef Roast, separable lean and fat, trimmed to 0\" fat, select, cooked, roasted",	LOW	0
Beef, chuck eye roast, boneless, America's Beef Roast, separable lean and fat, trimmed to 0\" fat, select, raw",	LOW	0
Beef, chuck eye roast, boneless, America's Beef Roast, separable lean only, trimmed to 0\" fat, all grades, cooked, roasted",	LOW	0
Beef, chuck eye roast, boneless, America's Beef Roast, separable lean only, trimmed to 0\" fat, all grades, raw",	LOW	0
Beef, chuck eye roast, boneless, America's Beef Roast, separable lean only, trimmed to 0\" fat, choice, cooked, roasted",	LOW	0
Beef, chuck eye roast, boneless, America's Beef Roast, separable lean only, trimmed to 0\" fat, choice, raw",	LOW	0
Beef, chuck eye roast, boneless, America's Beef Roast, separable lean only, trimmed to 0\" fat, select, cooked, roasted",	LOW	0
Beef, chuck eye roast, boneless, America's Beef Roast, separable lean only, trimmed to 0\" fat, select, raw",	LOW	0
Beef, chuck eye steak, boneless, separable lean and fat, trimmed to 0\" fat, all grades, cooked, grilled",	LOW	0
Beef, chuck eye steak, boneless, separable lean and fat, trimmed to 0\" fat, all grades, raw",	LOW	0
Beef, chuck eye steak, boneless, separable lean and fat, trimmed to 0\" fat, choice, cooked, grilled",	LOW	0
Beef, chuck eye steak, boneless, separable lean and fat, trimmed to 0\" fat, choice, raw",	LOW	0
Beef, chuck eye steak, boneless, separable lean and fat, trimmed to 0\" fat, select, cooked, grilled",	LOW	0
Beef, chuck eye steak, boneless, separable lean and fat, trimmed to 0\" fat, select, raw",	LOW	0
Beef, chuck eye steak, boneless, separable lean only, trimmed to 0\" fat, all grades, cooked, grilled",	LOW	0
Beef, chuck eye steak, boneless, separable lean only, trimmed to 0\" fat, all grades, raw",	LOW	0
Beef, chuck eye steak, boneless, separable lean only, trimmed to 0\" fat, choice, cooked, grilled",	LOW	0
Beef, chuck eye steak, boneless, separable lean only, trimmed to 0\" fat, choice, raw",	LOW	0
Beef, chuck eye steak, boneless, separable lean only, trimmed to 0\" fat, select, cooked, grilled",	LOW	0
Beef, chuck eye steak, boneless, separable lean only, trimmed to 0\" fat, select, raw",	LOW	0
Beef, chuck for stew, separable lean and fat, all grades, cooked, braised",	LOW	0

Food name/ Category (100 g)	Status	Carbs content in g
Beef, chuck for stew, separable lean and fat, all grades, raw",	LOW	0.16
Beef, chuck for stew, separable lean and fat, choice, cooked, braised",	LOW	0
Beef, chuck for stew, separable lean and fat, choice, raw",	LOW	0.12
Beef, chuck for stew, separable lean and fat, select, cooked, braised",	LOW	0
Beef, chuck for stew, separable lean and fat, select, raw",	LOW	0.21
Beef, chuck, arm pot roast, separable lean and fat, trimmed to 0\" fat, all grades, cooked, braised",	LOW	0
Beef, chuck, arm pot roast, separable lean and fat, trimmed to 0\" fat, select, cooked, braised",	LOW	0
Beef, chuck, arm pot roast, separable lean and fat, trimmed to 1\/8\" fat, all grades, cooked, braised",	LOW	0
Beef, chuck, arm pot roast, separable lean and fat, trimmed to 1\/8\" fat, all grades, raw",	LOW	0
Beef, chuck, arm pot roast, separable lean and fat, trimmed to 1\/8\" fat, choice, cooked, braised",	LOW	0
Beef, chuck, arm pot roast, separable lean and fat, trimmed to 1\/8\" fat, choice, raw",	LOW	0
Beef, chuck, arm pot roast, separable lean and fat, trimmed to 1\/8\" fat, select, cooked, braised",	LOW	0
Beef, chuck, arm pot roast, separable lean and fat, trimmed to 1\/8\" fat, select, raw",	LOW	0
Beef, chuck, arm pot roast, separable lean only, trimmed to 0\" fat, choice, cooked, braised",	LOW	0
Beef, chuck, arm pot roast, separable lean only, trimmed to 0\" fat, select, cooked, braised",	LOW	0
Beef, chuck, arm pot roast, separable lean only, trimmed to 1\/8\" fat, all grades, cooked, braised",	LOW	0
Beef, chuck, arm pot roast, separable lean only, trimmed to 1\/8\" fat, all grades, raw",	LOW	0
Beef, chuck, arm pot roast, separable lean only, trimmed to 1\/8\" fat, choice, cooked, braised",	LOW	0
Beef, chuck, arm pot roast, separable lean only, trimmed to 1\/8\" fat, choice, raw",	LOW	0
Beef, chuck, arm pot roast, separable lean only, trimmed to 1\/8\" fat, select, cooked, braised",	LOW	0
Beef, chuck, arm pot roast, separable lean only, trimmed to 1\/8\" fat, select, raw",	LOW	0
Beef, chuck, blade roast, separable lean and fat, trimmed to 0\" fat, all grades, cooked, braised",	LOW	0
Beef, chuck, blade roast, separable lean and fat, trimmed to 1\/8\" fat, all grades, cooked, braised",	LOW	0
Beef, chuck, blade roast, separable lean and fat, trimmed to 1\/8\" fat, all grades, raw",	LOW	0
Beef, chuck, blade roast, separable lean and fat, trimmed to 1\/8\" fat, choice, cooked, braised",	LOW	0
Beef, chuck, blade roast, separable lean and fat, trimmed to 1\/8\" fat, choice, raw",	LOW	0
Beef, chuck, blade roast, separable lean and fat, trimmed to 1\/8\" fat, select, cooked, braised",	LOW	0
Beef, chuck, blade roast, separable lean and fat, trimmed to 1\/8\" fat, select, raw",	LOW	0

Food name/ Category (100 g)	Status	Carbs content in g
Beef, chuck, blade roast, separable lean only, trimmed to 0\" fat, all grades, cooked, braised",	LOW	0
Beef, chuck, clod roast, separable lean and fat, trimmed to 0\" fat, all grades, cooked, roasted",	LOW	0
Beef, chuck, clod roast, separable lean and fat, trimmed to 0\" fat, choice, cooked, roasted",	LOW	0
Beef, chuck, clod roast, separable lean and fat, trimmed to 0\" fat, select, cooked, roasted",	LOW	0
Beef, chuck, clod roast, separable lean only, trimmed to 0\" fat, all grades, cooked, roasted",	LOW	0
Beef, chuck, clod roast, separable lean only, trimmed to 0\" fat, choice, cooked, roasted",	LOW	0
Beef, chuck, clod roast, separable lean only, trimmed to 0\" fat, select, cooked, roasted",	LOW	0
Beef, chuck, clod roast, separable lean only, trimmed to 1\/4\" fat, all grades, cooked, roasted",	LOW	0
Beef, chuck, clod roast, separable lean only, trimmed to 1\/4\" fat, all grades, raw",	LOW	0
Beef, chuck, clod steak, separable lean only, trimmed to 1\/4\" fat, all grades, cooked, braised",	LOW	0
Beef, chuck, mock tender steak, boneless, separable lean and fat, trimmed to 0\" fat, all grades, cooked, braised",	LOW	0
Beef, chuck, mock tender steak, boneless, separable lean and fat, trimmed to 0\" fat, all grades, raw",	LOW	0
Beef, chuck, mock tender steak, boneless, separable lean and fat, trimmed to 0\" fat, choice, cooked, braised",	LOW	0
Beef, chuck, mock tender steak, boneless, separable lean and fat, trimmed to 0\" fat, choice, raw",	LOW	0
Beef, chuck, mock tender steak, boneless, separable lean and fat, trimmed to 0\" fat, select, cooked, braised",	LOW	0
Beef, chuck, mock tender steak, boneless, separable lean and fat, trimmed to 0\" fat, select, raw",	LOW	0
Beef, chuck, mock tender steak, boneless, separable lean only, trimmed to 0\" fat, all grades, cooked, braised",	LOW	0
Beef, chuck, mock tender steak, boneless, separable lean only, trimmed to 0\" fat, all grades, raw",	LOW	0
Beef, chuck, mock tender steak, boneless, separable lean only, trimmed to 0\" fat, choice, cooked, braised",	LOW	0
Beef, chuck, mock tender steak, boneless, separable lean only, trimmed to 0\" fat, choice, raw",	LOW	0
Beef, chuck, mock tender steak, boneless, separable lean only, trimmed to 0\" fat, select, cooked, braised",	LOW	0
Beef, chuck, mock tender steak, boneless, separable lean only, trimmed to 0\" fat, select, raw",	LOW	0
Beef, chuck, mock tender steak, separable lean and fat, trimmed to 0\" fat, all grades, cooked, broiled",	LOW	0
Beef, chuck, mock tender steak, separable lean and fat, trimmed to 0\" fat, USDA choice, cooked, broiled",	LOW	0
Beef, chuck, mock tender steak, separable lean and fat, trimmed to 0\" fat, USDA select, cooked, broiled",	LOW	0
Beef, chuck, mock tender steak, separable lean only, trimmed to 0\" fat, all grades, cooked, broiled",	LOW	0
Beef, chuck, mock tender steak, separable lean only, trimmed to 0\" fat, choice, cooked, broiled",	LOW	0
Beef, chuck, mock tender steak, separable lean only, trimmed to 0\" fat, select, cooked, broiled",	LOW	0

Food name/ Category (100 g)	Status	Carbs content in g
Beef, chuck, short ribs, boneless, separable lean and fat, trimmed to 0\" fat, all grades, cooked, braised",	LOW	0
Beef, chuck, short ribs, boneless, separable lean and fat, trimmed to 0\" fat, all grades, raw",	LOW	0
Beef, chuck, short ribs, boneless, separable lean and fat, trimmed to 0\" fat, choice, cooked, braised",	LOW	0
Beef, chuck, short ribs, boneless, separable lean and fat, trimmed to 0\" fat, choice, raw",	LOW	0
Beef, chuck, short ribs, boneless, separable lean and fat, trimmed to 0\" fat, select, cooked, braised",	LOW	0
Beef, chuck, short ribs, boneless, separable lean and fat, trimmed to 0\" fat, select, raw",	LOW	0
Beef, chuck, short ribs, boneless, separable lean only, trimmed to 0\" fat, all grades, cooked, braised",	LOW	0
Beef, chuck, short ribs, boneless, separable lean only, trimmed to 0\" fat, all grades, raw",	LOW	0.05
Beef, chuck, short ribs, boneless, separable lean only, trimmed to 0\" fat, choice, cooked, braised",	LOW	0
Beef, chuck, short ribs, boneless, separable lean only, trimmed to 0\" fat, choice, raw",	LOW	0.29
Beef, chuck, short ribs, boneless, separable lean only, trimmed to 0\" fat, select, cooked, braised",	LOW	0
Beef, chuck, short ribs, boneless, separable lean only, trimmed to 0\" fat, select, raw",	LOW	0
Beef, chuck, shoulder clod, shoulder tender, medallion, separable lean and fat, trimmed to 0\" fat, all grades, cooked, grilled",	LOW	0
Beef, chuck, shoulder clod, shoulder tender, medallion, separable lean and fat, trimmed to 0\" fat, all grades, raw",	LOW	0
Beef, chuck, shoulder clod, shoulder tender, medallion, separable lean and fat, trimmed to 0\" fat, choice, cooked, grilled",	LOW	0
Beef, chuck, shoulder clod, shoulder tender, medallion, separable lean and fat, trimmed to 0\" fat, choice, raw",	LOW	0
Beef, chuck, shoulder clod, shoulder tender, medallion, separable lean and fat, trimmed to 0\" fat, select, cooked, grilled",	LOW	0
Beef, chuck, shoulder clod, shoulder tender, medallion, separable lean and fat, trimmed to 0\" fat, select, raw",	LOW	0
Beef, chuck, shoulder clod, shoulder top and center steaks, separable lean and fat, trimmed to 0\" fat, all grades, cooked, grilled",	LOW	0
Beef, chuck, shoulder clod, shoulder top and center steaks, separable lean and fat, trimmed to 0\" fat, all grades, raw",	LOW	0
Beef, chuck, shoulder clod, shoulder top and center steaks, separable lean and fat, trimmed to 0\" fat, choice, cooked, grilled",	LOW	0
Beef, chuck, shoulder clod, shoulder top and center steaks, separable lean and fat, trimmed to 0\" fat, choice, raw",	LOW	0
Beef, chuck, shoulder clod, shoulder top and center steaks, separable lean and fat, trimmed to 0\" fat, select, cooked, grilled",	LOW	0
Beef, chuck, shoulder clod, shoulder top and center steaks, separable lean and fat, trimmed to 0\" fat, select, raw",	LOW	0
Beef, chuck, shoulder clod, top blade, steak, separable lean and fat, trimmed to 0\" fat, all grades, cooked, grilled",	LOW	0
Beef, chuck, shoulder clod, top blade, steak, separable lean and fat, trimmed to 0\" fat, all grades, raw",	LOW	0
Beef, chuck, shoulder clod, top blade, steak, separable lean and fat, trimmed to 0\" fat, choice, cooked, grilled",	LOW	0
Beef, chuck, shoulder clod, top blade, steak, separable lean and fat, trimmed to 0\" fat, choice, raw",	LOW	0

Food name/ Category (100 g)	Status	Carbs content in g
Beef, chuck, shoulder clod, top blade, steak, separable lean and fat, trimmed to 0\" fat, select, cooked, grilled",	LOW	0
Beef, chuck, shoulder clod, top blade, steak, separable lean and fat, trimmed to 0\" fat, select, raw",	LOW	0
Beef, chuck, top blade, separable lean and fat, trimmed to 0\" fat, all grades, cooked, broiled",	LOW	0
Beef, chuck, top blade, separable lean and fat, trimmed to 0\" fat, choice, cooked, broiled",	LOW	0
Beef, chuck, top blade, separable lean and fat, trimmed to 0\" fat, select, cooked, broiled",	LOW	0
Beef, chuck, top blade, separable lean only, trimmed to 0\" fat, all grades, cooked, broiled",	LOW	0
Beef, chuck, top blade, separable lean only, trimmed to 0\" fat, choice, cooked, broiled",	LOW	0
Beef, chuck, top blade, separable lean only, trimmed to 0\" fat, select, cooked, broiled",	LOW	0
Beef, chuck, under blade center steak, boneless, Denver Cut, separable lean and fat, trimmed to 0\" fat, all grades, cooked, grilled",	LOW	0.21
Beef, chuck, under blade center steak, boneless, Denver Cut, separable lean and fat, trimmed to 0\" fat, all grades, raw",	LOW	0.36
Beef, chuck, under blade center steak, boneless, Denver Cut, separable lean and fat, trimmed to 0\" fat, choice, cooked, grilled",	LOW	0.4
Beef, chuck, under blade center steak, boneless, Denver Cut, separable lean and fat, trimmed to 0\" fat, choice, raw",	LOW	0.53
Beef, chuck, under blade center steak, boneless, Denver Cut, separable lean and fat, trimmed to 0\" fat, select, cooked, grilled",	LOW	0
Beef, chuck, under blade center steak, boneless, Denver Cut, separable lean and fat, trimmed to 0\" fat, select, raw",	LOW	0.09
Beef, chuck, under blade center steak, boneless, Denver Cut, separable lean only, trimmed to 0\" fat, all grades, cooked, grilled",	LOW	0.14
Beef, chuck, under blade center steak, boneless, Denver Cut, separable lean only, trimmed to 0\" fat, all grades, raw",	LOW	0.49
Beef, chuck, under blade center steak, boneless, Denver Cut, separable lean only, trimmed to 0\" fat, choice, cooked, grilled",	LOW	0.28
Beef, chuck, under blade center steak, boneless, Denver Cut, separable lean only, trimmed to 0\" fat, choice, raw",	LOW	0.67
Beef, chuck, under blade center steak, boneless, Denver Cut, separable lean only, trimmed to 0\" fat, select, cooked, grilled",	LOW	0
Beef, chuck, under blade center steak, boneless, Denver Cut, separable lean only, trimmed to 0\" fat, select, raw",	LOW	0.21
Beef, chuck, under blade pot roast or steak, boneless, separable lean and fat, trimmed to 0\" fat, all grades, raw",	LOW	0
Beef, chuck, under blade pot roast or steak, boneless, separable lean and fat, trimmed to 0\" fat, choice, raw",	LOW	0
Beef, chuck, under blade pot roast or steak, boneless, separable lean and fat, trimmed to 0\" fat, select, raw",	LOW	0
Beef, chuck, under blade pot roast or steak, boneless, separable lean only, trimmed to 0\" fat, all grades, raw",	LOW	0.31
Beef, chuck, under blade pot roast or steak, boneless, separable lean only, trimmed to 0\" fat, choice, raw",	LOW	0.39
Beef, chuck, under blade pot roast or steak, boneless, separable lean only, trimmed to 0\" fat, select, raw",	LOW	0.19
Beef, chuck, under blade pot roast, boneless, separable lean and fat, trimmed to 0\" fat, all grades, cooked, braised",	LOW	0
Beef, chuck, under blade pot roast, boneless, separable lean and fat, trimmed to 0\" fat, choice, cooked, braised",	LOW	0

Food name/ Category (100 g)	Status	Carbs content in g
Beef, chuck, under blade pot roast, boneless, separable lean and fat, trimmed to 0\" fat, select, cooked, braised",	LOW	0
Beef, chuck, under blade pot roast, boneless, separable lean only, trimmed to 0\" fat, all grades, cooked, braised",	LOW	0
Beef, chuck, under blade pot roast, boneless, separable lean only, trimmed to 0\" fat, choice, cooked, braised",	LOW	0
Beef, chuck, under blade pot roast, boneless, separable lean only, trimmed to 0\" fat, select, cooked, braised",	LOW	0
Beef, chuck, under blade steak, boneless, separable lean and fat, trimmed to 0\" fat, all grades, cooked, braised",	LOW	0
Beef, chuck, under blade steak, boneless, separable lean and fat, trimmed to 0\" fat, choice, cooked, braised",	LOW	0
Beef, chuck, under blade steak, boneless, separable lean and fat, trimmed to 0\" fat, select, cooked, braised",	LOW	0
Beef, chuck, under blade steak, boneless, separable lean only, trimmed to 0\" fat, all grades, cooked, braised",	LOW	0
Beef, chuck, under blade steak, boneless, separable lean only, trimmed to 0\" fat, choice, cooked, braised",	LOW	0
Beef, chuck, under blade steak, boneless, separable lean only, trimmed to 0\" fat, select, cooked, braised",	LOW	0
Beef, composite of trimmed retail cuts, separable lean and fat, trimmed to 0\" fat, all grades, cooked",	LOW	0
Beef, composite of trimmed retail cuts, separable lean and fat, trimmed to 0\" fat, all grades, raw",	LOW	0.05
Beef, composite of trimmed retail cuts, separable lean and fat, trimmed to 0\" fat, choice, cooked",	LOW	0
Beef, composite of trimmed retail cuts, separable lean and fat, trimmed to 0\" fat, choice, raw",	LOW	0.06
Beef, composite of trimmed retail cuts, separable lean and fat, trimmed to 0\" fat, select, cooked",	LOW	0
Beef, composite of trimmed retail cuts, separable lean and fat, trimmed to 0\" fat, select, raw",	LOW	0.04
Beef, composite of trimmed retail cuts, separable lean and fat, trimmed to 1\/8\" fat, all grades, cooked",	LOW	0
Beef, composite of trimmed retail cuts, separable lean and fat, trimmed to 1\/8\" fat, all grades, raw",	LOW	0
Beef, composite of trimmed retail cuts, separable lean and fat, trimmed to 1\/8\" fat, choice, cooked",	LOW	0
Beef, composite of trimmed retail cuts, separable lean and fat, trimmed to 1\/8\" fat, choice, raw",	LOW	0
Beef, composite of trimmed retail cuts, separable lean and fat, trimmed to 1\/8\" fat, select, cooked",	LOW	0
Beef, composite of trimmed retail cuts, separable lean and fat, trimmed to 1\/8\" fat, select, raw",	LOW	0
Beef, composite of trimmed retail cuts, separable lean only, trimmed to 0\" fat, all grades, cooked",	LOW	0
Beef, composite of trimmed retail cuts, separable lean only, trimmed to 0\" fat, all grades, raw",	LOW	0.08
Beef, composite of trimmed retail cuts, separable lean only, trimmed to 0\" fat, choice, cooked",	LOW	0
Beef, composite of trimmed retail cuts, separable lean only, trimmed to 0\" fat, choice, raw",	LOW	0
Beef, composite of trimmed retail cuts, separable lean only, trimmed to 0\" fat, select, cooked",	LOW	0
Beef, composite of trimmed retail cuts, separable lean only, trimmed to 0\" fat, select, raw",	LOW	0.05

Food name/ Category (100 g)	Status	Carbs content in g
Beef, composite of trimmed retail cuts, separable lean only, trimmed to 1\/8\" fat, all grades, cooked",	LOW	0
Beef, composite of trimmed retail cuts, separable lean only, trimmed to 1\/8\" fat, all grades, raw",	LOW	0
Beef, composite of trimmed retail cuts, separable lean only, trimmed to 1\/8\" fat, choice, raw",	LOW	0
Beef, composite of trimmed retail cuts, separable lean only, trimmed to 1\/8\" fat, select, cooked",	LOW	0
Beef, composite of trimmed retail cuts, separable lean only, trimmed to 1\/8\" fat, select, raw",	LOW	0
Beef, corned beef hash, with potato, canned",	LOW	9.27
Beef, cured, breakfast strips, cooked",	LOW	1.4
Beef, cured, breakfast strips, raw or unheated",	LOW	0.7
Beef, cured, corned beef, brisket, cooked",	LOW	0.47
Beef, cured, corned beef, brisket, raw",	LOW	0.14
Beef, cured, corned beef, canned",	LOW	0
Beef, cured, dried",	LOW	2.76
Beef, cured, luncheon meat, jellied",	LOW	0
Beef, cured, pastrami",	LOW	0.36
Beef, cured, sausage, cooked, smoked",	LOW	2.42
Beef, cured, smoked, chopped beef",	LOW	1.86
Beef, flank, steak, separable lean and fat, trimmed to 0\" fat, all grades, cooked, broiled",	LOW	0
Beef, flank, steak, separable lean and fat, trimmed to 0\" fat, all grades, raw",	LOW	0
Beef, flank, steak, separable lean and fat, trimmed to 0\" fat, choice, cooked, braised",	LOW	0
Beef, flank, steak, separable lean and fat, trimmed to 0\" fat, choice, cooked, broiled",	LOW	0
Beef, flank, steak, separable lean and fat, trimmed to 0\" fat, choice, raw",	LOW	0
Beef, flank, steak, separable lean and fat, trimmed to 0\" fat, select, cooked, broiled",	LOW	0
Beef, flank, steak, separable lean and fat, trimmed to 0\" fat, select, raw",	LOW	0
Beef, flank, steak, separable lean only, trimmed to 0\" fat, all grades, cooked, broiled",	LOW	0
Beef, flank, steak, separable lean only, trimmed to 0\" fat, all grades, raw",	LOW	0
Beef, flank, steak, separable lean only, trimmed to 0\" fat, choice, cooked, braised",	LOW	0
Beef, flank, steak, separable lean only, trimmed to 0\" fat, choice, cooked, broiled",	LOW	0
Beef, flank, steak, separable lean only, trimmed to 0\" fat, choice, raw",	LOW	0

Food name/ Category (100 g)	Status	Carbs content in g
Beef, flank, steak, separable lean only, trimmed to 0\" fat, select, cooked, broiled",	LOW	0
Beef, flank, steak, separable lean only, trimmed to 0\" fat, select, raw",	LOW	0
Beef, grass-fed, ground, raw",	LOW	0
Beef, grass-fed, strip steaks, lean only, raw",	LOW	0
Beef, ground, 70% lean meat \/ 30% fat, crumbles, cooked, pan-browned",	LOW	0
Beef, ground, 70% lean meat \/ 30% fat, loaf, cooked, baked",	LOW	0
Beef, ground, 70% lean meat \/ 30% fat, patty cooked, pan-broiled",	LOW	0
Beef, ground, 70% lean meat \/ 30% fat, patty, cooked, broiled",	LOW	0
Beef, ground, 70% lean meat \/ 30% fat, raw",	LOW	0
Beef, ground, 75% lean meat \/ 25% fat, crumbles, cooked, pan-browned",	LOW	0
Beef, ground, 75% lean meat \/ 25% fat, loaf, cooked, baked",	LOW	0
Beef, ground, 75% lean meat \/ 25% fat, patty, cooked, broiled",	LOW	0
Beef, ground, 75% lean meat \/ 25% fat, patty, cooked, pan-broiled",	LOW	0
Beef, ground, 75% lean meat \/ 25% fat, raw",	LOW	0
Beef, ground, 80% lean meat \/ 20% fat, crumbles, cooked, pan-browned",	LOW	0
Beef, ground, 80% lean meat \/ 20% fat, loaf, cooked, baked",	LOW	0
Beef, ground, 80% lean meat \/ 20% fat, patty, cooked, pan-broiled",	LOW	0
Beef, ground, 80% lean meat \/ 20% fat, raw",	LOW	0
Beef, ground, 85% lean meat \/ 15% fat, crumbles, cooked, pan-browned",	LOW	0
Beef, ground, 85% lean meat \/ 15% fat, loaf, cooked, baked",	LOW	0
Beef, ground, 85% lean meat \/ 15% fat, patty, cooked, broiled",	LOW	0
Beef, ground, 85% lean meat \/ 15% fat, patty, cooked, pan-broiled",	LOW	0
Beef, ground, 85% lean meat \/ 15% fat, raw",	LOW	0
Beef, ground, 90% lean meat \/ 10% fat, crumbles, cooked, pan-browned",	LOW	0
Beef, ground, 90% lean meat \/ 10% fat, loaf, cooked, baked",	LOW	0
Beef, ground, 90% lean meat \/ 10% fat, patty, cooked, broiled",	LOW	0
Beef, ground, 90% lean meat \/ 10% fat, patty, cooked, pan-broiled",	LOW	0
Beef, ground, 90% lean meat \/ 10% fat, raw",	LOW	0

Food name/ Category (100 g)	Status	Carbs content in g
Beef, ground, 93% lean meat \/ 7% fat, crumbles, cooked, pan-browned",	LOW	0
Beef, ground, 93% lean meat \/ 7% fat, loaf, cooked, baked",	LOW	0
Beef, ground, 93% lean meat \/ 7% fat, patty, cooked, broiled",	LOW	0
Beef, ground, 93% lean meat \/ 7% fat, raw",	LOW	0
Beef, ground, 93% lean meat \/7% fat, patty, cooked, pan-broiled",	LOW	0.06
Beef, ground, 95% lean meat \/ 5% fat, crumbles, cooked, pan-browned",	LOW	0
Beef, ground, 95% lean meat \/ 5% fat, loaf, cooked, baked",	LOW	0
Beef, ground, 95% lean meat \/ 5% fat, patty, cooked, broiled",	LOW	0
Beef, ground, 95% lean meat \/ 5% fat, patty, cooked, pan-broiled",	LOW	0
Beef, ground, 95% lean meat \/ 5% fat, raw",	LOW	0
Beef, ground, 97% lean meat \/ 3% fat, crumbles, cooked, pan-browned",	LOW	0
Beef, ground, 97% lean meat \/ 3% fat, loaf, cooked, baked",	LOW	0
Beef, ground, 97% lean meat \/ 3% fat, patty, cooked, broiled",	LOW	0
Beef, ground, 97% lean meat \/ 3% fat, raw",	LOW	0
Beef, ground, 97% lean meat \/3% fat, patty, cooked, pan-broiled",	LOW	0
Beef, ground, patties, frozen, cooked, broiled",	LOW	0
Beef, ground, unspecified fat content, cooked",	LOW	0.62
Beef, loin, bottom sirloin butt, tri-tip roast, separable lean only, trimmed to 0\" fat, all grades, cooked, roasted",	LOW	0
Beef, loin, bottom sirloin butt, tri-tip steak, separable lean and fat, trimmed to 0\" fat, all grades, cooked, broiled",	LOW	0
Beef, loin, tenderloin roast, boneless, separable lean and fat, trimmed to 0\" fat, all grades, cooked, roasted",	LOW	0
Beef, loin, tenderloin roast, boneless, separable lean and fat, trimmed to 0\" fat, all grades, raw",	LOW	0
Beef, loin, tenderloin roast, boneless, separable lean and fat, trimmed to 0\" fat, choice, cooked, roasted",	LOW	0
Beef, loin, tenderloin roast, boneless, separable lean and fat, trimmed to 0\" fat, choice, raw",	LOW	0
Beef, loin, tenderloin roast, boneless, separable lean and fat, trimmed to 0\" fat, select, cooked, roasted",	LOW	0
Beef, loin, tenderloin roast, boneless, separable lean and fat, trimmed to 0\" fat, select, raw",	LOW	0
Beef, loin, tenderloin roast, boneless, separable lean only, trimmed to 0\" fat, all grades, cooked, roasted",	LOW	0
Beef, loin, tenderloin roast, boneless, separable lean only, trimmed to 0\" fat, all grades, raw",	LOW	0
Beef, loin, tenderloin roast, boneless, separable lean only, trimmed to 0\" fat, choice, cooked, roasted",	LOW	0

Food name/ Category (100 g)	Status	Carbs content in g
Beef, loin, tenderloin roast, boneless, separable lean only, trimmed to 0\" fat, choice, raw",	LOW	0
Beef, loin, tenderloin roast, boneless, separable lean only, trimmed to 0\" fat, select, raw",	LOW	0
Beef, loin, tenderloin roast, separable lean only, boneless, trimmed to 0\" fat, select, cooked, roasted",	LOW	0
Beef, loin, tenderloin steak, boneless, separable lean and fat, trimmed to 0\" fat, all grades, cooked, grilled",	LOW	0
Beef, loin, tenderloin steak, boneless, separable lean and fat, trimmed to 0\" fat, all grades, raw",	LOW	0
Beef, loin, tenderloin steak, boneless, separable lean and fat, trimmed to 0\" fat, choice, cooked, grilled",	LOW	0
Beef, loin, tenderloin steak, boneless, separable lean and fat, trimmed to 0\" fat, choice, raw",	LOW	0
Beef, loin, tenderloin steak, boneless, separable lean and fat, trimmed to 0\" fat, select, cooked, grilled",	LOW	0
Beef, loin, tenderloin steak, boneless, separable lean and fat, trimmed to 0\" fat, select, raw",	LOW	0
Beef, loin, tenderloin steak, boneless, separable lean only, trimmed to 0\" fat, all grades, cooked, grilled",	LOW	0
Beef, loin, tenderloin steak, boneless, separable lean only, trimmed to 0\" fat, all grades, raw",	LOW	0
Beef, loin, tenderloin steak, boneless, separable lean only, trimmed to 0\" fat, choice, cooked, grilled",	LOW	0
Beef, loin, tenderloin steak, boneless, separable lean only, trimmed to 0\" fat, choice, raw",	LOW	0
Beef, loin, tenderloin steak, boneless, separable lean only, trimmed to 0\" fat, select, cooked, grilled",	LOW	0
Beef, loin, tenderloin steak, boneless, separable lean only, trimmed to 0\" fat, select, raw",	LOW	0
Beef, loin, top loin steak, boneless, lip off, separable lean and fat, trimmed to 0\" fat, all grades, cooked, grilled",	LOW	0
Beef, loin, top loin steak, boneless, lip off, separable lean and fat, trimmed to 0\" fat, all grades, raw",	LOW	0
Beef, loin, top loin steak, boneless, lip off, separable lean and fat, trimmed to 0\" fat, choice, cooked, grilled",	LOW	0
Beef, loin, top loin steak, boneless, lip off, separable lean and fat, trimmed to 0\" fat, choice, raw",	LOW	0
Beef, loin, top loin steak, boneless, lip off, separable lean and fat, trimmed to 0\" fat, select, cooked, grilled",	LOW	0
Beef, loin, top loin steak, boneless, lip off, separable lean and fat, trimmed to 0\" fat, select, raw",	LOW	0
Beef, loin, top loin steak, boneless, lip off, separable lean only, trimmed to 0\" fat, all grades, cooked, grilled",	LOW	0
Beef, loin, top loin steak, boneless, lip off, separable lean only, trimmed to 0\" fat, all grades, raw",	LOW	0
Beef, loin, top loin steak, boneless, lip off, separable lean only, trimmed to 0\" fat, choice, cooked, grilled",	LOW	0
Beef, loin, top loin steak, boneless, lip off, separable lean only, trimmed to 0\" fat, choice, raw",	LOW	0
Beef, loin, top loin steak, boneless, lip off, separable lean only, trimmed to 0\" fat, select, cooked, grilled",	LOW	0
Beef, loin, top loin steak, boneless, lip off, separable lean only, trimmed to 0\" fat, select, raw",	LOW	0
Beef, loin, top loin steak, boneless, lip-on, separable lean and fat, trimmed to 1\/8\" fat, all grades, cooked, grilled",	LOW	0

Food name/ Category (100 g)	Status	Carbs content in g
Beef, loin, top loin steak, boneless, lip-on, separable lean and fat, trimmed to 1\/8\" fat, all grades, raw",	LOW	0
Beef, loin, top loin steak, boneless, lip-on, separable lean and fat, trimmed to 1\/8\" fat, choice, cooked, grilled",	LOW	0
Beef, loin, top loin steak, boneless, lip-on, separable lean and fat, trimmed to 1\/8\" fat, choice, raw",	LOW	0
Beef, loin, top loin steak, boneless, lip-on, separable lean and fat, trimmed to 1\/8\" fat, select, cooked, grilled",	LOW	0
Beef, loin, top loin steak, boneless, lip-on, separable lean and fat, trimmed to 1\/8\" fat, select, raw",	LOW	0
Beef, loin, top loin steak, boneless, lip-on, separable lean only, trimmed to 1\/8\" fat, all grades, cooked, grilled",	LOW	0
Beef, loin, top loin steak, boneless, lip-on, separable lean only, trimmed to 1\/8\" fat, all grades, raw",	LOW	0
Beef, loin, top loin steak, boneless, lip-on, separable lean only, trimmed to 1\/8\" fat, choice, cooked, grilled",	LOW	0
Beef, loin, top loin steak, boneless, lip-on, separable lean only, trimmed to 1\/8\" fat, choice, raw",	LOW	0
Beef, loin, top loin steak, boneless, lip-on, separable lean only, trimmed to 1\/8\" fat, select, cooked, grilled",	LOW	0
Beef, loin, top loin steak, boneless, lip-on, separable lean only, trimmed to 1\/8\" fat, select, raw",	LOW	0
Beef, loin, top loin, separable lean and fat, trimmed to 1\/8\" fat, all grades, cooked, grilled",	LOW	0
Beef, loin, top loin, separable lean and fat, trimmed to 1\/8\" fat, choice, raw",	LOW	0
Beef, loin, top loin, separable lean and fat, trimmed to 1\/8\" fat, select, cooked, grilled",	LOW	0
Beef, loin, top loin, separable lean and fat, trimmed to 1\/8\" fat, select, raw",	LOW	0
Beef, loin, top sirloin cap steak, boneless, separable lean and fat, trimmed to 1\/8\" fat, all grades, cooked, grilled",	LOW	0.8
Beef, loin, top sirloin cap steak, boneless, separable lean and fat, trimmed to 1\/8\" fat, all grades, raw",	LOW	0
Beef, loin, top sirloin cap steak, boneless, separable lean and fat, trimmed to 1\/8\" fat, choice, cooked, grilled",	LOW	1.1
Beef, loin, top sirloin cap steak, boneless, separable lean and fat, trimmed to 1\/8\" fat, choice, raw",	LOW	0
Beef, loin, top sirloin cap steak, boneless, separable lean and fat, trimmed to 1\/8\" fat, select, cooked, grilled",	LOW	0.4
Beef, loin, top sirloin cap steak, boneless, separable lean and fat, trimmed to 1\/8\" fat, select, raw",	LOW	0
Beef, loin, top sirloin cap steak, boneless, separable lean only, trimmed to 1\/8\" fat, all grades, cooked, grilled",	LOW	0.73
Beef, loin, top sirloin cap steak, boneless, separable lean only, trimmed to 1\/8\" fat, all grades, raw",	LOW	0
Beef, loin, top sirloin cap steak, boneless, separable lean only, trimmed to 1\/8\" fat, choice, cooked, grilled",	LOW	1.07
Beef, loin, top sirloin cap steak, boneless, separable lean only, trimmed to 1\/8\" fat, choice, raw",	LOW	0
Beef, loin, top sirloin cap steak, boneless, separable lean only, trimmed to 1\/8\" fat, select, cooked, grilled",	LOW	0.22
Beef, loin, top sirloin cap steak, boneless, separable lean only, trimmed to 1\/8\" fat, select, raw",	LOW	0
Beef, loin, top sirloin filet, boneless, separable lean only, trimmed to 0\" fat, all grades, cooked, grilled",	LOW	0

Food name/ Category (100 g)	Status	Carbs content in g
Beef, loin, top sirloin filet, boneless, separable lean only, trimmed to 0\" fat, choice, cooked, grilled",	LOW	0
Beef, loin, top sirloin filet, boneless, separable lean only, trimmed to 0\" fat, select, cooked, grilled",	LOW	0
Beef, loin, top sirloin petite roast, boneless, separable lean only, trimmed to 0\" fat, all grades, cooked, roasted",	LOW	0
Beef, loin, top sirloin petite roast, boneless, separable lean only, trimmed to 0\" fat, choice, cooked, roasted",	LOW	0
Beef, loin, top sirloin petite roast, boneless, separable lean only, trimmed to 0\" fat, select, cooked, roasted",	LOW	0
Beef, loin, top sirloin petite roast\/filet, boneless, separable lean only, trimmed to 0\" fat, all grades, raw",	LOW	0
Beef, loin, top sirloin petite roast\/filet, boneless, separable lean only, trimmed to 0\" fat, choice, raw",	LOW	0
Beef, loin, top sirloin petite roast\/filet, boneless, separable lean only, trimmed to 0\" fat, select, raw",	LOW	0
Beef, New Zealand, imported, bolar blade, separable lean and fat, raw",	LOW	0
Beef, New Zealand, imported, bolar blade, separable lean only, raw",	LOW	0
Beef, New Zealand, imported, brisket navel end, separable lean and fat, raw",	LOW	0
Beef, New Zealand, imported, brisket navel end, separable lean only, cooked, braised",	LOW	0
Beef, New Zealand, imported, brisket navel end, separable lean only, raw",	LOW	0
Beef, New Zealand, imported, brisket point end, separable lean and fat, raw",	LOW	0
Beef, New Zealand, imported, brisket point end, separable lean only, raw",	LOW	0
Beef, New Zealand, imported, chuck eye roll, separable lean and fat, cooked, braised",	LOW	0
Beef, New Zealand, imported, chuck eye roll, separable lean and fat, raw",	LOW	0
Beef, New Zealand, imported, chuck eye roll, separable lean only, cooked, braised",	LOW	0
Beef, New Zealand, imported, cube roll, separable lean and fat, cooked, fast roasted",	LOW	0.03
Beef, New Zealand, imported, cube roll, separable lean and fat, raw",	LOW	1.31
Beef, New Zealand, imported, cube roll, separable lean only, cooked, fast roasted",	LOW	0
Beef, New Zealand, imported, cube roll, separable lean only, raw",	LOW	1.38
Beef, New Zealand, imported, eye round, separable lean and fat, cooked, slow roasted",	LOW	0
Beef, New Zealand, imported, eye round, separable lean and fat, raw",	LOW	1.32
Beef, New Zealand, imported, eye round, separable lean only, cooked, slow roasted",	LOW	0
Beef, New Zealand, imported, eye round, separable lean only, raw",	LOW	1.35
Beef, New Zealand, imported, flank, separable lean and fat, raw",	LOW	0
Beef, New Zealand, imported, flank, separable lean only, raw",	LOW	0

Food name/ Category (100 g)	Status	Carbs content in g
Beef, New Zealand, imported, flat, separable lean and fat, raw",	LOW	0
Beef, New Zealand, imported, flat, separable lean only, raw",	LOW	0
Beef, New Zealand, imported, hind shin, separable lean and fat, cooked, braised",	LOW	0.07
Beef, New Zealand, imported, hind shin, separable lean and fat, raw",	LOW	0
Beef, New Zealand, imported, hind shin, separable lean only, cooked, braised",	LOW	0
Beef, New Zealand, imported, hind shin, separable lean only, raw",	LOW	0
Beef, New Zealand, imported, inside, raw",	LOW	0.1
Beef, New Zealand, imported, knuckle, cooked, fast fried",	LOW	0
Beef, New Zealand, imported, manufacturing beef, raw",	LOW	0.23
Beef, New Zealand, imported, oyster blade, separable lean and fat, raw",	LOW	0
Beef, New Zealand, imported, oyster blade, separable lean only, raw",	LOW	0
Beef, New Zealand, imported, ribs prepared, cooked, fast roasted",	LOW	0.09
Beef, New Zealand, imported, ribs prepared, raw",	LOW	0
Beef, New Zealand, imported, rump centre, separable lean and fat, cooked, fast fried",	LOW	0
Beef, New Zealand, imported, rump centre, separable lean and fat, raw",	LOW	0
Beef, New Zealand, imported, rump centre, separable lean only, cooked, fast fried",	LOW	0
Beef, New Zealand, imported, rump centre, separable lean only, raw",	LOW	0
Beef, New Zealand, imported, striploin, separable lean and fat, cooked, fast fried",	LOW	0.02
Beef, New Zealand, imported, striploin, separable lean and fat, raw",	LOW	0.6
Beef, New Zealand, imported, striploin, separable lean only, cooked, fast fried",	LOW	0
Beef, New Zealand, imported, striploin, separable lean only, raw",	LOW	0.74
Beef, New Zealand, imported, sweetbread, cooked, boiled",	LOW	0
Beef, New Zealand, imported, sweetbread, raw",	LOW	0
Beef, New Zealand, imported, tenderloin, separable lean and fat, cooked, fast fried",	LOW	0.27
Beef, New Zealand, imported, tenderloin, separable lean and fat, raw",	LOW	0
Beef, New Zealand, imported, tenderloin, separable lean only, cooked, fast fried",	LOW	0.27
Beef, New Zealand, imported, tenderloin, separable lean only, raw",	LOW	0
Beef, New Zealand, imported, variety meats and by-products liver, cooked, boiled",	LOW	3.78

Food name/ Category (100 g)	Status	Carbs content in g
Beef, New Zealand, imported, variety meats and by-products, heart, cooked, boiled",	LOW	0
Beef, New Zealand, imported, variety meats and by-products, heart, raw",	LOW	0
Beef, New Zealand, imported, variety meats and by-products, kidney, cooked, boiled",	LOW	0
Beef, New Zealand, imported, variety meats and by-products, kidney, raw",	LOW	0
Beef, New Zealand, imported, variety meats and by-products, liver, raw",	LOW	3.6
Beef, New Zealand, imported, variety meats and by-products, tongue, cooked, boiled",	LOW	3.68
Beef, New Zealand, imported, variety meats and by-products, tongue, raw",	LOW	0
Beef, New Zealand, imported, variety meats and by-products, tripe cooked, boiled",	LOW	0
Beef, New Zealand, imported, variety meats and by-products, tripe uncooked, raw",	LOW	0
Beef, plate steak, boneless, inside skirt, separable lean and fat, trimmed to 0\" fat, all grades, cooked, grilled",	LOW	0
Beef, plate steak, boneless, inside skirt, separable lean and fat, trimmed to 0\" fat, all grades, raw",	LOW	0
Beef, plate steak, boneless, inside skirt, separable lean and fat, trimmed to 0\" fat, choice, cooked, grilled",	LOW	0
Beef, plate steak, boneless, inside skirt, separable lean and fat, trimmed to 0\" fat, choice, raw",	LOW	0
Beef, plate steak, boneless, inside skirt, separable lean and fat, trimmed to 0\" fat, select, cooked, grilled",	LOW	0
Beef, plate steak, boneless, inside skirt, separable lean and fat, trimmed to 0\" fat, select, raw",	LOW	0
Beef, plate steak, boneless, inside skirt, separable lean only, trimmed to 0\" fat, all grades, cooked, grilled",	LOW	0
Beef, plate steak, boneless, inside skirt, separable lean only, trimmed to 0\" fat, all grades, raw",	LOW	0
Beef, plate steak, boneless, inside skirt, separable lean only, trimmed to 0\" fat, choice, cooked, grilled",	LOW	0
Beef, plate steak, boneless, inside skirt, separable lean only, trimmed to 0\" fat, choice, raw",	LOW	0
Beef, plate steak, boneless, inside skirt, separable lean only, trimmed to 0\" fat, select, cooked, grilled",	LOW	0
Beef, plate steak, boneless, inside skirt, separable lean only, trimmed to 0\" fat, select, raw",	LOW	0
Beef, plate steak, boneless, outside skirt, separable lean and fat, trimmed to 0\" fat, all grades, cooked, grilled",	LOW	0
Beef, plate steak, boneless, outside skirt, separable lean and fat, trimmed to 0\" fat, all grades, raw",	LOW	0.35
Beef, plate steak, boneless, outside skirt, separable lean and fat, trimmed to 0\" fat, choice, cooked, grilled",	LOW	0
Beef, plate steak, boneless, outside skirt, separable lean and fat, trimmed to 0\" fat, choice, raw",	LOW	0.35
Beef, plate steak, boneless, outside skirt, separable lean and fat, trimmed to 0\" fat, select, cooked, grilled",	LOW	0
Beef, plate steak, boneless, outside skirt, separable lean and fat, trimmed to 0\" fat, select, raw",	LOW	0.36
Beef, plate steak, boneless, outside skirt, separable lean only, trimmed to 0\" fat, all grades, cooked, grilled",	LOW	0

Food name/ Category (100 g)	Status	Carbs content in g
Beef, plate steak, boneless, outside skirt, separable lean only, trimmed to 0\" fat, all grades, raw",	LOW	**0.19**
Beef, plate steak, boneless, outside skirt, separable lean only, trimmed to 0\" fat, choice, cooked, grilled",	LOW	0
Beef, plate steak, boneless, outside skirt, separable lean only, trimmed to 0\" fat, choice, raw",	LOW	**0.17**
Beef, plate steak, boneless, outside skirt, separable lean only, trimmed to 0\" fat, select, cooked, grilled",	LOW	0
Beef, plate steak, boneless, outside skirt, separable lean only, trimmed to 0\" fat, select, raw",	LOW	**0.23**
Beef, plate, inside skirt steak, separable lean and fat, trimmed to 0\" fat, all grades, cooked, broiled",	LOW	0
Beef, plate, inside skirt steak, separable lean only, trimmed to 0\" fat, all grades, cooked, broiled",	LOW	0
Beef, plate, outside skirt steak, separable lean and fat, trimmed to 0\" fat, all grades, cooked, broiled",	LOW	0
Beef, plate, outside skirt steak, separable lean only, trimmed to 0\" fat, all grades, cooked, broiled",	LOW	0
Beef, rib eye roast, bone-in, lip-on, separable lean and fat, trimmed to 1\/8\" fat, all grades, cooked, roasted",	LOW	0
Beef, rib eye roast, bone-in, lip-on, separable lean and fat, trimmed to 1\/8\" fat, choice, cooked, roasted",	LOW	0
Beef, rib eye roast, bone-in, lip-on, separable lean and fat, trimmed to 1\/8\" fat, select, cooked, roasted",	LOW	0
Beef, rib eye roast, bone-in, lip-on, separable lean only, trimmed to 1\/8\" fat, all grades, cooked, roasted",	LOW	0
Beef, rib eye roast, bone-in, lip-on, separable lean only, trimmed to 1\/8\" fat, choice, cooked, roasted",	LOW	0
Beef, rib eye roast, bone-in, lip-on, separable lean only, trimmed to 1\/8\" fat, select, cooked, roasted",	LOW	0
Beef, rib eye roast, boneless, lip-on, separable lean and fat, trimmed to 1\/8\" fat, all grades, cooked, roasted",	LOW	0
Beef, rib eye roast, boneless, lip-on, separable lean and fat, trimmed to 1\/8\" fat, choice, cooked, roasted",	LOW	0
Beef, rib eye roast, boneless, lip-on, separable lean and fat, trimmed to 1\/8\" fat, select, cooked, roasted",	LOW	0
Beef, rib eye roast, boneless, lip-on, separable lean only, trimmed to 1\/8\" fat, all grades, cooked, roasted",	LOW	0
Beef, rib eye roast, boneless, lip-on, separable lean only, trimmed to 1\/8\" fat, choice, cooked, roasted",	LOW	0
Beef, rib eye roast, boneless, lip-on, separable lean only, trimmed to 1\/8\" fat, select, cooked, roasted",	LOW	0
Beef, rib eye steak, bone-in, lip-on, separable lean and fat, trimmed to 1\/8\" fat, all grades, cooked, grilled",	LOW	0
Beef, rib eye steak, bone-in, lip-on, separable lean and fat, trimmed to 1\/8\" fat, choice, cooked, grilled",	LOW	0
Beef, rib eye steak, bone-in, lip-on, separable lean and fat, trimmed to 1\/8\" fat, select, cooked, grilled",	LOW	0
Beef, rib eye steak, bone-in, lip-on, separable lean only, trimmed to 1\/8\" fat, all grades, cooked, grilled",	LOW	0
Beef, rib eye steak, bone-in, lip-on, separable lean only, trimmed to 1\/8\" fat, choice, cooked, grilled",	LOW	0
Beef, rib eye steak, bone-in, lip-on, separable lean only, trimmed to 1\/8\" fat, select, cooked, grilled",	LOW	0
Beef, rib eye steak, boneless, lip off, separable lean and fat, trimmed to 0\" fat, all grades, cooked, grilled",	LOW	0

Food name/ Category (100 g)	Status	Carbs content in g
Beef, rib eye steak, boneless, lip off, separable lean and fat, trimmed to 0\" fat, all grades, raw",	LOW	0.12
Beef, rib eye steak, boneless, lip off, separable lean and fat, trimmed to 0\" fat, choice, cooked, grilled",	LOW	0
Beef, rib eye steak, boneless, lip off, separable lean and fat, trimmed to 0\" fat, choice, raw",	LOW	0.2
Beef, rib eye steak, boneless, lip off, separable lean and fat, trimmed to 0\" fat, select, cooked, grilled",	LOW	0
Beef, rib eye steak, boneless, lip off, separable lean and fat, trimmed to 0\" fat, select, raw",	LOW	0
Beef, rib eye steak, boneless, lip off, separable lean only, trimmed to 0\" fat, all grades, cooked, grilled",	LOW	0
Beef, rib eye steak, boneless, lip off, separable lean only, trimmed to 0\" fat, all grades, raw",	LOW	0
Beef, rib eye steak, boneless, lip off, separable lean only, trimmed to 0\" fat, choice, cooked, grilled",	LOW	0
Beef, rib eye steak, boneless, lip off, separable lean only, trimmed to 0\" fat, choice, raw",	LOW	0
Beef, rib eye steak, boneless, lip off, separable lean only, trimmed to 0\" fat, select, cooked, grilled",	LOW	0
Beef, rib eye steak, boneless, lip off, separable lean only, trimmed to 0\" fat, select, raw",	LOW	0
Beef, rib eye steak, boneless, lip-on, separable lean and fat, trimmed to 1\/8\" fat, all grades, cooked, grilled",	LOW	0
Beef, rib eye steak, boneless, lip-on, separable lean and fat, trimmed to 1\/8\" fat, choice, cooked, grilled",	LOW	0
Beef, rib eye steak, boneless, lip-on, separable lean and fat, trimmed to 1\/8\" fat, select, cooked, grilled",	LOW	0
Beef, rib eye steak, boneless, lip-on, separable lean only, trimmed to 1\/8\" fat, all grades, cooked, grilled",	LOW	0
Beef, rib eye steak, boneless, lip-on, separable lean only, trimmed to 1\/8\" fat, choice, cooked, grilled",	LOW	0
Beef, rib eye steak, boneless, lip-on, separable lean only, trimmed to 1\/8\" fat, select, cooked, grilled",	LOW	0
Beef, rib eye steak\/roast, bone-in, lip-on, separable lean and fat, trimmed to 1\/8\" fat, all grades, raw",	LOW	0
Beef, rib eye steak\/roast, bone-in, lip-on, separable lean and fat, trimmed to 1\/8\" fat, choice, raw",	LOW	0
Beef, rib eye steak\/roast, bone-in, lip-on, separable lean and fat, trimmed to 1\/8\" fat, select, raw",	LOW	0
Beef, rib eye steak\/roast, bone-in, lip-on, separable lean only, trimmed to 1\/8\" fat, all grades, raw",	LOW	0
Beef, rib eye steak\/roast, bone-in, lip-on, separable lean only, trimmed to 1\/8\" fat, choice, raw",	LOW	0
Beef, rib eye steak\/roast, bone-in, lip-on, separable lean only, trimmed to 1\/8\" fat, select, raw",	LOW	0
Beef, rib eye steak\/roast, boneless, lip-on, separable lean and fat, trimmed to 1\/8\" fat, all grades, raw",	LOW	0
Beef, rib eye steak\/roast, boneless, lip-on, separable lean and fat, trimmed to 1\/8\" fat, choice, raw",	LOW	0
Beef, rib eye steak\/roast, boneless, lip-on, separable lean and fat, trimmed to 1\/8\" fat, select, raw",	LOW	0
Beef, rib eye steak\/roast, boneless, lip-on, separable lean only, trimmed to 1\/8\" fat, all grades, raw",	LOW	0
Beef, rib eye steak\/roast, boneless, lip-on, separable lean only, trimmed to 1\/8\" fat, choice, raw",	LOW	0

Food name/ Category (100 g)	Status	Carbs content in g
Beef, rib eye steak\/roast, boneless, lip-on, separable lean only, trimmed to 1\/8\" fat, select, raw",	LOW	0
Beef, rib eye, small end (ribs 10-12), separable lean and fat, trimmed to 0\" fat, all grades, cooked, broiled",	LOW	0
Beef, rib eye, small end (ribs 10-12), separable lean and fat, trimmed to 0\" fat, select, cooked, broiled",	LOW	0
Beef, rib eye, small end (ribs 10-12), separable lean only, trimmed to 0\" fat, select, raw",	LOW	0
Beef, rib, back ribs, bone-in, separable lean and fat, trimmed to 0\" fat, all grades, cooked, braised",	LOW	0
Beef, rib, back ribs, bone-in, separable lean and fat, trimmed to 0\" fat, all grades, raw",	LOW	0.78
Beef, rib, back ribs, bone-in, separable lean and fat, trimmed to 0\" fat, choice, cooked, braised",	LOW	0
Beef, rib, back ribs, bone-in, separable lean and fat, trimmed to 0\" fat, choice, raw",	LOW	0.9
Beef, rib, back ribs, bone-in, separable lean and fat, trimmed to 0\" fat, select, cooked, braised",	LOW	0
Beef, rib, back ribs, bone-in, separable lean and fat, trimmed to 0\" fat, select, raw",	LOW	0.6
Beef, rib, back ribs, bone-in, separable lean only, trimmed to 0\" fat, all grades, cooked, braised",	LOW	0
Beef, rib, back ribs, bone-in, separable lean only, trimmed to 0\" fat, all grades, raw",	LOW	0.46
Beef, rib, back ribs, bone-in, separable lean only, trimmed to 0\" fat, choice, cooked, braised",	LOW	0
Beef, rib, back ribs, bone-in, separable lean only, trimmed to 0\" fat, choice, raw",	LOW	0.64
Beef, rib, back ribs, bone-in, separable lean only, trimmed to 0\" fat, select, cooked, braised",	LOW	0
Beef, rib, back ribs, bone-in, separable lean only, trimmed to 0\" fat, select, raw",	LOW	0.2
Beef, rib, eye, small end (ribs 10- 12) separable lean only, trimmed to 0\" fat, select, cooked, broiled",	LOW	0
Beef, rib, eye, small end (ribs 10-12), separable lean and fat, trimmed to 0\" fat, choice, cooked, broiled",	LOW	0
Beef, rib, eye, small end (ribs 10-12), separable lean and fat, trimmed to 0\" fat, choice, raw",	LOW	0
Beef, rib, eye, small end (ribs 10-12), separable lean only, trimmed to 0\" fat, choice, cooked, broiled",	LOW	0
Beef, rib, eye, small end (ribs 10-12), separable lean only, trimmed to 0\" fat, choice, raw",	LOW	0
Beef, rib, large end (ribs 6-9), separable lean and fat, trimmed to 0\" fat, choice, cooked, roasted",	LOW	0
Beef, rib, large end (ribs 6-9), separable lean and fat, trimmed to 0\" fat, select, cooked, roasted",	LOW	0
Beef, rib, large end (ribs 6-9), separable lean and fat, trimmed to 1\/8\" fat, all grades, cooked, broiled",	LOW	0
Beef, rib, large end (ribs 6-9), separable lean and fat, trimmed to 1\/8\" fat, all grades, cooked, roasted",	LOW	0
Beef, rib, large end (ribs 6-9), separable lean and fat, trimmed to 1\/8\" fat, all grades, raw",	LOW	0
Beef, rib, large end (ribs 6-9), separable lean and fat, trimmed to 1\/8\" fat, choice, cooked, broiled",	LOW	0
Beef, rib, large end (ribs 6-9), separable lean and fat, trimmed to 1\/8\" fat, choice, cooked, roasted",	LOW	0

Food name/ Category (100 g)	Status	Carbs content in g
Beef, rib, large end (ribs 6-9), separable lean and fat, trimmed to 1\/8\" fat, choice, raw",	LOW	0
Beef, rib, large end (ribs 6-9), separable lean and fat, trimmed to 1\/8\" fat, prime, cooked, broiled",	LOW	0
Beef, rib, large end (ribs 6-9), separable lean and fat, trimmed to 1\/8\" fat, prime, cooked, roasted",	LOW	0
Beef, rib, large end (ribs 6-9), separable lean and fat, trimmed to 1\/8\" fat, prime, raw",	LOW	0
Beef, rib, large end (ribs 6-9), separable lean and fat, trimmed to 1\/8\" fat, select, cooked, broiled",	LOW	0
Beef, rib, large end (ribs 6-9), separable lean and fat, trimmed to 1\/8\" fat, select, cooked, roasted",	LOW	0
Beef, rib, large end (ribs 6-9), separable lean and fat, trimmed to 1\/8\" fat, select, raw",	LOW	0
Beef, rib, large end (ribs 6-9), separable lean only, trimmed to 0\" fat, all grades, cooked, roasted",	LOW	0
Beef, rib, large end (ribs 6-9), separable lean only, trimmed to 0\" fat, choice, cooked, roasted",	LOW	0
Beef, rib, large end (ribs 6-9), separable lean only, trimmed to 0\" fat, select, cooked, roasted",	LOW	0
Beef, rib, shortribs, separable lean and fat, choice, cooked, braised",	LOW	0
Beef, rib, shortribs, separable lean and fat, choice, raw",	LOW	0
Beef, rib, shortribs, separable lean only, choice, cooked, braised",	LOW	0
Beef, rib, shortribs, separable lean only, choice, raw",	LOW	0
Beef, rib, small end (ribs 10-12), separable lean and fat, trimmed to 0\" fat, all grades, cooked, broiled",	LOW	0
Beef, rib, small end (ribs 10-12), separable lean and fat, trimmed to 0\" fat, choice, cooked, broiled",	LOW	0
Beef, rib, small end (ribs 10-12), separable lean and fat, trimmed to 0\" fat, select, cooked, broiled",	LOW	0
Beef, rib, small end (ribs 10-12), separable lean and fat, trimmed to 1\/8\" fat, all grades, cooked, broiled",	LOW	0
Beef, rib, small end (ribs 10-12), separable lean and fat, trimmed to 1\/8\" fat, all grades, cooked, roasted",	LOW	0
Beef, rib, small end (ribs 10-12), separable lean and fat, trimmed to 1\/8\" fat, all grades, raw",	LOW	0
Beef, rib, small end (ribs 10-12), separable lean and fat, trimmed to 1\/8\" fat, choice, cooked, broiled",	LOW	0
Beef, rib, small end (ribs 10-12), separable lean and fat, trimmed to 1\/8\" fat, choice, cooked, roasted",	LOW	0
Beef, rib, small end (ribs 10-12), separable lean and fat, trimmed to 1\/8\" fat, choice, raw",	LOW	0
Beef, rib, small end (ribs 10-12), separable lean and fat, trimmed to 1\/8\" fat, prime, cooked, broiled",	LOW	0
Beef, rib, small end (ribs 10-12), separable lean and fat, trimmed to 1\/8\" fat, prime, cooked, roasted",	LOW	0
Beef, rib, small end (ribs 10-12), separable lean and fat, trimmed to 1\/8\" fat, prime, raw",	LOW	0
Beef, rib, small end (ribs 10-12), separable lean and fat, trimmed to 1\/8\" fat, select, cooked, broiled",	LOW	0
Beef, rib, small end (ribs 10-12), separable lean and fat, trimmed to 1\/8\" fat, select, cooked, roasted",	LOW	0

Food name/ Category (100 g)	Status	Carbs content in g
Beef, rib, small end (ribs 10-12), separable lean and fat, trimmed to 1\/8\" fat, select, raw",	LOW	0
Beef, rib, small end (ribs 10-12), separable lean only, trimmed to 0\" fat, all grades, cooked, broiled",	LOW	0
Beef, rib, small end (ribs 10-12), separable lean only, trimmed to 0\" fat, choice, cooked, broiled",	LOW	0
Beef, rib, small end (ribs 10-12), separable lean only, trimmed to 0\" fat, select, cooked, broiled",	LOW	0
Beef, rib, small end (ribs 10-12), separable lean only, trimmed to 1\/8\" fat, all grades, cooked, broiled",	LOW	0
Beef, rib, small end (ribs 10-12), separable lean only, trimmed to 1\/8\" fat, all grades, raw",	LOW	0
Beef, rib, small end (ribs 10-12), separable lean only, trimmed to 1\/8\" fat, choice, raw",	LOW	0
Beef, rib, small end (ribs 10-12), separable lean only, trimmed to 1\/8\" fat, select, cooked, broiled",	LOW	0
Beef, rib, small end (ribs 10-12), separable lean only, trimmed to 1\/8\" fat, select, raw",	LOW	0
Beef, rib, small end (ribs 10-12), separable lean only, trimmed to 1\/8\"fat, choice, cooked, broiled",	LOW	0
Beef, rib, whole (ribs 6-12), separable lean and fat, trimmed to 1\/8\" fat, all grades, cooked, broiled",	LOW	0
Beef, rib, whole (ribs 6-12), separable lean and fat, trimmed to 1\/8\" fat, all grades, cooked, roasted",	LOW	0
Beef, rib, whole (ribs 6-12), separable lean and fat, trimmed to 1\/8\" fat, all grades, raw",	LOW	0
Beef, rib, whole (ribs 6-12), separable lean and fat, trimmed to 1\/8\" fat, choice, cooked, broiled",	LOW	0
Beef, rib, whole (ribs 6-12), separable lean and fat, trimmed to 1\/8\" fat, choice, cooked, roasted",	LOW	0
Beef, rib, whole (ribs 6-12), separable lean and fat, trimmed to 1\/8\" fat, choice, raw",	LOW	0
Beef, rib, whole (ribs 6-12), separable lean and fat, trimmed to 1\/8\" fat, prime, cooked, broiled",	LOW	0
Beef, rib, whole (ribs 6-12), separable lean and fat, trimmed to 1\/8\" fat, prime, cooked, roasted",	LOW	0
Beef, rib, whole (ribs 6-12), separable lean and fat, trimmed to 1\/8\" fat, prime, raw",	LOW	0
Beef, rib, whole (ribs 6-12), separable lean and fat, trimmed to 1\/8\" fat, select, cooked, broiled",	LOW	0
Beef, rib, whole (ribs 6-12), separable lean and fat, trimmed to 1\/8\" fat, select, cooked, roasted",	LOW	0
Beef, rib, whole (ribs 6-12), separable lean and fat, trimmed to 1\/8\" fat, select, raw",	LOW	0
Beef, ribeye cap steak, boneless, separable lean only, trimmed to 0\" fat, all grades, cooked, grilled",	LOW	1.53
Beef, ribeye cap steak, boneless, separable lean only, trimmed to 0\" fat, all grades, raw",	LOW	1.51
Beef, ribeye cap steak, boneless, separable lean only, trimmed to 0\" fat, choice, cooked, grilled",	LOW	1.81
Beef, ribeye cap steak, boneless, separable lean only, trimmed to 0\" fat, choice, raw",	LOW	1.75
Beef, ribeye cap steak, boneless, separable lean only, trimmed to 0\" fat, select, cooked, grilled",	LOW	1.1
Beef, ribeye cap steak, boneless, separable lean only, trimmed to 0\" fat, select, raw",	LOW	1.15

Food name/ Category (100 g)	Status	Carbs content in g
Beef, ribeye filet, boneless, separable lean only, trimmed to 0\" fat, all grades, cooked, grilled",	LOW	0.17
Beef, ribeye filet, boneless, separable lean only, trimmed to 0\" fat, choice, cooked, grilled",	LOW	0.51
Beef, ribeye filet, boneless, separable lean only, trimmed to 0\" fat, select, cooked, grilled",	LOW	0
Beef, ribeye petite roast, boneless, separable lean only, trimmed to 0\" fat, all grades, cooked, roasted",	LOW	0
Beef, ribeye petite roast, boneless, separable lean only, trimmed to 0\" fat, choice, cooked, roasted",	LOW	0
Beef, ribeye petite roast, boneless, separable lean only, trimmed to 0\" fat, select, cooked, roasted",	LOW	0
Beef, ribeye petite roast\/filet, boneless, separable lean only, trimmed to 0\" fat, all grades, raw",	LOW	0.04
Beef, ribeye petite roast\/filet, boneless, separable lean only, trimmed to 0\" fat, choice, raw",	LOW	0.18
Beef, ribeye petite roast\/filet, boneless, separable lean only, trimmed to 0\" fat, select, raw",	LOW	0
Beef, round, bottom round , roast, separable lean only, trimmed to 1\/8\" fat, select, cooked, roasted",	LOW	0
Beef, round, bottom round roast, separable lean only, trimmed to 0\" fat, select, cooked, roasted",	LOW	0
Beef, round, bottom round, roast, separable lean and fat, trimmed to 0\" fat, all grades, cooked, roasted",	LOW	0
Beef, round, bottom round, roast, separable lean and fat, trimmed to 0\" fat, select, cooked, roasted",	LOW	0
Beef, round, bottom round, roast, separable lean only, trimmed to 0\" fat, all grades, cooked, roasted",	LOW	0
Beef, round, bottom round, roast, separable lean only, trimmed to 0\" fat, choice, cooked, roasted",	LOW	0
Beef, round, bottom round, roast, separable lean only, trimmed to 1\/8\" fat, all grades, cooked",	LOW	0
Beef, round, bottom round, roast, separable lean only, trimmed to 1\/8\" fat, all grades, raw",	LOW	0
Beef, round, bottom round, roast, separable lean only, trimmed to 1\/8\" fat, choice, cooked, roasted",	LOW	0
Beef, round, bottom round, roast, separable lean only, trimmed to 1\/8\" fat, choice, raw",	LOW	0
Beef, round, bottom round, roast, separable lean only, trimmed to 1\/8\" fat, select, raw",	LOW	0
Beef, round, bottom round, steak, separable lean and fat, trimmed to 0\" fat, all grades, cooked, braised",	LOW	0
Beef, round, bottom round, steak, separable lean and fat, trimmed to 0\" fat, choice, cooked, braised",	LOW	0
Beef, round, bottom round, steak, separable lean and fat, trimmed to 0\" fat, select, cooked, braised",	LOW	0
Beef, round, bottom round, steak, separable lean and fat, trimmed to 1\/8\" fat, all grades, cooked, braised",	LOW	0
Beef, round, bottom round, steak, separable lean and fat, trimmed to 1\/8\" fat, all grades, raw",	LOW	0
Beef, round, bottom round, steak, separable lean and fat, trimmed to 1\/8\" fat, choice, cooked, braised",	LOW	0
Beef, round, bottom round, steak, separable lean and fat, trimmed to 1\/8\" fat, choice, raw",	LOW	0
Beef, round, bottom round, steak, separable lean and fat, trimmed to 1\/8\" fat, select, cooked, braised",	LOW	0

Food name/ Category (100 g)	Status	Carbs content in g
Beef, round, bottom round, steak, separable lean and fat, trimmed to 1\/8\" fat, select, raw",	LOW	0
Beef, round, bottom round, steak, separable lean only, trimmed to 0\" fat, all grades, cooked, braised",	LOW	0
Beef, round, bottom round, steak, separable lean only, trimmed to 0\" fat, choice, cooked, braised",	LOW	0
Beef, round, bottom round, steak, separable lean only, trimmed to 0\" fat, select, cooked, braised",	LOW	0
Beef, round, bottom round, steak, separable lean only, trimmed to 1\/8\" fat, all grades, cooked, braised",	LOW	0
Beef, round, bottom round, steak, separable lean only, trimmed to 1\/8\" fat, choice, cooked, braised",	LOW	0
Beef, round, bottom round, steak, separable lean only, trimmed to 1\/8\" fat, select, cooked, braised",	LOW	0
Beef, round, eye of round roast, boneless, separable lean and fat, trimmed to 0\" fat, all grades, cooked, roasted",	LOW	0
Beef, round, eye of round roast, boneless, separable lean and fat, trimmed to 0\" fat, all grades, raw",	LOW	0
Beef, round, eye of round roast, boneless, separable lean and fat, trimmed to 0\" fat, choice, cooked, roasted",	LOW	0
Beef, round, eye of round roast, boneless, separable lean and fat, trimmed to 0\" fat, choice, raw",	LOW	0
Beef, round, eye of round roast, boneless, separable lean and fat, trimmed to 0\" fat, select, cooked, roasted",	LOW	0
Beef, round, eye of round roast, boneless, separable lean and fat, trimmed to 0\" fat, select, raw",	LOW	0
Beef, round, eye of round roast, boneless, separable lean only, trimmed to 0\" fat, all grades, cooked, roasted",	LOW	0
Beef, round, eye of round roast, boneless, separable lean only, trimmed to 0\" fat, all grades, raw",	LOW	0
Beef, round, eye of round roast, boneless, separable lean only, trimmed to 0\" fat, choice, cooked, roasted",	LOW	0
Beef, round, eye of round roast, boneless, separable lean only, trimmed to 0\" fat, choice, raw",	LOW	0
Beef, round, eye of round roast, boneless, separable lean only, trimmed to 0\" fat, select, cooked, roasted",	LOW	0
Beef, round, eye of round roast, boneless, separable lean only, trimmed to 0\" fat, select, raw",	LOW	0
Beef, round, eye of round steak, boneless separable lean and fat, trimmed to 0\" fat, choice, raw",	LOW	0
Beef, round, eye of round steak, boneless, separable lean and fat, trimmed to 0\" fat, all grades, cooked, grilled",	LOW	0
Beef, round, eye of round steak, boneless, separable lean and fat, trimmed to 0\" fat, all grades, raw",	LOW	0
Beef, round, eye of round steak, boneless, separable lean and fat, trimmed to 0\" fat, choice, cooked, grilled",	LOW	0
Beef, round, eye of round steak, boneless, separable lean and fat, trimmed to 0\" fat, select, cooked, grilled",	LOW	0
Beef, round, eye of round steak, boneless, separable lean and fat, trimmed to 0\" fat, select, raw",	LOW	0
Beef, round, eye of round steak, boneless, separable lean only, trimmed to 0\" fat, all grades, cooked, grilled",	LOW	0
Beef, round, eye of round steak, boneless, separable lean only, trimmed to 0\" fat, all grades, raw",	LOW	0
Beef, round, eye of round steak, boneless, separable lean only, trimmed to 0\" fat, choice, cooked, grilled",	LOW	0

Food name/ Category (100 g)	Status	Carbs content in g
Beef, round, eye of round steak, boneless, separable lean only, trimmed to 0\" fat, choice, raw",	LOW	0
Beef, round, eye of round steak, boneless, separable lean only, trimmed to 0\" fat, select, cooked, grilled",	LOW	0
Beef, round, eye of round steak, boneless, separable lean only, trimmed to 0\" fat, select, raw",	LOW	0
Beef, round, eye of round, roast, separable lean and fat, trimmed to 1\/8\" fat, all grades, cooked, roasted",	LOW	0
Beef, round, eye of round, roast, separable lean and fat, trimmed to 1\/8\" fat, all grades, raw",	LOW	0
Beef, round, eye of round, roast, separable lean and fat, trimmed to 1\/8\" fat, choice, cooked, roasted",	LOW	0
Beef, round, eye of round, roast, separable lean and fat, trimmed to 1\/8\" fat, choice, raw",	LOW	0
Beef, round, eye of round, roast, separable lean and fat, trimmed to 1\/8\" fat, select, cooked, roasted",	LOW	0
Beef, round, eye of round, roast, separable lean and fat, trimmed to 1\/8\" fat, select, raw",	LOW	0
Beef, round, eye of round, roast, separable lean only, trimmed to 1\/8\" fat, all grades, cooked, roasted",	LOW	0
Beef, round, eye of round, roast, separable lean only, trimmed to 1\/8\" fat, all grades, raw",	LOW	0
Beef, round, eye of round, roast, separable lean only, trimmed to 1\/8\" fat, choice, cooked, roasted",	LOW	0
Beef, round, eye of round, roast, separable lean only, trimmed to 1\/8\" fat, choice, raw",	LOW	0
Beef, round, eye of round, roast, separable lean only, trimmed to 1\/8\" fat, select, cooked, roasted",	LOW	0
Beef, round, eye of round, roast, separable lean only, trimmed to 1\/8\" fat, select, raw",	LOW	0
Beef, round, full cut, separable lean and fat, trimmed to 1\/8\" fat, choice, cooked, broiled",	LOW	0
Beef, round, full cut, separable lean and fat, trimmed to 1\/8\" fat, choice, raw",	LOW	0
Beef, round, full cut, separable lean and fat, trimmed to 1\/8\" fat, select, cooked, broiled",	LOW	0
Beef, round, full cut, separable lean and fat, trimmed to 1\/8\" fat, select, raw",	LOW	0
Beef, round, full cut, separable lean only, trimmed to 1\/4\" fat, choice, cooked, broiled",	LOW	0
Beef, round, full cut, separable lean only, trimmed to 1\/4\" fat, select, cooked, broiled",	LOW	0
Beef, round, knuckle, tip center, steak, separable lean and fat, trimmed to 0\" fat, all grades, cooked, grilled",	LOW	0
Beef, round, knuckle, tip center, steak, separable lean and fat, trimmed to 0\" fat, all grades, raw",	LOW	0
Beef, round, knuckle, tip center, steak, separable lean and fat, trimmed to 0\" fat, choice, cooked, grilled",	LOW	0
Beef, round, knuckle, tip center, steak, separable lean and fat, trimmed to 0\" fat, choice, raw",	LOW	0
Beef, round, knuckle, tip center, steak, separable lean and fat, trimmed to 0\" fat, select, cooked, grilled",	LOW	0
Beef, round, knuckle, tip center, steak, separable lean and fat, trimmed to 0\" fat, select, raw",	LOW	0
Beef, round, knuckle, tip side, steak, separable lean and fat , trimmed to 0\" fat, select, raw",	LOW	0

Food name/ Category (100 g)	Status	Carbs content in g
Beef, round, knuckle, tip side, steak, separable lean and fat, trimmed to 0\" fat, all grades, cooked, grilled",	LOW	0
Beef, round, knuckle, tip side, steak, separable lean and fat, trimmed to 0\" fat, all grades, raw",	LOW	0
Beef, round, knuckle, tip side, steak, separable lean and fat, trimmed to 0\" fat, choice, cooked, grilled",	LOW	0
Beef, round, knuckle, tip side, steak, separable lean and fat, trimmed to 0\" fat, choice, raw",	LOW	0
Beef, round, knuckle, tip side, steak, separable lean and fat, trimmed to 0\" fat, select, cooked, grilled",	LOW	0
Beef, round, outside round, bottom round, steak, separable lean and fat, trimmed to 0\" fat, all grades, cooked, grilled",	LOW	0
Beef, round, outside round, bottom round, steak, separable lean and fat, trimmed to 0\" fat, all grades, raw",	LOW	0
Beef, round, outside round, bottom round, steak, separable lean and fat, trimmed to 0\" fat, choice, cooked, grilled",	LOW	0
Beef, round, outside round, bottom round, steak, separable lean and fat, trimmed to 0\" fat, choice, raw",	LOW	0
Beef, round, outside round, bottom round, steak, separable lean and fat, trimmed to 0\" fat, select, cooked, grilled",	LOW	0
Beef, round, outside round, bottom round, steak, separable lean and fat, trimmed to 0\" fat, select, raw",	LOW	0
Beef, round, tip round, roast, separable lean and fat, trimmed to 0\" fat, all grades, raw",	LOW	0
Beef, round, tip round, roast, separable lean and fat, trimmed to 0\" fat, choice, raw",	LOW	0
Beef, round, tip round, roast, separable lean and fat, trimmed to 0\" fat, select, raw",	LOW	0
Beef, round, tip round, roast, separable lean and fat, trimmed to 1\/8\" fat, all grades, cooked, roasted",	LOW	0
Beef, round, tip round, roast, separable lean and fat, trimmed to 1\/8\" fat, choice, cooked, roasted",	LOW	0
Beef, round, tip round, roast, separable lean and fat, trimmed to 1\/8\" fat, select, cooked, roasted",	LOW	0
Beef, round, tip round, roast, separable lean only, trimmed to 0\" fat, all grades, cooked, roasted",	LOW	0
Beef, round, tip round, roast, separable lean only, trimmed to 0\" fat, all grades, raw",	LOW	0
Beef, round, tip round, roast, separable lean only, trimmed to 0\" fat, choice, cooked, roasted",	LOW	0
Beef, round, tip round, roast, separable lean only, trimmed to 0\" fat, choice, raw",	LOW	0
Beef, round, tip round, roast, separable lean only, trimmed to 0\" fat, select, cooked, roasted",	LOW	0
Beef, round, tip round, roast, separable lean only, trimmed to 0\" fat, select, raw",	LOW	0
Beef, round, tip round, separable lean and fat, trimmed to 1\/8\" fat, all grades, raw",	LOW	0
Beef, round, tip round, separable lean and fat, trimmed to 1\/8\" fat, choice, raw",	LOW	0
Beef, round, tip round, separable lean and fat, trimmed to 1\/8\" fat, select, raw",	LOW	0
Beef, round, top round roast, boneless, separable lean and fat, trimmed to 0\" fat, all grades, cooked, roasted",	LOW	0
Beef, round, top round roast, boneless, separable lean and fat, trimmed to 0\" fat, all grades, raw",	LOW	0

Food name/ Category (100 g)	Status	Carbs content in g
Beef, round, top round roast, boneless, separable lean and fat, trimmed to 0\" fat, choice, cooked, roasted",	LOW	0
Beef, round, top round roast, boneless, separable lean and fat, trimmed to 0\" fat, choice, raw",	LOW	0
Beef, round, top round roast, boneless, separable lean and fat, trimmed to 0\" fat, select, cooked, roasted",	LOW	0
Beef, round, top round roast, boneless, separable lean and fat, trimmed to 0\" fat, select, raw",	LOW	0
Beef, round, top round roast, boneless, separable lean only, trimmed to 0\" fat, all grades, cooked, roasted",	LOW	0
Beef, round, top round roast, boneless, separable lean only, trimmed to 0\" fat, all grades, raw",	LOW	0
Beef, round, top round roast, boneless, separable lean only, trimmed to 0\" fat, choice, cooked, roasted",	LOW	0.06
Beef, round, top round roast, boneless, separable lean only, trimmed to 0\" fat, choice, raw",	LOW	0
Beef, round, top round roast, boneless, separable lean only, trimmed to 0\" fat, select, cooked, roasted",	LOW	0
Beef, round, top round roast, boneless, separable lean only, trimmed to 0\" fat, select, raw",	LOW	0
Beef, round, top round steak, boneless, separable lean and fat, trimmed to 0\" fat, all grades, cooked, grilled",	LOW	0
Beef, round, top round steak, boneless, separable lean and fat, trimmed to 0\" fat, all grades, raw",	LOW	0
Beef, round, top round steak, boneless, separable lean and fat, trimmed to 0\" fat, choice, cooked, grilled",	LOW	0
Beef, round, top round steak, boneless, separable lean and fat, trimmed to 0\" fat, choice, raw",	LOW	0
Beef, round, top round steak, boneless, separable lean and fat, trimmed to 0\" fat, select, cooked, grilled",	LOW	0
Beef, round, top round steak, boneless, separable lean and fat, trimmed to 0\" fat, select, raw",	LOW	0
Beef, round, top round steak, boneless, separable lean only, trimmed to 0\" fat, all grades, cooked, grilled",	LOW	0
Beef, round, top round steak, boneless, separable lean only, trimmed to 0\" fat, all grades, raw",	LOW	0
Beef, round, top round steak, boneless, separable lean only, trimmed to 0\" fat, choice, cooked, grilled",	LOW	0
Beef, round, top round steak, boneless, separable lean only, trimmed to 0\" fat, choice, raw",	LOW	0
Beef, round, top round steak, boneless, separable lean only, trimmed to 0\" fat, select, cooked, grilled",	LOW	0
Beef, round, top round steak, boneless, separable lean only, trimmed to 0\" fat, select, raw",	LOW	0
Beef, round, top round steak, separable lean and fat, trimmed to 1\/8\" fat, all grades, cooked, broiled",	LOW	0
Beef, round, top round, separable lean and fat, trimmed to 0\" fat, all grades, cooked, braised",	LOW	0
Beef, round, top round, separable lean and fat, trimmed to 0\" fat, choice, cooked, braised",	LOW	0
Beef, round, top round, separable lean and fat, trimmed to 0\" fat, select, cooked, braised",	LOW	0
Beef, round, top round, separable lean and fat, trimmed to 1\/8\" fat, all grades, cooked, braised",	LOW	0
Beef, round, top round, separable lean and fat, trimmed to 1\/8\" fat, choice, cooked, braised",	LOW	0

Food name/ Category (100 g)	Status	Carbs content in g
Beef, round, top round, separable lean and fat, trimmed to 1\/8\" fat, choice, cooked, pan-fried",	LOW	0
Beef, round, top round, separable lean and fat, trimmed to 1\/8\" fat, prime, raw",	LOW	0
Beef, round, top round, separable lean and fat, trimmed to 1\/8\" fat, select, cooked, braised",	LOW	0
Beef, round, top round, separable lean only, trimmed to 0\" fat, choice, cooked, braised",	LOW	0
Beef, round, top round, separable lean only, trimmed to 0\" fat, select, cooked, braised",	LOW	0
Beef, round, top round, separable lean only, trimmed to 1\/8\" fat, choice, cooked, pan-fried",	LOW	2.03
Beef, round, top round, steak, separable lean and fat, trimmed to 1\/8\" fat, all grades, raw",	LOW	0
Beef, round, top round, steak, separable lean and fat, trimmed to 1\/8\" fat, choice, cooked, broiled",	LOW	0
Beef, round, top round, steak, separable lean and fat, trimmed to 1\/8\" fat, choice, raw",	LOW	0
Beef, round, top round, steak, separable lean and fat, trimmed to 1\/8\" fat, prime, cooked, broiled",	LOW	0
Beef, round, top round, steak, separable lean and fat, trimmed to 1\/8\" fat, select, cooked, broiled",	LOW	0
Beef, round, top round, steak, separable lean and fat, trimmed to 1\/8\" fat, select, raw",	LOW	0
Beef, round, top round, steak, separable lean only, trimmed to 1\/8\" fat, all grades, cooked, broiled",	LOW	0
Beef, round, top round, steak, separable lean only, trimmed to 1\/8\" fat, all grades, raw",	LOW	0
Beef, round, top round, steak, separable lean only, trimmed to 1\/8\" fat, choice, cooked, broiled",	LOW	0
Beef, round, top round, steak, separable lean only, trimmed to 1\/8\" fat, choice, raw",	LOW	0
Beef, round, top round, steak, separable lean only, trimmed to 1\/8\" fat, select, cooked, broiled",	LOW	0
Beef, round, top round, steak, separable lean only, trimmed to 1\/8\" fat, select, raw",	LOW	0
Beef, sandwich steaks, flaked, chopped, formed and thinly sliced, raw",	LOW	0
Beef, shank crosscuts, separable lean only, trimmed to 1\/4\" fat, choice, cooked, simmered",	LOW	0
Beef, shank crosscuts, separable lean only, trimmed to 1\/4\" fat, choice, raw",	LOW	0
Beef, short loin, porterhouse steak, separable lean and fat, trimmed to 0\" fat, all grades, cooked, broiled",	LOW	0
Beef, short loin, porterhouse steak, separable lean and fat, trimmed to 0\" fat, USDA choice, cooked, broiled",	LOW	0
Beef, short loin, porterhouse steak, separable lean and fat, trimmed to 0\" fat, USDA select, cooked, broiled",	LOW	0
Beef, short loin, porterhouse steak, separable lean and fat, trimmed to 1\/8\" fat, all grades, cooked, grilled",	LOW	0
Beef, short loin, porterhouse steak, separable lean and fat, trimmed to 1\/8\" fat, all grades, raw",	LOW	0
Beef, short loin, porterhouse steak, separable lean and fat, trimmed to 1\/8\" fat, choice, cooked, grilled",	LOW	0
Beef, short loin, porterhouse steak, separable lean and fat, trimmed to 1\/8\" fat, choice, raw",	LOW	0

Food name/ Category (100 g)	Status	Carbs content in g
Beef, short loin, porterhouse steak, separable lean and fat, trimmed to 1\/8\" fat, select, cooked, grilled",	LOW	0
Beef, short loin, porterhouse steak, separable lean and fat, trimmed to 1\/8\" fat, select, raw",	LOW	0
Beef, short loin, porterhouse steak, separable lean only, trimmed to 0\" fat, all grades, cooked, broiled",	LOW	0
Beef, short loin, porterhouse steak, separable lean only, trimmed to 0\" fat, choice, cooked, broiled",	LOW	0
Beef, short loin, porterhouse steak, separable lean only, trimmed to 0\" fat, select, cooked, broiled",	LOW	0
Beef, short loin, porterhouse steak, separable lean only, trimmed to 1\/8\" fat, all grades, cooked, grilled",	LOW	0
Beef, short loin, porterhouse steak, separable lean only, trimmed to 1\/8\" fat, all grades, raw",	LOW	0
Beef, short loin, porterhouse steak, separable lean only, trimmed to 1\/8\" fat, choice, cooked, grilled",	LOW	0
Beef, short loin, porterhouse steak, separable lean only, trimmed to 1\/8\" fat, choice, raw",	LOW	0
Beef, short loin, porterhouse steak, separable lean only, trimmed to 1\/8\" fat, select, cooked, grilled",	LOW	0
Beef, short loin, porterhouse steak, separable lean only, trimmed to 1\/8\" fat, select, raw",	LOW	0
Beef, short loin, t-bone steak, bone-in, separable lean only, trimmed to 1\/8\" fat, all grades, cooked, grilled",	LOW	0
Beef, short loin, t-bone steak, bone-in, separable lean only, trimmed to 1\/8\" fat, all grades, raw",	LOW	0
Beef, short loin, t-bone steak, bone-in, separable lean only, trimmed to 1\/8\" fat, choice, cooked, grilled",	LOW	0
Beef, short loin, t-bone steak, bone-in, separable lean only, trimmed to 1\/8\" fat, select, cooked, grilled",	LOW	0
Beef, short loin, t-bone steak, bone-in, separable lean only, trimmed to 1\/8\" fat, select, raw",	LOW	0
Beef, short loin, t-bone steak, separable lean and fat, trimmed to 0\" fat, all grades, cooked, broiled",	LOW	0
Beef, short loin, t-bone steak, separable lean and fat, trimmed to 0\" fat, USDA choice, cooked, broiled",	LOW	0
Beef, short loin, t-bone steak, separable lean and fat, trimmed to 0\" fat, USDA select, cooked, broiled",	LOW	0
Beef, short loin, t-bone steak, separable lean and fat, trimmed to 1\/8\" fat, all grades, cooked, grilled",	LOW	0
Beef, short loin, t-bone steak, separable lean and fat, trimmed to 1\/8\" fat, all grades, raw",	LOW	0
Beef, short loin, t-bone steak, separable lean and fat, trimmed to 1\/8\" fat, choice, cooked, grilled",	LOW	0
Beef, short loin, t-bone steak, separable lean and fat, trimmed to 1\/8\" fat, select, cooked, grilled",	LOW	0
Beef, short loin, t-bone steak, separable lean and fat, trimmed to 1\/8\" fat, select, raw",	LOW	0
Beef, short loin, t-bone steak, separable lean only, trimmed to 0\" fat, choice, cooked, broiled",	LOW	0
Beef, short loin, t-bone steak, separable lean only, trimmed to 0\" fat, select, cooked, broiled",	LOW	0
Beef, short loin, top loin steak, separable lean only, trimmed to 1\/8\" fat, all grades, raw",	LOW	0
Beef, short loin, top loin, separable lean and fat, trimmed to 1\/8\" fat, prime, cooked, broiled",	LOW	0

Food name/ Category (100 g)	Status	Carbs content in g
Beef, short loin, top loin, steak, separable lean and fat, trimmed to 1\/8\" fat, all grades, raw",	LOW	0
Beef, short loin, top loin, steak, separable lean and fat, trimmed to 1\/8\" fat, choice, cooked, grilled",	LOW	0
Beef, short loin, top loin, steak, separable lean and fat, trimmed to 1\/8\" fat, prime, raw",	LOW	0
Beef, short loin, top loin, steak, separable lean only, trimmed to 1\/8\" fat, all grades, cooked, broiled",	LOW	0
Beef, short loin, top loin, steak, separable lean only, trimmed to 1\/8\" fat, choice, cooked, broiled",	LOW	0
Beef, short loin, top loin, steak, separable lean only, trimmed to 1\/8\" fat, choice, raw",	LOW	0
Beef, short loin, top loin, steak, separable lean only, trimmed to 1\/8\" fat, select, cooked, grilled",	LOW	0
Beef, short loin, top loin, steak, separable lean only, trimmed to 1\/8\" fat, select, raw",	LOW	0
Beef, shoulder pot roast or steak, boneless, separable lean and fat, trimmed to 0\" fat, all grades, raw",	LOW	0
Beef, shoulder pot roast or steak, boneless, separable lean and fat, trimmed to 0\" fat, choice, raw",	LOW	0.07
Beef, shoulder pot roast or steak, boneless, separable lean and fat, trimmed to 0\" fat, select, raw",	LOW	0
Beef, shoulder pot roast or steak, boneless, separable lean only, trimmed to 0\" fat, all grades, raw",	LOW	0
Beef, shoulder pot roast or steak, boneless, separable lean only, trimmed to 0\" fat, choice, raw",	LOW	0.11
Beef, shoulder pot roast or steak, boneless, separable lean only, trimmed to 0\" fat, select, raw",	LOW	0
Beef, shoulder pot roast, boneless, separable lean and fat, trimmed to 0\" fat, all grades, cooked, braised",	LOW	0
Beef, shoulder pot roast, boneless, separable lean and fat, trimmed to 0\" fat, choice, cooked, braised",	LOW	0
Beef, shoulder pot roast, boneless, separable lean and fat, trimmed to 0\" fat, select, cooked, braised",	LOW	0
Beef, shoulder pot roast, boneless, separable lean only, trimmed to 0\" fat, all grades, cooked, braised",	LOW	0
Beef, shoulder pot roast, boneless, separable lean only, trimmed to 0\" fat, choice, cooked, braised",	LOW	0
Beef, shoulder pot roast, boneless, separable lean only, trimmed to 0\" fat, select, cooked, braised",	LOW	0
Beef, shoulder steak, boneless, separable lean and fat, trimmed to 0\" fat, all grades, cooked, grilled",	LOW	0
Beef, shoulder steak, boneless, separable lean and fat, trimmed to 0\" fat, select, cooked, grilled",	LOW	0
Beef, shoulder steak, boneless, separable lean only, trimmed to 0\" fat, all grades, cooked, grilled",	LOW	0
Beef, shoulder steak, boneless, separable lean only, trimmed to 0\" fat, choice, cooked, grilled",	LOW	0
Beef, shoulder steak, boneless, separable lean only, trimmed to 0\" fat, select, cooked, grilled",	LOW	0
Beef, shoulder top blade steak, boneless, separable lean and fat, trimmed to 0\" fat, all grades, cooked, grilled",	LOW	0
Beef, shoulder top blade steak, boneless, separable lean and fat, trimmed to 0\" fat, all grades, raw",	LOW	0
Beef, shoulder top blade steak, boneless, separable lean and fat, trimmed to 0\" fat, choice, cooked, grilled",	LOW	0

Food name/ Category (100 g)	Status	Carbs content in g
Beef, shoulder top blade steak, boneless, separable lean and fat, trimmed to 0\" fat, choice, raw",	LOW	0
Beef, shoulder top blade steak, boneless, separable lean and fat, trimmed to 0\" fat, select, cooked, grilled",	LOW	0
Beef, shoulder top blade steak, boneless, separable lean and fat, trimmed to 0\" fat, select, raw",	LOW	0
Beef, shoulder top blade steak, boneless, separable lean only, trimmed to 0\" fat, all grades, cooked, grilled",	LOW	0
Beef, shoulder top blade steak, boneless, separable lean only, trimmed to 0\" fat, all grades, raw",	LOW	0
Beef, shoulder top blade steak, boneless, separable lean only, trimmed to 0\" fat, choice, cooked, grilled",	LOW	0
Beef, shoulder top blade steak, boneless, separable lean only, trimmed to 0\" fat, choice, raw",	LOW	0
Beef, shoulder top blade steak, boneless, separable lean only, trimmed to 0\" fat, select, cooked, grilled",	LOW	0
Beef, shoulder top blade steak, boneless, separable lean only, trimmed to 0\" fat, select, raw",	LOW	0
Beef, tenderloin, roast, separable lean and fat, trimmed to 1\/8\" fat, all grades, cooked, roasted",	LOW	0
Beef, tenderloin, roast, separable lean and fat, trimmed to 1\/8\" fat, choice, cooked, roasted",	LOW	0
Beef, tenderloin, roast, separable lean and fat, trimmed to 1\/8\" fat, prime, cooked, roasted",	LOW	0
Beef, tenderloin, roast, separable lean and fat, trimmed to 1\/8\" fat, select, cooked, roasted",	LOW	0
Beef, tenderloin, separable lean and fat, trimmed to 1\/8\" fat, prime, raw",	LOW	0
Beef, tenderloin, steak, separable lean and fat, trimmed to 1\/8\" fat, all grades, cooked, broiled",	LOW	0
Beef, tenderloin, steak, separable lean and fat, trimmed to 1\/8\" fat, all grades, raw",	LOW	0
Beef, tenderloin, steak, separable lean and fat, trimmed to 1\/8\" fat, choice, cooked, broiled",	LOW	0
Beef, tenderloin, steak, separable lean and fat, trimmed to 1\/8\" fat, choice, raw",	LOW	0
Beef, tenderloin, steak, separable lean and fat, trimmed to 1\/8\" fat, prime, cooked, broiled",	LOW	0
Beef, tenderloin, steak, separable lean and fat, trimmed to 1\/8\" fat, select, cooked, broiled",	LOW	0
Beef, tenderloin, steak, separable lean and fat, trimmed to 1\/8\" fat, select, raw",	LOW	0
Beef, tenderloin, steak, separable lean only, trimmed to 1\/8\" fat, all grades, cooked, broiled",	LOW	0
Beef, tenderloin, steak, separable lean only, trimmed to 1\/8\" fat, all grades, raw",	LOW	0
Beef, tenderloin, steak, separable lean only, trimmed to 1\/8\" fat, choice, cooked, broiled",	LOW	0
Beef, tenderloin, steak, separable lean only, trimmed to 1\/8\" fat, choice, raw",	LOW	0
Beef, tenderloin, steak, separable lean only, trimmed to 1\/8\" fat, select, cooked, broiled",	LOW	0
Beef, tenderloin, steak, separable lean only, trimmed to 1\/8\" fat, select, raw",	LOW	0
Beef, top loin filet, boneless, separable lean and fat, trimmed to 1\/8\" fat, all grades, cooked, grilled",	LOW	0.6

Food name/ Category (100 g)	Status	Carbs content in g
Beef, top loin filet, boneless, separable lean and fat, trimmed to 1\/8\" fat, choice, cooked, grilled",	LOW	**0.6**
Beef, top loin filet, boneless, separable lean and fat, trimmed to 1\/8\" fat, select, cooked, grilled",	LOW	**0.4**
Beef, top loin filet, boneless, separable lean only, trimmed to 1\/8\" fat, all grades, cooked, grilled",	LOW	**0.3**
Beef, top loin filet, boneless, separable lean only, trimmed to 1\/8\" fat, choice, cooked, grilled",	LOW	**0.36**
Beef, top loin filet, boneless, separable lean only, trimmed to 1\/8\" fat, select, cooked, grilled",	LOW	**0.2**
Beef, top loin petite roast, boneless, separable lean and fat, trimmed to 1\/8\" fat, all grades, cooked, roasted",	LOW	**1**
Beef, top loin petite roast, boneless, separable lean and fat, trimmed to 1\/8\" fat, choice, cooked, roasted",	LOW	**1.1**
Beef, top loin petite roast, boneless, separable lean and fat, trimmed to 1\/8\" fat, select, cooked, roasted",	LOW	**0.9**
Beef, top loin petite roast, boneless, separable lean only, trimmed to 1\/8\" fat, all grades, cooked, roasted",	LOW	**0.82**
Beef, top loin petite roast, boneless, separable lean only, trimmed to 1\/8\" fat, choice, cooked, roasted",	LOW	**0.88**
Beef, top loin petite roast, boneless, separable lean only, trimmed to 1\/8\" fat, select, cooked, roasted",	LOW	**0.74**
Beef, top loin petite roast\/filet, boneless, separable lean and fat, trimmed to 1\/8\" fat, all grades, raw",	LOW	**0.3**
Beef, top loin petite roast\/filet, boneless, separable lean and fat, trimmed to 1\/8\" fat, choice, raw",	LOW	**0.6**
Beef, top loin petite roast\/filet, boneless, separable lean and fat, trimmed to 1\/8\" fat, select, raw",	LOW	**0**
Beef, top loin petite roast\/filet, boneless, separable lean only, trimmed to 1\/8\" fat, all grades, raw",	LOW	**0**
Beef, top loin petite roast\/filet, boneless, separable lean only, trimmed to 1\/8\" fat, choice, raw",	LOW	**0.23**
Beef, top loin petite roast\/filet, boneless, separable lean only, trimmed to 1\/8\" fat, select, raw",	LOW	**0**
Beef, top sirloin, steak, separable lean and fat, trimmed to 0\" fat, all grades, cooked, broiled",	LOW	**0**
Beef, top sirloin, steak, separable lean and fat, trimmed to 0\" fat, choice, cooked, broiled",	LOW	**0**
Beef, top sirloin, steak, separable lean and fat, trimmed to 0\" fat, select, cooked, broiled",	LOW	**0**
Beef, top sirloin, steak, separable lean and fat, trimmed to 1\/8\" fat, all grades, cooked, broiled",	LOW	**0**
Beef, top sirloin, steak, separable lean and fat, trimmed to 1\/8\" fat, all grades, raw",	LOW	**0**
Beef, top sirloin, steak, separable lean and fat, trimmed to 1\/8\" fat, choice, cooked, broiled",	LOW	**0**
Beef, top sirloin, steak, separable lean and fat, trimmed to 1\/8\" fat, choice, cooked, pan-fried",	LOW	**0**
Beef, top sirloin, steak, separable lean and fat, trimmed to 1\/8\" fat, choice, raw",	LOW	**0**
Beef, top sirloin, steak, separable lean and fat, trimmed to 1\/8\" fat, select, cooked, broiled",	LOW	**0**
Beef, top sirloin, steak, separable lean and fat, trimmed to 1\/8\" fat, select, raw",	LOW	**0**
Beef, top sirloin, steak, separable lean only, trimmed to 0\" fat, all grades, cooked, broiled",	LOW	**0**

Food name/ Category (100 g)	Status	Carbs content in g
Beef, top sirloin, steak, separable lean only, trimmed to 0\" fat, choice, cooked, broiled",	LOW	0
Beef, top sirloin, steak, separable lean only, trimmed to 0\" fat, select, cooked, broiled",	LOW	0
Beef, top sirloin, steak, separable lean only, trimmed to 1\/8\" fat, all grades, cooked, broiled",	LOW	0
Beef, top sirloin, steak, separable lean only, trimmed to 1\/8\" fat, all grades, raw",	LOW	0
Beef, top sirloin, steak, separable lean only, trimmed to 1\/8\" fat, choice, cooked, broiled",	LOW	0
Beef, top sirloin, steak, separable lean only, trimmed to 1\/8\" fat, choice, raw",	LOW	0
Beef, top sirloin, steak, separable lean only, trimmed to 1\/8\" fat, select, cooked, broiled",	LOW	0
Beef, top sirloin, steak, separable lean only, trimmed to 1\/8\" fat, select, raw",	LOW	0
Beef, variety meats and by-products, brain, cooked, pan-fried",	LOW	0
Beef, variety meats and by-products, brain, cooked, simmered",	LOW	1.48
Beef, variety meats and by-products, brain, raw",	LOW	1.05
Beef, variety meats and by-products, heart, cooked, simmered",	LOW	0.15
Beef, variety meats and by-products, heart, raw",	LOW	0.14
Beef, variety meats and by-products, kidneys, cooked, simmered",	LOW	0
Beef, variety meats and by-products, kidneys, raw",	LOW	0.29
Beef, variety meats and by-products, liver, cooked, braised",	LOW	5.13
Beef, variety meats and by-products, liver, cooked, pan-fried",	LOW	5.16
Beef, variety meats and by-products, liver, raw",	LOW	3.89
Beef, variety meats and by-products, lungs, cooked, braised",	LOW	0
Beef, variety meats and by-products, lungs, raw",	LOW	0
Beef, variety meats and by-products, mechanically separated beef, raw",	LOW	0
Beef, variety meats and by-products, pancreas, cooked, braised",	LOW	0
Beef, variety meats and by-products, pancreas, raw",	LOW	0
Beef, variety meats and by-products, spleen, cooked, braised",	LOW	0
Beef, variety meats and by-products, spleen, raw",	LOW	0
Beef, variety meats and by-products, thymus, cooked, braised",	LOW	0
Beef, variety meats and by-products, thymus, raw",	LOW	0
Beef, variety meats and by-products, tongue, cooked, simmered",	LOW	0

Food name/ Category (100 g)	Status	Carbs content in g
Beef, variety meats and by-products, tongue, raw",	LOW	3.68
Beef, variety meats and by-products, tripe, cooked, simmered",	LOW	1.99
Beef, variety meats and by-products, tripe, raw",	LOW	0
Beet greens, cooked, boiled, drained, with salt",	LOW	5.46
Beet greens, cooked, boiled, drained, without salt",	LOW	5.46
Beet greens, raw",	LOW	4.33
Beets, canned, drained solids",	LOW	7.21
Beets, canned, regular pack, solids and liquids",	LOW	7.14
Beets, cooked, boiled, drained",	LOW	9.96
Beets, cooked, boiled. drained, with salt",	LOW	9.96
Beets, harvard, canned, solids and liquids",	LOW	18.18
Beets, pickled, canned, solids and liquids",	LOW	16.28
Beets, raw",	LOW	9.56
Beverage, instant breakfast powder, chocolate, not reconstituted",	HIGH	66.2
Beverage, instant breakfast powder, chocolate, sugar-free, not reconstituted",	MEDIUM	41
Beverage, milkshake mix, dry, not chocolate",	MEDIUM	52.9
Beverages, ABBOTT, EAS soy protein powder",	MEDIUM	43.94
Beverages, ABBOTT, EAS whey protein powder",	LOW	17.95
Beverages, ABBOTT, ENSURE PLUS, ready-to-drink",	LOW	19.88
Beverages, ABBOTT, ENSURE, Nutritional Shake, Ready-to-Drink",	LOW	16.88
Beverages, almond milk, chocolate, ready-to-drink",	LOW	9.38
Beverages, almond milk, sweetened, vanilla flavor, ready-to-drink",	LOW	6.59
Beverages, almond milk, unsweetened, shelf stable",	LOW	0.58
Beverages, AMBER, hard cider",	LOW	5.92
Beverages, ARIZONA, tea, ready-to-drink, lemon",	LOW	9.77
Beverages, carbonated, cola, fast-food cola",	LOW	9.56
Beverages, carbonated, cola, regular",	LOW	10.36
Beverages, carbonated, cola, without caffeine",	LOW	10.58
Beverages, carbonated, limeade, high caffeine",	LOW	4.16
Beverages, carbonated, low calorie, cola or pepper-type, with aspartame, without caffeine",	LOW	0.12

Food name/ Category (100 g)	Status	Carbs content in g
Beverages, carbonated, reduced sugar, cola, contains caffeine and sweeteners",	LOW	5.16
Beverages, Carob-flavor beverage mix, powder, prepared with whole milk",	LOW	8.68
Beverages, Carob-flavor beverage mix, powder",	HIGH	93.3
Beverages, chocolate almond milk, unsweetened, shelf-stable, fortified with vitamin D2 and E",	LOW	1.25
Beverages, chocolate drink, milk and soy based, ready to drink, fortified",	LOW	17.3
Beverages, chocolate malt powder, prepared with 1% milk, fortified",	LOW	8.81
Beverages, chocolate malt, powder, prepared with fat free milk",	LOW	8.64
Beverages, chocolate powder, no sugar added",	HIGH	63.64
Beverages, chocolate syrup, prepared with whole milk",	LOW	12.78
Beverages, chocolate syrup",	HIGH	65.1
Beverages, chocolate-flavor beverage mix for milk, powder, with added nutrients, prepared with whole milk",	LOW	11.87
Beverages, chocolate-flavor beverage mix for milk, powder, with added nutrients",	HIGH	90.28
Beverages, chocolate-flavor beverage mix, powder, prepared with whole milk",	LOW	11.91
Beverages, Chocolate-flavored drink, whey and milk based",	LOW	10.68
Beverages, citrus fruit juice drink, frozen concentrate, prepared with water",	LOW	11.42
Beverages, citrus fruit juice drink, frozen concentrate",	MEDIUM	40.2
Beverages, Clam and tomato juice, canned",	LOW	10.95
Beverages, COCA-COLA, POWERADE, lemon-lime flavored, ready-to-drink",	LOW	7.84
Beverages, Cocktail mix, non-alcoholic, concentrated, frozen",	HIGH	71.6
Beverages, Cocoa mix, low calorie, powder, with added calcium, phosphorus, aspa	HIGH	58
Beverages, Cocoa mix, NESTLE, Hot Cocoa Mix Rich Chocolate With Marshmallov	HIGH	75
Beverages, Cocoa mix, no sugar added, powder",	HIGH	71.93
Beverages, Cocoa mix, powder, prepared with water",	LOW	11.54
Beverages, Cocoa mix, powder",	HIGH	83.73
Beverages, cocoa mix, with aspartame, powder, prepared with water",	LOW	5.61
Beverages, coffee and cocoa, instant, decaffeinated, with whitener and low calorie	HIGH	71.4
Beverages, coffee substitute, cereal grain beverage, powder, prepared with whole milk",	LOW	5.6
Beverages, coffee substitute, cereal grain beverage, powder",	HIGH	78.42
Beverages, coffee substitute, cereal grain beverage, prepared with water",	LOW	1.3
Beverages, coffee, brewed, breakfast blend",	LOW	0.23
Beverages, coffee, brewed, prepared with tap water, decaffeinated",	LOW	0
Beverages, coffee, brewed, prepared with tap water",	LOW	0
Beverages, coffee, instant, decaffeinated, prepared with water",	LOW	0.43
Beverages, coffee, instant, mocha, sweetened",	HIGH	74.04
Beverages, coffee, instant, regular, half the caffeine",	HIGH	73.18

Food name/ Category (100 g)	Status	Carbs content in g
Beverages, coffee, instant, regular, powder",	HIGH	75.4
Beverages, coffee, instant, regular, prepared with water",	LOW	0.34
Beverages, coffee, instant, vanilla, sweetened, decaffeinated, with non dairy cream	HIGH	86.28
Beverages, coffee, instant, with chicory",	HIGH	78.9
Beverages, coffee, instant, with whitener, reduced calorie",	HIGH	59.94
Beverages, Cranberry juice cocktail",	LOW	12.25
Beverages, cranberry-apple juice drink, bottled",	LOW	15.85
Beverages, cranberry-apple juice drink, low calorie, with vitamin C added",	LOW	4.7
Beverages, cranberry-apricot juice drink, bottled",	LOW	16.2
Beverages, cranberry-grape juice drink, bottled",	LOW	14
Beverages, CYTOSPORT, Muscle Milk, ready-to-drink",	LOW	2.06
Beverages, dairy drink mix, chocolate, reduced calorie, with aspartame, powder, prepared with water and ice",	LOW	4.51
Beverages, Dairy drink mix, chocolate, reduced calorie, with low-calorie sweeteners	MEDIUM	51.4
Beverages, drink mix, QUAKER OATS, GATORADE, orange flavor, powder",	HIGH	94.11
Beverages, Eggnog-flavor mix, powder, prepared with whole milk",	LOW	14.2
Beverages, Energy Drink with carbonated water and high fructose corn syrup",	LOW	15
Beverages, Energy Drink, Monster, fortified with vitamins C, B2, B3, B6, B12",	LOW	11.28
Beverages, Energy drink, RED BULL, sugar free, with added caffeine, niacin, pantothenic acid, vitamins B6 and B12",	LOW	0.7
Beverages, Energy drink, RED BULL",	LOW	10.23
Beverages, Energy drink, ROCKSTAR, sugar free",	LOW	0.7
Beverages, Energy Drink, sugar free",	LOW	0.42
Beverages, Fruit flavored drink containing less than 3% fruit juice, with high vitamin C",	LOW	6.67
Beverages, Fruit flavored drink, less than 3% juice, not fortified with vitamin C",	LOW	16.03
Beverages, fruit juice drink, greater than 3% fruit juice, high vitamin C and added thiamin",	LOW	13.16
Beverages, fruit juice drink, reduced sugar, with vitamin E added",	LOW	10
Beverages, Fruit punch drink, frozen concentrate, prepared with water",	LOW	11.66
Beverages, Fruit punch drink, with added nutrients, canned",	LOW	11.94
Beverages, fruit punch juice drink, frozen concentrate, prepared with water",	LOW	11.4
Beverages, fruit-flavored drink, dry powdered mix, low calorie, with aspartame",	HIGH	87.38
Beverages, Horchata, dry mix, unprepared, variety of brands, all with morro seeds",	HIGH	79.05
Beverages, ICELANDIC, Glacial Natural spring water",	LOW	0
Beverages, KELLOGG'S SPECIAL K20 protein powder",	HIGH	58.4

Food name/ Category (100 g)	Status	Carbs content in g
Beverages, KELLOGG'S, SPECIAL K Protein Shake",	LOW	9.2
Beverages, KRAFT, coffee, instant, French Vanilla Cafe",	HIGH	74.6
Beverages, Lemonade fruit juice drink light, fortified with vitamin E and C",	LOW	5
Beverages, lemonade-flavor drink, powder",	HIGH	97.9
Beverages, lemonade, frozen concentrate, pink, prepared with water",	LOW	10.81
Beverages, Lemonade, powder",	HIGH	97.57
Beverages, Malt liquor beverage",	LOW	0
Beverages, Malted drink mix, chocolate, powder, prepared with whole milk",	LOW	11.2
Beverages, malted drink mix, chocolate, powder",	HIGH	86.94
Beverages, Malted drink mix, chocolate, with added nutrients, powder, prepared with whole milk",	LOW	11.19
Beverages, Malted drink mix, natural, powder, dairy based.",	HIGH	71.21
Beverages, Malted drink mix, natural, powder, prepared with whole milk",	LOW	10.23
Beverages, Malted drink mix, natural, with added nutrients, powder, prepared with whole milk",	LOW	10.67
Beverages, Meal supplement drink, canned, peanut flavor",	LOW	14.74
Beverages, milk beverage, reduced fat, flavored and sweetened, Ready-to-drink, added calcium, vitamin A and vitamin D",	LOW	12.08
Beverages, MONSTER energy drink, low carb",	LOW	1.38
Beverages, NESTLE, Boost plus, nutritional drink, ready-to-drink",	LOW	17.29
Beverages, nutritional shake mix, high protein, powder",	LOW	20.38
Beverages, OCEAN SPRAY, Cran Lemonade",	LOW	11.12
Beverages, OCEAN SPRAY, Light Cranberry and Raspberry Flavored Juice",	LOW	5.77
Beverages, OCEAN SPRAY, White Cranberry Strawberry Flavored Juice Drink",	LOW	11.98
Beverages, orange and apricot juice drink, canned",	LOW	12.7
Beverages, orange breakfast drink, ready-to-drink, with added nutrients",	LOW	13.2
Beverages, orange drink, canned, with added vitamin C",	LOW	12.34
Beverages, Orange juice drink",	LOW	13.41
Beverages, Orange juice, light, No pulp",	LOW	5.42
Beverages, Orange-flavor drink, breakfast type, low calorie, powder",	HIGH	85.9
Beverages, orange-flavor drink, breakfast type, powder, prepared with water",	LOW	12.65
Beverages, OVALTINE, chocolate malt powder",	HIGH	92.96
Beverages, OVALTINE, Classic Malt powder",	HIGH	93.33
Beverages, PEPSICO QUAKER, Gatorade G2, low calorie",	LOW	1.94
Beverages, PEPSICO QUAKER, Gatorade, G performance O 2, ready-to-drink.",	LOW	6.43

Food name/ Category (100 g)	Status	Carbs content in g
Beverages, pineapple and orange juice drink, canned",	LOW	11.8
Beverages, Powerade Zero Ion4, calorie-free, assorted flavors",	LOW	0
Beverages, POWERADE, Zero, Mixed Berry",	LOW	0.14
Beverages, Protein powder soy based",	LOW	28.89
Beverages, Protein powder whey based",	LOW	6.25
Beverages, rice milk, unsweetened",	LOW	9.17
Beverages, rich chocolate, powder",	HIGH	92.96
Beverages, shake, fast food, strawberry",	LOW	18.9
Beverages, SLIMFAST, Meal replacement, High Protein Shake, Ready-To-Drink, 3-2-1 plan",	LOW	0.85
Beverages, Strawberry-flavor beverage mix, powder, prepared with whole milk",	LOW	12.3
Beverages, tea, black, brewed, prepared with distilled water",	LOW	0.3
Beverages, tea, black, brewed, prepared with tap water, decaffeinated",	LOW	0.3
Beverages, tea, black, brewed, prepared with tap water",	LOW	0.3
Beverages, tea, black, ready to drink, decaffeinated, diet",	LOW	0.83
Beverages, tea, black, ready to drink",	LOW	0
Beverages, tea, black, ready-to-drink, lemon, sweetened",	LOW	10.8
Beverages, tea, black, ready-to-drink, peach, diet",	LOW	0.25
Beverages, tea, green, brewed, decaffeinated",	LOW	0
Beverages, tea, green, brewed, regular",	LOW	0
Beverages, tea, green, instant, decaffeinated, lemon, unsweetened, fortified with vit	HIGH	94.45
Beverages, tea, green, ready to drink, ginseng and honey, sweetened",	LOW	7.16
Beverages, tea, hibiscus, brewed",	LOW	0
Beverages, tea, instant, decaffeinated, lemon, diet",	HIGH	85.4
Beverages, tea, instant, decaffeinated, lemon, sweetened",	HIGH	98.55
Beverages, tea, instant, decaffeinated, unsweetened",	HIGH	58.66
Beverages, tea, instant, lemon, sweetened, powder",	HIGH	98.55
Beverages, tea, instant, lemon, sweetened, prepared with water",	LOW	8.61
Beverages, tea, instant, lemon, unsweetened",	HIGH	78.52
Beverages, tea, instant, lemon, with added ascorbic acid",	HIGH	97.6
Beverages, tea, instant, sweetened with sodium saccharin, lemon-flavored, powder'	HIGH	85.4
Beverages, tea, instant, unsweetened, powder",	HIGH	58.66
Beverages, tea, instant, unsweetened, prepared with water",	LOW	0.17
Beverages, tea, ready-to-drink, lemon, diet",	LOW	0.41

Food name/ Category (100 g)	Status	Carbs content in g
Beverages, The COCA-COLA company, DASANI, water, bottled, non-carbonated",	LOW	0
Beverages, The COCA-COLA company, Glaceau Vitamin Water, Revive Fruit Punch, fortified",	LOW	0
Beverages, THE COCA-COLA COMPANY, NOS energy drink, Original, grape, loaded cherry, charged citrus, fortified with vitamins B6 and B12",	LOW	11.25
Beverages, THE COCA-COLA COMPANY, NOS Zero, energy drink, sugar-free with guarana, fortified with vitamins B6 and B12",	LOW	1.03
Beverages, UNILEVER, SLIMFAST Shake Mix, high protein, whey powder, 3-2-1 P	MEDIUM	50
Beverages, UNILEVER, SLIMFAST Shake Mix, powder, 3-2-1 Plan",	HIGH	73.92
Beverages, UNILEVER, SLIMFAST, meal replacement, regular, ready-to-drink, 3-2-1 Plan",	LOW	7.74
Beverages, Water with added vitamins and minerals, bottles, sweetened, assorted fruit flavors",	LOW	5.49
Beverages, water, bottled, non-carbonated, CALISTOGA",	LOW	0
Beverages, water, bottled, non-carbonated, CRYSTAL GEYSER",	LOW	0
Beverages, water, bottled, non-carbonated, DANNON Fluoride To Go",	LOW	0.03
Beverages, water, bottled, non-carbonated, DANNON",	LOW	0
Beverages, water, bottled, non-carbonated, EVIAN",	LOW	0
Beverages, water, bottled, non-carbonated, PEPSI, AQUAFINA",	LOW	0
Beverages, water, bottled, PERRIER",	LOW	0
Beverages, water, bottled, POLAND SPRING",	LOW	0
Beverages, water, tap, drinking",	LOW	0
Beverages, water, tap, municipal",	LOW	0
Beverages, water, tap, well",	LOW	0
Beverages, WENDY'S, tea, ready-to-drink, unsweetened",	LOW	0
Beverages, Whey protein powder isolate",	LOW	29.07
Beverages, Whiskey sour mix, bottled",	LOW	21.4
Beverages, Whiskey sour mix, powder",	HIGH	97.3
Biscuits, mixed grain, refrigerated dough",	MEDIUM	47.4
Biscuits, plain or buttermilk, dry mix, prepared",	MEDIUM	48.4
Biscuits, plain or buttermilk, dry mix",	HIGH	63.4
Biscuits, plain or buttermilk, frozen, baked",	MEDIUM	53.87
Biscuits, plain or buttermilk, prepared from recipe",	MEDIUM	44.6
Biscuits, plain or buttermilk, refrigerated dough, higher fat, baked",	MEDIUM	49.05
Biscuits, plain or buttermilk, refrigerated dough, higher fat",	MEDIUM	46.32
Biscuits, plain or buttermilk, refrigerated dough, lower fat, baked",	MEDIUM	51.6
Biscuits, plain or buttermilk, refrigerated dough, lower fat",	MEDIUM	43.7
Bison, ground, grass-fed, cooked",	LOW	0
Bison, ground, grass-fed, raw",	LOW	0.05

Food name/ Category (100 g)	Status	Carbs content in g
Blackberries, canned, heavy syrup, solids and liquids",	LOW	23.1
Blackberries, frozen, unsweetened",	LOW	15.67
Blackberries, raw",	LOW	9.61
Blackberry juice, canned",	LOW	7.8
Blood sausage",	LOW	1.29
Blueberries, canned, heavy syrup, solids and liquids",	LOW	22.06
Blueberries, canned, light syrup, drained",	LOW	22.66
Blueberries, dried, sweetened",	HIGH	80
Blueberries, frozen, sweetened",	LOW	21.95
Blueberries, frozen, unsweetened",	LOW	12.17
Blueberries, raw",	LOW	14.49
Blueberries, wild, canned, heavy syrup, drained",	LOW	28.32
Blueberries, wild, frozen",	LOW	13.85
Bologna, beef, low fat",	LOW	5.2
Bologna, beef",	LOW	4.29
Bologna, meat and poultry",	LOW	6.31
Bologna, turkey",	LOW	4.68
Borage, raw",	LOW	3.06
Boysenberries, canned, heavy syrup",	LOW	22.31
Boysenberries, frozen, unsweetened",	LOW	12.19
Bratwurst, chicken, cooked",	LOW	0
Bratwurst, veal, cooked",	LOW	0
Bread crumbs, dry, grated, plain",	HIGH	71.98
Bread crumbs, dry, grated, seasoned",	HIGH	68.49
Bread sticks, plain",	HIGH	68.4
Bread stuffing, bread, dry mix, prepared",	LOW	18.84
Bread stuffing, bread, dry mix",	HIGH	76.2
Bread stuffing, cornbread, dry mix, prepared",	LOW	21.9
Bread stuffing, cornbread, dry mix",	HIGH	76.7
Bread, banana, prepared from recipe, made with margarine",	MEDIUM	54.6
Bread, boston brown, canned",	MEDIUM	43.3
Bread, chapati or roti, plain, commercially prepared",	MEDIUM	46.36
Bread, chapati or roti, whole wheat, commercially prepared, frozen",	MEDIUM	46.13

Food name/ Category (100 g)	Status	Carbs content in g
Bread, cheese",	MEDIUM	44.83
Bread, cinnamon",	MEDIUM	44.38
Bread, cornbread, dry mix, enriched (includes corn muffin mix)",	HIGH	69.5
Bread, cornbread, dry mix, prepared with 2% milk, 80% margarine, and eggs",	MEDIUM	54.46
Bread, cornbread, dry mix, unenriched (includes corn muffin mix)",	HIGH	69.5
Bread, cornbread, prepared from recipe, made with low fat (2%) milk",	MEDIUM	43.5
Bread, cracked-wheat",	MEDIUM	49.5
Bread, egg, toasted",	MEDIUM	52.6
Bread, egg",	MEDIUM	47.8
Bread, french or vienna (includes sourdough)",	MEDIUM	51.88
Bread, french or vienna, toasted (includes sourdough)",	HIGH	61.93
Bread, french or vienna, whole wheat",	MEDIUM	49.1
Bread, gluten-free, white, made with potato extract, rice starch, and rice flour",	MEDIUM	52.83
Bread, gluten-free, white, made with rice flour, corn starch, and\/or tapioca",	MEDIUM	45.78
Bread, gluten-free, white, made with tapioca starch and brown rice flour",	MEDIUM	51.15
Bread, gluten-free, whole grain, made with tapioca starch and brown rice flour",	MEDIUM	49.09
Bread, irish soda, prepared from recipe",	MEDIUM	56
Bread, italian",	MEDIUM	50.1
Bread, kneel down (Navajo)",	LOW	39.47
Bread, multi-grain (includes whole-grain)",	MEDIUM	43.34
Bread, multi-grain, toasted (includes whole-grain)",	MEDIUM	47.11
Bread, naan, plain, commercially prepared, refrigerated",	MEDIUM	50.43
Bread, naan, whole wheat, commercially prepared, refrigerated",	MEDIUM	46.21
Bread, oat bran, toasted",	MEDIUM	43.7
Bread, oat bran",	LOW	39.8
Bread, oatmeal, toasted",	MEDIUM	52.7
Bread, oatmeal",	MEDIUM	48.5
Bread, pan dulce, sweet yeast bread",	MEDIUM	56.38
Bread, paratha, whole wheat, commercially prepared, frozen",	MEDIUM	45.35
Bread, pita, white, enriched",	MEDIUM	55.7
Bread, pita, white, unenriched",	MEDIUM	55.7
Bread, pita, whole-wheat",	MEDIUM	55.89
Bread, potato",	MEDIUM	47.07
Bread, pound cake type, pan de torta salvadoran",	MEDIUM	51.29
Bread, protein (includes gluten)",	MEDIUM	43.8
Bread, protein, (includes gluten), toasted",	MEDIUM	48.1
Bread, pumpernickel, toasted",	MEDIUM	52.2
Bread, pumpernickel",	MEDIUM	47.5
Bread, raisin, enriched, toasted",	MEDIUM	56.9
Bread, raisin, enriched",	MEDIUM	52.3
Bread, raisin, unenriched",	MEDIUM	52.3
Bread, reduced-calorie, oat bran, toasted",	MEDIUM	49.2
Bread, reduced-calorie, oat bran",	MEDIUM	41.3
Bread, reduced-calorie, oatmeal",	MEDIUM	43.3
Bread, reduced-calorie, rye",	MEDIUM	40.5
Bread, reduced-calorie, wheat",	MEDIUM	42.47
Bread, reduced-calorie, white",	MEDIUM	44.3
Bread, rice bran, toasted",	MEDIUM	47.3
Bread, rice bran",	MEDIUM	43.5
Bread, roll, Mexican, bollilo",	MEDIUM	55.77
Bread, rye, toasted",	MEDIUM	53.1
Bread, rye",	MEDIUM	48.3
Bread, salvadoran sweet cheese (quesadilla salvadorena)",	MEDIUM	47.84
Bread, wheat bran",	MEDIUM	47.8
Bread, wheat germ, toasted",	MEDIUM	54.3

Food name/ Category (100 g)	Status	Carbs content in g
Bread, wheat, sprouted, toasted",	LOW	36.82
Bread, wheat, sprouted",	LOW	33.88
Bread, wheat, toasted",	MEDIUM	55.77
Bread, wheat",	MEDIUM	48.68
Bread, white wheat",	MEDIUM	43.91
Bread, white, commercially prepared (includes soft bread crumbs)",	MEDIUM	49.42
Bread, white, commercially prepared, low sodium, no salt",	MEDIUM	49.6
Bread, white, commercially prepared, toasted, low sodium no salt",	MEDIUM	54.4
Bread, white, commercially prepared, toasted",	MEDIUM	54.5
Bread, white, prepared from recipe, made with low fat (2%) milk",	MEDIUM	49.6
Bread, white, prepared from recipe, made with nonfat dry milk",	MEDIUM	53.6
Bread, whole-wheat, commercially prepared, toasted",	MEDIUM	51.16
Bread, whole-wheat, commercially prepared",	MEDIUM	42.71
Bread, whole-wheat, prepared from recipe, toasted",	MEDIUM	56.4
Bread, whole-wheat, prepared from recipe",	MEDIUM	51.4
Breadfruit, raw",	LOW	27.12
Breakfast bar, corn flake crust with fruit",	HIGH	72.9
Breakfast bars, oats, sugar, raisins, coconut (include granola bar)",	HIGH	66.7
Breakfast tart, low fat",	HIGH	76.8
Broadbeans (fava beans), mature seeds, canned",	LOW	12.41
Broadbeans (fava beans), mature seeds, cooked, boiled, with salt",	LOW	19.65
Broadbeans (fava beans), mature seeds, cooked, boiled, without salt",	LOW	19.65
Broadbeans, immature seeds, raw",	LOW	11.7
Broccoli raab, cooked",	LOW	3.12
Broccoli, cooked, boiled, drained, with salt",	LOW	7.18
Broccoli, cooked, boiled, drained, without salt",	LOW	7.18
Broccoli, frozen, chopped, cooked, boiled, drained, with salt",	LOW	5.35
Broccoli, frozen, spears, cooked, boiled, drained, with salt",	LOW	5.35
Brussels sprouts, cooked, boiled, drained, with salt",	LOW	7.1
Brussels sprouts, frozen, cooked, boiled, drained, with salt",	LOW	8.32
Buckwheat groats, roasted, cooked",	LOW	19.94
Buckwheat",	HIGH	71.5
Bulgur, cooked",	LOW	18.58
Burdock root, cooked, boiled, drained, with salt",	LOW	21.15
Burdock root, cooked, boiled, drained, without salt",	LOW	21.15
Burdock root, raw",	LOW	17.34

Food name/ Category (100 g)	Status	Carbs content in g
BURGER KING, Cheeseburger",	LOW	23.71
BURGER KING, Chicken Strips",	LOW	20.49
BURGER KING, CROISSAN'WICH with Egg and Cheese",	LOW	24.79
BURGER KING, CROISSAN'WICH with Sausage and Cheese",	LOW	23
BURGER KING, CROISSAN'WICH with Sausage, Egg and Cheese",	LOW	15.9
BURGER KING, Double Cheeseburger",	LOW	17.43
BURGER KING, DOUBLE WHOPPER, no cheese",	LOW	13.74
BURGER KING, DOUBLE WHOPPER, with cheese",	LOW	13.52
BURGER KING, french fries",	LOW	38.7
BURGER KING, french toast sticks",	MEDIUM	41.21
BURGER KING, Hash Brown Rounds",	LOW	29.37
BURGER KING, Onion Rings",	MEDIUM	43.58
BURGER KING, Original Chicken Sandwich",	LOW	26.22
BURGER KING, Premium Fish Sandwich",	LOW	26.69
BURGER KING, Vanilla Shake",	LOW	19.03
BURGER KING, WHOPPER, no cheese",	LOW	18.55
BURGER KING, WHOPPER, with cheese",	LOW	16.7
Burrito, bean and cheese, frozen",	LOW	34.01
Burrito, beef and bean, frozen",	LOW	30.84
Burrito, beef and bean, microwaved",	LOW	38.95
Butter oil, anhydrous",	LOW	0
Butter replacement, without fat, powder",	HIGH	89
Butter, light, stick, with salt",	LOW	0
Butter, light, stick, without salt",	LOW	0
Butter, salted",	LOW	0.06
Butter, whipped, with salt",	LOW	2.87
Butterbur, canned",	LOW	0.38
Cabbage, chinese (pak-choi), cooked, boiled, drained, with salt",	LOW	1.78
Cabbage, chinese (pak-choi), raw",	LOW	2.18

Food name/ Category (100 g)	Status	Carbs content in g
Cabbage, chinese (pe-tsai), cooked, boiled, drained, with salt",	LOW	2.41
Cabbage, common, cooked, boiled, drained, with salt",	LOW	5.51
Cabbage, japanese style, fresh, pickled",	LOW	5.67
Cabbage, kimchi",	LOW	2.4
Cabbage, mustard, salted",	LOW	5.63
Cabbage, red, cooked, boiled, drained, with salt",	LOW	6.94
Cabbage, savoy, cooked, boiled, drained, with salt",	LOW	5.41
Cake, angelfood, commercially prepared",	HIGH	57.8
Cake, angelfood, dry mix, prepared",	HIGH	58.7
Cake, angelfood, dry mix",	HIGH	86.13
Cake, boston cream pie, commercially prepared",	MEDIUM	42.9
Cake, cherry fudge with chocolate frosting",	LOW	38
Cake, chocolate, commercially prepared with chocolate frosting, in-store bakery",	MEDIUM	52.84
Cake, chocolate, prepared from recipe without frosting",	MEDIUM	53.4
Cake, fruitcake, commercially prepared",	HIGH	61.6
Cake, gingerbread, dry mix",	HIGH	74.6
Cake, gingerbread, prepared from recipe",	MEDIUM	49.2
Cake, pineapple upside-down, prepared from recipe",	MEDIUM	50.5
Cake, pound, BIMBO Bakeries USA, Panque Casero, home baked style",	MEDIUM	48.94
Cake, pound, commercially prepared, butter (includes fresh and frozen)",	MEDIUM	53.64
Cake, pound, commercially prepared, fat-free",	HIGH	61
Cake, pound, commercially prepared, other than all butter, enriched",	MEDIUM	52.5
Cake, pound, commercially prepared, other than all butter, unenriched",	MEDIUM	52.5
Cake, pudding-type, carrot, dry mix",	HIGH	79.2
Cake, pudding-type, chocolate, dry mix",	HIGH	80.16
Cake, pudding-type, german chocolate, dry mix",	HIGH	81.25
Cake, pudding-type, marble, dry mix",	HIGH	79.5
Cake, pudding-type, white, enriched, dry mix",	HIGH	80.9
Cake, pudding-type, white, unenriched, dry mix",	HIGH	81
Cake, pudding-type, yellow, dry mix",	HIGH	80
Cake, shortcake, biscuit-type, prepared from recipe",	MEDIUM	48.5
Cake, snack cakes, creme-filled, chocolate with frosting, low-fat, with added fiber",	HIGH	69.37
Cake, snack cakes, creme-filled, chocolate with frosting",	HIGH	60.31
Cake, snack cakes, creme-filled, sponge",	HIGH	64.03
Cake, snack cakes, not chocolate, with icing or filling, low-fat, with added fiber",	HIGH	74.3
Cake, sponge, commercially prepared",	HIGH	61
Cake, sponge, prepared from recipe",	HIGH	57.7
Cake, white, dry mix, special dietary (includes lemon-flavored)",	HIGH	79.6
Cake, white, prepared from recipe with coconut frosting",	HIGH	63.2
Cake, white, prepared from recipe without frosting",	HIGH	57.2
Cake, yellow, commercially prepared, with chocolate frosting, in-store bakery",	MEDIUM	55.36
Cake, yellow, commercially prepared, with vanilla frosting",	MEDIUM	56.2
Cake, yellow, enriched, dry mix",	HIGH	81.92
Cake, yellow, light, dry mix",	HIGH	84.1
Cake, yellow, prepared from recipe without frosting",	MEDIUM	53
Cake, yellow, unenriched, dry mix",	HIGH	78.1
CAMPBELL'S CHUNKY Microwavable Bowls, Beef with Country Vegetables Soup, ready-to-serve",	LOW	8.57

Food name/ Category (100 g)	Status	Carbs content in g
CAMPBELL'S CHUNKY Microwavable Bowls, Chicken and Dumplings Soup, ready-to-serve",	LOW	7.35
CAMPBELL'S CHUNKY Microwavable Bowls, Classic Chicken Noodle, ready-to-serve",	LOW	5.71
CAMPBELL'S CHUNKY Microwavable Bowls, Grilled Chicken and Sausage Gumbo, ready-to-serve",	LOW	7.35
CAMPBELL'S CHUNKY Microwavable Bowls, New England Clam Chowder, ready-to-serve",	LOW	6.94
CAMPBELL'S CHUNKY Microwavable Bowls, Old Fashioned Vegetable Beef Soup, ready-to-serve",	LOW	5.71
CAMPBELL'S CHUNKY Microwavable Bowls, Sirloin Burger with Country Vegetables Soup, ready-to-serve",	LOW	7.35
CAMPBELL'S CHUNKY Soups, Baked Potato with Steak & Cheese Soup",	LOW	8.57
CAMPBELL'S CHUNKY Soups, Beef Rib Roast with Potatoes & Herbs Soup",	LOW	6.94
CAMPBELL'S CHUNKY Soups, Beef with Country Vegetables Soup",	LOW	7.35
CAMPBELL'S CHUNKY Soups, Beef with White and Wild Rice Soup",	LOW	9.8
CAMPBELL'S CHUNKY Soups, Chicken Broccoli Cheese & Potato Soup",	LOW	8.16
CAMPBELL'S CHUNKY Soups, Chicken Corn Chowder",	LOW	8.16
CAMPBELL'S CHUNKY Soups, Fajita Chicken with Rice & Beans Soup",	LOW	9.39
CAMPBELL'S CHUNKY Soups, Firehouse - Hot & Spicy Beef & Bean Chili",	LOW	10.2
CAMPBELL'S CHUNKY Soups, Grilled Chicken & Sausage Gumbo Soup",	LOW	8.57
CAMPBELL'S CHUNKY Soups, Grilled Chicken with Vegetables & Pasta Soup",	LOW	5.71
CAMPBELL'S CHUNKY Soups, Grilled Sirloin Steak with Hearty Vegetables Soup",	LOW	7.76
CAMPBELL'S CHUNKY Soups, Grilled Steak- Steak Chili with Beans",	LOW	11.02
CAMPBELL'S CHUNKY Soups, HEALTHY REQUEST Microwavable Bowls, Chicken Noodle Soup",	LOW	6.94
CAMPBELL'S CHUNKY Soups, HEALTHY REQUEST Microwavable Bowls, Grilled Chicken & Sausage Gumbo Soup",	LOW	7.35
CAMPBELL'S CHUNKY Soups, HEALTHY REQUEST New England Clam Chowder",	LOW	8.16
CAMPBELL'S CHUNKY Soups, HEALTHY REQUEST Vegetable Soup",	LOW	9.8
CAMPBELL'S CHUNKY Soups, Hearty Beef Barley Soup",	LOW	8.98
CAMPBELL'S CHUNKY Soups, Hearty Chicken with Vegetables Soup",	LOW	6.94
CAMPBELL'S CHUNKY Soups, Manhattan Clam Chowder",	LOW	7.76
CAMPBELL'S CHUNKY Soups, Old Fashioned Vegetable Beef Soup",	LOW	6.24
CAMPBELL'S CHUNKY Soups, Roadhouse - Beef & Bean Chili",	LOW	10.2
CAMPBELL'S CHUNKY Soups, Salisbury Steak with Mushrooms & Onions Soup",	LOW	7.76

Food name/ Category (100 g)	Status	Carbs content in g
CAMPBELL'S CHUNKY Soups, Savory Chicken with White & Wild Rice Soup",	LOW	7.35
CAMPBELL'S CHUNKY Soups, Savory Pot Roast Soup",	LOW	8.16
CAMPBELL'S CHUNKY Soups, Savory Vegetable Soup",	LOW	8.98
CAMPBELL'S CHUNKY Soups, Slow Roasted Beef with Mushrooms Soup",	LOW	7.35
CAMPBELL'S CHUNKY Soups, Steak 'N' Potato Soup",	LOW	7.35
CAMPBELL'S CHUNKY, Classic Chicken Noodle Soup",	LOW	5.41
CAMPBELL'S CHUNKY, Creamy Chicken and Dumplings Soup",	LOW	7.09
CAMPBELL'S CHUNKY, HEALTHY REQUEST Chicken Noodle Soup",	LOW	5.88
CAMPBELL'S CHUNKY, New England Clam Chowder",	LOW	9.01
CAMPBELL'S HEALTHY REQUEST, Chicken Noodle Soup, condensed",	LOW	6.51
CAMPBELL'S HEALTHY REQUEST, Cream of Mushroom Soup, condensed",	LOW	8.6
CAMPBELL'S HEALTHY REQUEST, Homestyle Chicken Noodle Soup, condensed",	LOW	7.8
CAMPBELL'S Homestyle Chicken with White & Wild Rice Soup",	LOW	6.94
CAMPBELL'S Homestyle Harvest Tomato with Basil Soup",	LOW	9.39
CAMPBELL'S Homestyle HEALTHY REQUEST Chicken with Whole Grain Pasta Soup",	LOW	4.28
CAMPBELL'S Homestyle HEALTHY REQUEST Mexican Style Chicken Tortilla",	LOW	7.76
CAMPBELL'S Homestyle Italian-Style Wedding Soup",	LOW	6.12
CAMPBELL'S Homestyle Light Italian-Style Wedding Soup",	LOW	4.49
CAMPBELL'S Homestyle Light New England Clam Chowder",	LOW	6.12
CAMPBELL'S Homestyle Mexican Style Chicken Tortilla Soup",	LOW	8.16
CAMPBELL'S Homestyle Microwaveable Bowls, HEALTHY REQUEST Italian Wedding Soup",	LOW	5.31
CAMPBELL'S Homestyle Microwaveable Bowls, HEALTHY REQUEST Mexican Style Tortilla",	LOW	7.76
CAMPBELL'S Homestyle Minestrone Soup",	LOW	7.35
CAMPBELL'S Homestyle New England Clam Chowder",	LOW	5.68
CAMPBELL'S Homestyle Potato Broccoli Cheese Soup",	LOW	6.94
CAMPBELL'S Homestyle Vegetable Medley Soup",	LOW	7.35
CAMPBELL'S Low Sodium Soups, Chicken Broth",	LOW	0.34
CAMPBELL'S Low Sodium Soups, Chicken with Noodles Soup",	LOW	5.57

Food name/ Category (100 g)	Status	Carbs content in g
CAMPBELL'S Red and White - Microwaveable Bowls, Chicken Noodle Soup",	LOW	4.08
CAMPBELL'S Red and White - Microwaveable Bowls, Chicken Rice Soup",	LOW	5.71
CAMPBELL'S Red and White - Microwaveable Bowls, Creamy Tomato Soup",	LOW	10.2
CAMPBELL'S Red and White - Microwaveable Bowls, Tomato Soup",	LOW	9.8
CAMPBELL'S Red and White - Microwaveable Bowls, Vegetable Beef Soup",	LOW	6.12
CAMPBELL'S Red and White, 25% Less Sodium Tomato Soup, condensed",	LOW	16.13
CAMPBELL'S Red and White, Beef Broth, condensed",	LOW	0.81
CAMPBELL'S Red and White, Beef Consomme, condensed",	LOW	0.81
CAMPBELL'S Red and White, Beef Noodle Soup, condensed",	LOW	6.35
CAMPBELL'S Red and White, Beef with Vegetables and Barley Soup, condensed",	LOW	11.9
CAMPBELL'S Red and White, Beefy Mushroom Soup, condensed",	LOW	4.76
CAMPBELL'S Red and White, Broccoli Cheese Soup, condensed",	LOW	9.68
CAMPBELL'S Red and White, Chicken Alphabet Soup, condensed",	LOW	9.52
CAMPBELL'S Red and White, Chicken and Dumplings Soup, condensed",	LOW	7.94
CAMPBELL'S Red and White, Chicken and Stars Soup, condensed",	LOW	8.73
CAMPBELL'S Red and White, Chicken Barley with Mushrooms Soup, condensed",	LOW	12.7
CAMPBELL'S Red and White, Chicken Broth, condensed",	LOW	0.81
CAMPBELL'S Red and White, Chicken Gumbo Soup, condensed",	LOW	7.94
CAMPBELL'S Red and White, Chicken NOODLEO's Soup, condensed",	LOW	11.9
CAMPBELL'S Red and White, Chicken Vegetable Soup, condensed",	LOW	11.9
CAMPBELL'S Red and White, Chicken Won Ton Soup, condensed",	LOW	6.35
CAMPBELL'S Red and White, Cream of Asparagus Soup, condensed",	LOW	7.26
CAMPBELL'S Red and White, Cream of Broccoli Soup, condensed",	LOW	9.68
CAMPBELL'S Red and White, Cream of Celery Soup, condensed",	LOW	7.26
CAMPBELL'S Red and White, Cream of Onion Soup, condensed",	LOW	8.06
CAMPBELL'S Red and White, Cream of Shrimp Soup, condensed",	LOW	6.45
CAMPBELL'S Red and White, Creamy Chicken Noodle Soup, condensed",	LOW	8.87
CAMPBELL'S Red and White, DOUBLE NOODLE in Chicken Broth Soup, condensed",	LOW	15.87

Food name/ Category (100 g)	Status	Carbs content in g
CAMPBELL'S Red and White, Fiesta Nacho Cheese Soup, condensed",	LOW	8.06
CAMPBELL'S Red and White, French Onion Soup, condensed",	LOW	4.76
CAMPBELL'S Red and White, Golden Mushroom Soup, condensed",	LOW	8.06
CAMPBELL'S Red and White, GOLDFISH Pasta with Chicken in Chicken Broth, condensed",	LOW	9.52
CAMPBELL'S Red and White, Green Pea Soup, condensed",	LOW	21.88
CAMPBELL'S Red and White, Italian Style Wedding Soup, condensed",	LOW	9.52
CAMPBELL'S Red and White, Lentil Soup, condensed",	LOW	19.05
CAMPBELL'S Red and White, Manhattan Clam Chowder, condensed",	LOW	9.52
CAMPBELL'S Red and White, Mega Noodle in Chicken Broth, condensed",	LOW	11.9
CAMPBELL'S Red and White, Minestrone Soup, condensed",	LOW	13.49
CAMPBELL'S Red and White, New England Clam Chowder, condensed",	LOW	10.32
CAMPBELL'S Red and White, Old Fashioned Tomato Rice Soup, condensed",	LOW	18.25
CAMPBELL'S Red and White, PHINEAS and FERB Soup, condensed",	LOW	8.73
CAMPBELL'S Red and White, SCOOBY-DOO Soup, condensed",	LOW	8.73
CAMPBELL'S Red and White, Tomato Bisque, condensed",	LOW	18.25
CAMPBELL'S Red and White, Vegetable Soup, condensed",	LOW	16.67
CAMPBELL'S Red and White, Vegetarian Vegetable Soup, condensed",	LOW	14.29
CAMPBELL'S Soup on the Go, Chicken & Stars Soup",	LOW	3.28
CAMPBELL'S Soup on the Go, Chicken with Mini Noodles Soup",	LOW	3.61
CAMPBELL'S Soup on the Go, Classic Tomato Soup",	LOW	10.16
CAMPBELL'S Soup on the Go, Creamy Broccoli Soup",	LOW	4.26
CAMPBELL'S Soup on the Go, Creamy Chicken Soup",	LOW	3.28
CAMPBELL'S Soup on the Go, Creamy Tomato Soup",	LOW	9.84
CAMPBELL'S Soup on the GO, HEALTHY REQUEST Chicken with Mini Noodles Soup",	LOW	2.62
CAMPBELL'S Soup on the Go, HEALTHY REQUEST Classic Tomato Soup",	LOW	9.18
CAMPBELL'S Soup on the Go, New England Clam Chowder",	LOW	4.26
CAMPBELL'S Soup on the Go, Vegetable Beef Soup",	LOW	3.28
CAMPBELL'S Soup on the Go, Vegetable with Mini Round Noodles Soup",	LOW	6.89

Food name/ Category (100 g)	Status	Carbs content in g
CAMPBELL'S, 25% Less Sodium Chicken Noodle Soup, condensed",	LOW	6.3
CAMPBELL'S, 25% Less Sodium Cream of Mushroom Soup, condensed",	LOW	6.45
CAMPBELL'S, 98% Fat Free Broccoli Cheese Soup, condensed",	LOW	9.68
CAMPBELL'S, 98% Fat Free Cream of Broccoli Soup, condensed",	LOW	8.06
CAMPBELL'S, 98% Fat Free Cream of Celery Soup, condensed",	LOW	7.26
CAMPBELL'S, 98% Fat Free Cream of Chicken Soup, condensed",	LOW	7.46
CAMPBELL'S, 98% Fat Free Cream of Mushroom Soup, condensed",	LOW	7.63
CAMPBELL'S, Cheddar Cheese Soup, condensed",	LOW	11.44
CAMPBELL'S, Chicken with Rice Soup, condensed",	LOW	11.28
CAMPBELL'S, Cream of Chicken Soup, condensed",	LOW	6.03
CAMPBELL'S, Cream of Chicken with Herbs Soup, condensed",	LOW	7.26
CAMPBELL'S, Cream of Mushroom Soup, condensed",	LOW	6.59
CAMPBELL'S, Cream of Mushroom with Roasted Garlic Soup, condensed",	LOW	8.06
CAMPBELL'S, Cream of Potato Soup, condensed",	LOW	13.25
CAMPBELL'S, HEALTHY REQUEST, chicken with rice, condensed",	LOW	7.19
CAMPBELL'S, HEALTHY REQUEST, cream of chicken soup, condensed",	LOW	7.5
CAMPBELL'S, Homestyle Chicken Noodle Soup, condensed",	LOW	7.53
CAMPBELL'S, Organic Tomato juice",	LOW	4.12
CAMPBELL'S, Red and White, Chicken Noodle Soup, condensed",	LOW	5.97
CAMPBELL'S, Tomato juice, low sodium",	LOW	4.12
CAMPBELL'S, Tomato juice",	LOW	4.12
CAMPBELL'S, Tomato Soup, condensed",	LOW	15.22
CAMPBELL'S, V8 100% Vegetable Juice",	LOW	4.12
CAMPBELL'S, V8 60% Vegetable Juice, V8 V-Lite",	LOW	2.88
CAMPBELL'S, V8 Vegetable Juice, Calcium Enriched V8",	LOW	4.53
CAMPBELL'S, V8 Vegetable Juice, Essential Antioxidants V8",	LOW	4.53
CAMPBELL'S, V8 Vegetable Juice, High Fiber V8",	LOW	5.39
CAMPBELL'S, V8 Vegetable Juice, Low Sodium Spicy Hot",	LOW	4.53

Food name/ Category (100 g)	Status	Carbs content in g
CAMPBELL'S, V8 Vegetable Juice, Low Sodium V8",	LOW	4.12
CAMPBELL'S, V8 Vegetable Juice, Organic V8",	LOW	4.53
CAMPBELL'S, V8 Vegetable Juice, Spicy Hot V8",	LOW	4.12
CAMPBELL'S, Vegetable Beef Soup, condensed",	LOW	11.8
Canada Goose, breast meat, skinless, raw",	LOW	0
Candies, 5TH AVENUE Candy Bar",	HIGH	62.68
Candies, ALMOND JOY Candy Bar",	HIGH	59.51
Candies, butterscotch",	HIGH	90.4
Candies, CARAMELLO Candy Bar",	HIGH	63.81
Candies, caramels, chocolate-flavor roll",	HIGH	87.73
Candies, caramels",	HIGH	77
Candies, carob, unsweetened",	MEDIUM	56.29
Candies, chocolate covered, caramel with nuts",	HIGH	60.67
Candies, confectioner's coating, butterscotch",	HIGH	67.1
Candies, confectioner's coating, peanut butter",	MEDIUM	46.88
Candies, confectioner's coating, yogurt",	HIGH	63.94
Candies, crispy bar with peanut butter filling",	MEDIUM	55.53
Candies, fudge, chocolate marshmallow, prepared-from-recipe",	HIGH	71.34
Candies, fudge, chocolate marshmallow, with nuts, prepared-by-recipe",	HIGH	67.69
Candies, fudge, chocolate, prepared-from-recipe",	HIGH	76.44
Candies, fudge, chocolate, with nuts, prepared-from-recipe",	HIGH	67.93
Candies, fudge, peanut butter, prepared-from-recipe",	HIGH	77.75
Candies, fudge, vanilla with nuts",	HIGH	74.61
Candies, fudge, vanilla, prepared-from-recipe",	HIGH	82.15
Candies, gumdrops, starch jelly pieces",	HIGH	98.9
Candies, halavah, plain",	HIGH	60.49
Candies, hard, dietetic or low calorie (sorbitol)",	HIGH	98.6
Candies, hard",	HIGH	98
Candies, HEATH BITES",	HIGH	63.39
Candies, HERSHEY, KIT KAT BIG KAT Bar",	HIGH	63.64
Candies, HERSHEY, REESESTICKS crispy wafers, peanut butter, milk chocolate"	MEDIUM	55.38
Candies, HERSHEY'S GOLDEN ALMOND SOLITAIRES",	MEDIUM	46.85
Candies, HERSHEY'S MILK CHOCOLATE WITH ALMOND BITES",	MEDIUM	51.72
Candies, HERSHEY'S POT OF GOLD Almond Bar",	MEDIUM	44.89
Candies, HERSHEY'S SKOR Toffee Bar",	HIGH	63.73
Candies, HERSHEY'S, ALMOND JOY BITES",	HIGH	57.54
Candies, jellybeans",	HIGH	93.55
Candies, KIT KAT Wafer Bar",	HIGH	64.59
Candies, KRACKEL Chocolate Bar",	HIGH	63.96
Candies, M&M MARS 3 MUSKETEERS Truffle Crisp",	HIGH	63.15
Candies, M&M MARS Pretzel Chocolate Candies",	HIGH	72.94
Candies, MARS SNACKFOOD US, 3 MUSKETEERS Bar",	HIGH	77.77
Candies, MARS SNACKFOOD US, COCOAVIA Crispy Chocolate Bar",	HIGH	62.06
Candies, MARS SNACKFOOD US, DOVE Dark Chocolate",	HIGH	59.4
Candies, MARS SNACKFOOD US, DOVE Milk Chocolate",	HIGH	59.78
Candies, MARS SNACKFOOD US, M&M's Almond Chocolate Candies",	HIGH	60.5
Candies, MARS SNACKFOOD US, M&M's Crispy Chocolate Candies",	HIGH	72.4
Candies, MARS SNACKFOOD US, M&M's Milk Chocolate Candies",	HIGH	71.19
Candies, MARS SNACKFOOD US, M&M's MINIs Milk Chocolate Candies",	HIGH	68.4
Candies, MARS SNACKFOOD US, M&M's Peanut Butter Chocolate Candies",	MEDIUM	56.89
Candies, MARS SNACKFOOD US, M&M's Peanut Chocolate Candies",	HIGH	60.48
Candies, MARS SNACKFOOD US, MARS Almond Bar",	HIGH	62.7

Food name/ Category (100 g)	Status	Carbs content in g
Candies, MARS SNACKFOOD US, MILKY WAY Bar",	HIGH	71.17
Candies, MARS SNACKFOOD US, MILKY WAY Caramels, milk chocolate covered	HIGH	68.49
Candies, MARS SNACKFOOD US, MILKY WAY Caramels. dark chocolate covered	HIGH	67.56
Candies, MARS SNACKFOOD US, MILKY WAY Midnight Bar",	HIGH	71.22
Candies, MARS SNACKFOOD US, POP'ABLES 3 MUSKETEERS Brand Bite Size	HIGH	75.94
Candies, MARS SNACKFOOD US, POP'ABLES MILKY WAY Brand Bite Size Can	HIGH	71.85
Candies, MARS SNACKFOOD US, POP'ABLES SNICKERS Brand Bite Size Cand	HIGH	61.07
Candies, MARS SNACKFOOD US, SNICKERS Almond bar",	HIGH	64.67
Candies, MARS SNACKFOOD US, SNICKERS Bar",	HIGH	61.51
Candies, MARS SNACKFOOD US, SNICKERS CRUNCHER",	HIGH	62.85
Candies, MARS SNACKFOOD US, SNICKERS MUNCH bar",	MEDIUM	43.64
Candies, MARS SNACKFOOD US, STARBURST Fruit Chews, Fruit and Creme",	HIGH	82.43
Candies, MARS SNACKFOOD US, STARBURST Fruit Chews, Original fruits",	HIGH	82.57
Candies, MARS SNACKFOOD US, STARBURST Fruit Chews, Tropical fruits",	HIGH	82.76
Candies, MARS SNACKFOOD US, STARBURST Sour Fruit Chews",	HIGH	79.73
Candies, MARS SNACKFOOD US, TWIX Caramel Cookie Bars",	HIGH	64.8
Candies, MARS SNACKFOOD US, TWIX chocolate fudge cookie bars",	MEDIUM	56
Candies, MARS SNACKFOOD US, TWIX Peanut Butter Cookie Bars",	MEDIUM	54.15
Candies, marshmallows",	HIGH	81.3
Candies, milk chocolate coated coffee beans",	MEDIUM	55.25
Candies, milk chocolate coated peanuts",	MEDIUM	49.7
Candies, milk chocolate, with almonds",	MEDIUM	53.4
Candies, milk chocolate, with rice cereal",	HIGH	59.67
Candies, milk chocolate",	HIGH	59.4
Candies, MOUNDS Candy Bar",	HIGH	58.59
Candies, MR. GOODBAR Chocolate Bar",	MEDIUM	54.34
Candies, NESTLE, 100 GRAND Bar",	HIGH	70.97
Candies, NESTLE, AFTER EIGHT Mints",	HIGH	79.53
Candies, NESTLE, BABY RUTH Bar",	HIGH	64.8
Candies, NESTLE, BIT-O'-HONEY Candy Chews",	HIGH	80.89
Candies, NESTLE, BUTTERFINGER Bar",	HIGH	72.9
Candies, NESTLE, CHUNKY Bar",	HIGH	60
Candies, NESTLE, CRUNCH Bar and Dessert Topping",	HIGH	67
Candies, NESTLE, GOOBERS Chocolate Covered Peanuts",	MEDIUM	53
Candies, NESTLE, OH HENRY! Bar",	HIGH	65.5
Candies, peanut bar",	MEDIUM	47.4
Candies, peanut brittle, prepared-from-recipe",	HIGH	71.24
Candies, praline, prepared-from-recipe",	HIGH	59.59
Candies, REESE'S BITES",	MEDIUM	55.18
Candies, REESE's Fast Break, milk chocolate, peanut butter, soft nougats, candy	HIGH	63.9
Candies, REESE'S NUTRAGEOUS Candy Bar",	MEDIUM	52.8
Candies, REESE'S Peanut Butter Cups",	MEDIUM	55.36
Candies, REESE'S PIECES Candy",	HIGH	59.86
Candies, REESE'S, FAST BREAK, milk chocolate peanut butter and soft nougats"	HIGH	61.6
Candies, ROLO Caramels in Milk Chocolate",	HIGH	67.95
Candies, sesame crunch",	MEDIUM	50.3
Candies, soft fruit and nut squares",	HIGH	73.81
Candies, SYMPHONY Milk Chocolate Bar",	HIGH	58.01
Candies, taffy, prepared-from-recipe",	HIGH	91.56
Candies, TOBLERONE, milk chocolate with honey and almond nougat",	HIGH	61.21
Candies, toffee, prepared-from-recipe",	HIGH	64.72
Candies, TOOTSIE ROLL, chocolate-flavor roll",	HIGH	87.73
Candies, truffles, prepared-from-recipe",	MEDIUM	44.88
Candies, TWIZZLERS CHERRY BITES",	HIGH	79.38
Candies, TWIZZLERS NIBS CHERRY BITS",	HIGH	79.37
Candies, TWIZZLERS Strawberry Twists Candy",	HIGH	79.16
Candies, white chocolate",	HIGH	59.24

Food name/ Category (100 g)	Status	Carbs content in g
Candies, YORK BITES",	HIGH	81.64
Capers, canned",	LOW	4.89
Carambola, (starfruit), raw",	LOW	6.73
Carbonated beverage, chocolate-flavored soda",	LOW	10.7
Cardoon, raw",	LOW	4.07
Caribou, hind quarter, meat, cooked (Alaska Native)",	LOW	0
Carissa, (natal-plum), raw",	LOW	13.63
CARRABBA'S ITALIAN GRILL, cheese ravioli with marinara sauce",	LOW	17.62
CARRABBA'S ITALIAN GRILL, chicken parmesan without cavatappi pasta",	LOW	7.8
CARRABBA'S ITALIAN GRILL, lasagne",	LOW	12.36
CARRABBA'S ITALIAN GRILL, spaghetti with meat sauce",	LOW	15.71
CARRABBA'S ITALIAN GRILL, spaghetti with pomodoro sauce",	LOW	18.63
Carrot juice, canned",	LOW	9.28
Carrot, dehydrated",	HIGH	79.57
Carrots, baby, raw",	LOW	8.24
Carrots, canned, no salt added, drained solids",	LOW	5.54
Carrots, canned, regular pack, drained solids",	LOW	5.54
Carrots, canned, regular pack, solids and liquids",	LOW	5.37
Carrots, cooked, boiled, drained, with salt",	LOW	8.22
Carrots, cooked, boiled, drained, without salt",	LOW	8.22
Carrots, frozen, cooked, boiled, drained, with salt",	LOW	7.73
Carrots, frozen, cooked, boiled, drained, without salt",	LOW	7.73
Carrots, frozen, unprepared",	LOW	7.9
Carrots, raw",	LOW	9.58
Catsup",	LOW	27.4
Cattail, Narrow Leaf Shoots (Northern Plains Indians)",	LOW	5.14
Cauliflower, cooked, boiled, drained, with salt",	LOW	4.11
Cauliflower, frozen, cooked, boiled, drained, with salt",	LOW	3.16
Cauliflower, green, cooked, with salt",	LOW	6.28

Food name/ Category (100 g)	Status	Carbs content in g
Celeriac, cooked, boiled, drained, with salt",	LOW	5.9
Celeriac, cooked, boiled, drained, without salt",	LOW	5.9
Celeriac, raw",	LOW	9.2
Celery, cooked, boiled, drained, with salt",	LOW	4
Celery, cooked, boiled, drained, without salt",	LOW	4
Celery, raw",	LOW	2.97
Cereals ready-to-eat, BARBARA'S PUFFINS, original",	HIGH	84
Cereals ready-to-eat, CASCADIAN FARM, Cinnamon Crunch",	HIGH	81.59
Cereals ready-to-eat, CASCADIAN FARM, Honey Nut O's",	HIGH	83.09
Cereals ready-to-eat, CASCADIAN FARM, Multi-Grain Squares",	HIGH	83
Cereals ready-to-eat, chocolate-flavored frosted puffed corn",	HIGH	87.2
Cereals ready-to-eat, frosted oat cereal with marshmallows",	HIGH	84.7
Cereals ready-to-eat, GENERAL MILLS, 25% Less Sugar CINNAMON TOAST CRU	HIGH	78.19
Cereals ready-to-eat, GENERAL MILLS, 25% Less Sugar TRIX",	HIGH	85.5
Cereals ready-to-eat, GENERAL MILLS, APPLE CINNAMON CHEERIOS",	HIGH	79.9
Cereals ready-to-eat, GENERAL MILLS, Apple Cinnamon CHEX",	HIGH	82.8
Cereals ready-to-eat, GENERAL MILLS, BASIC 4",	HIGH	79.09
Cereals ready-to-eat, GENERAL MILLS, BERRY BERRY KIX",	HIGH	83.9
Cereals ready-to-eat, GENERAL MILLS, Berry Burst CHEERIOS, Triple Berry",	HIGH	80.5
Cereals ready-to-eat, GENERAL MILLS, BOO BERRY",	HIGH	85.4
Cereals ready-to-eat, GENERAL MILLS, CHEERIOS, Banana Nut",	HIGH	84.69
Cereals ready-to-eat, GENERAL MILLS, CHEERIOS, Chocolate",	HIGH	83.5
Cereals ready-to-eat, GENERAL MILLS, CHEERIOS, Yogurt Burst, strawberry",	HIGH	81.75
Cereals ready-to-eat, GENERAL MILLS, CHEERIOS",	HIGH	73.23
Cereals ready-to-eat, GENERAL MILLS, Chocolate CHEX",	HIGH	81.09
Cereals ready-to-eat, GENERAL MILLS, CHOCOLATE LUCKY CHARMS",	HIGH	84.4
Cereals ready-to-eat, GENERAL MILLS, Cinnamon Burst CHEERIOS",	HIGH	83.2
Cereals ready-to-eat, GENERAL MILLS, Cinnamon CHEX",	HIGH	82.4
Cereals ready-to-eat, GENERAL MILLS, CINNAMON TOAST CRUNCH",	HIGH	77.99
Cereals ready-to-eat, GENERAL MILLS, COCOA PUFFS, 25% Reduced Sugar",	HIGH	82.69
Cereals ready-to-eat, GENERAL MILLS, COCOA PUFFS",	HIGH	83.7
Cereals ready-to-eat, GENERAL MILLS, COOKIE CRISP",	HIGH	84.5
Cereals ready-to-eat, GENERAL MILLS, Corn CHEX",	HIGH	85
Cereals ready-to-eat, GENERAL MILLS, COUNT CHOCULA",	HIGH	84.5
Cereals ready-to-eat, GENERAL MILLS, DORA THE EXPLORER",	HIGH	82.8
Cereals ready-to-eat, GENERAL MILLS, Dulce De Leche CHEERIOS",	HIGH	82
Cereals ready-to-eat, GENERAL MILLS, FIBER ONE 80 Calories, Chocolate Squar	HIGH	84
Cereals ready-to-eat, GENERAL MILLS, FIBER ONE 80 Calories, Honey Squares",	HIGH	85.19
Cereals ready-to-eat, GENERAL MILLS, FIBER ONE Bran Cereal",	HIGH	84.3
Cereals ready-to-eat, GENERAL MILLS, FIBER ONE, Caramel Delight",	HIGH	82.69
Cereals ready-to-eat, GENERAL MILLS, FIBER ONE, HONEY CLUSTERS",	HIGH	83.9
Cereals ready-to-eat, GENERAL MILLS, FIBER ONE, Nutty Clusters & Almonds",	HIGH	79.5
Cereals ready-to-eat, GENERAL MILLS, FIBER ONE, RAISIN BRAN CLUSTERS",	HIGH	83.4
Cereals ready-to-eat, GENERAL MILLS, FRANKENBERRY",	HIGH	85.4
Cereals ready-to-eat, GENERAL MILLS, FROSTED CHEERIOS",	HIGH	79.8
Cereals ready-to-eat, GENERAL MILLS, FROSTED TOAST CRUNCH",	HIGH	78.59
Cereals ready-to-eat, GENERAL MILLS, Fruity CHEERIOS",	HIGH	84.19
Cereals ready-to-eat, GENERAL MILLS, Honey KIX",	HIGH	83
Cereals ready-to-eat, GENERAL MILLS, HONEY NUT CHEERIOS, MEDLEY CRUN	HIGH	79.5
Cereals ready-to-eat, GENERAL MILLS, HONEY NUT CHEERIOS",	HIGH	79.69
Cereals ready-to-eat, GENERAL MILLS, Honey Nut CHEX",	HIGH	86.67

Food name/ Category (100 g)	Status	Carbs content in g
Cereals ready-to-eat, GENERAL MILLS, HONEY NUT CLUSTERS",	HIGH	85.2
Cereals ready-to-eat, GENERAL MILLS, KIX",	HIGH	82.82
Cereals ready-to-eat, GENERAL MILLS, LUCKY CHARMS",	HIGH	80.89
Cereals ready-to-eat, GENERAL MILLS, Multi Grain CHEERIOS, Peanut Butter",	HIGH	82
Cereals ready-to-eat, GENERAL MILLS, Multi-Grain CHEERIOS",	HIGH	81.4
Cereals ready-to-eat, GENERAL MILLS, NATURE VALLEY LOW FAT FRUIT GRA	HIGH	79.4
Cereals ready-to-eat, GENERAL MILLS, Oat Cluster CHEERIOS Crunch",	HIGH	80.7
Cereals ready-to-eat, GENERAL MILLS, OATMEAL CRISP, Crunchy Almond",	HIGH	78.09
Cereals ready-to-eat, GENERAL MILLS, OATMEAL CRISP, Hearty Raisin",	HIGH	80.8
Cereals ready-to-eat, GENERAL MILLS, PEANUT BUTTER TOAST CRUNCH",	HIGH	76.19
Cereals ready-to-eat, GENERAL MILLS, RAISIN NUT BRAN",	HIGH	80
Cereals ready-to-eat, GENERAL MILLS, REESE'S PUFFS",	HIGH	75.6
Cereals ready-to-eat, GENERAL MILLS, Rice CHEX",	HIGH	85.09
Cereals ready-to-eat, GENERAL MILLS, RICE CRUNCHINS",	HIGH	80.95
Cereals ready-to-eat, GENERAL MILLS, TOTAL Raisin Bran",	HIGH	76.8
Cereals ready-to-eat, GENERAL MILLS, TRIX",	HIGH	86.19
Cereals ready-to-eat, GENERAL MILLS, Wheat CHEX",	HIGH	82.2
Cereals ready-to-eat, GENERAL MILLS, WHEATIES",	HIGH	83.3
Cereals ready-to-eat, GENERAL MILLS, Whole Grain TOTAL",	HIGH	74.7
Cereals ready-to-eat, HEALTH VALLEY, FIBER 7 Flakes",	HIGH	78.15
Cereals ready-to-eat, KASHI 7 Whole Grain Flakes",	HIGH	81.4
Cereals ready-to-eat, KASHI 7 Whole Grain Nuggets",	HIGH	81
Cereals ready-to-eat, KASHI Berry Blossom",	HIGH	83.09
Cereals ready-to-eat, KASHI GO LEAN CRUNCH!, Honey Almond Flax",	HIGH	66.9
Cereals ready-to-eat, KASHI GOLEAN CRISP Cinnamon Crumble",	HIGH	62.59
Cereals ready-to-eat, KASHI GOLEAN CRISP Toasted Berry Crumble",	HIGH	66.69
Cereals ready-to-eat, KASHI GOLEAN CRUNCH!",	HIGH	71.4
Cereals ready-to-eat, KASHI GOLEAN",	HIGH	67.19
Cereals ready-to-eat, KASHI GOOD FRIENDS",	HIGH	79.3
Cereals ready-to-eat, KASHI HEART TO HEART, Honey Toasted Oat",	HIGH	78.69
Cereals ready-to-eat, KASHI HEART TO HEART, Warm Cinnamon",	HIGH	78.5
Cereals ready-to-eat, KASHI Honey Sunshine",	HIGH	82
Cereals ready-to-eat, KASHI INDIGO MORNING",	HIGH	82.8
Cereals ready-to-eat, KASHI ORGANIC PROMISE, Berry Fruitful",	HIGH	76.2
Cereals ready-to-eat, KASHI ORGANIC PROMISE, CINNAMON HARVEST",	HIGH	79
Cereals ready-to-eat, KASHI ORGANIC PROMISE, RAISIN VINEYARD",	HIGH	79.9
Cereals ready-to-eat, KASHI ORGANIC PROMISE, STRAWBERRY FIELDS",	HIGH	83.5
Cereals ready-to-eat, KASHI Simply Maize",	HIGH	83.3
Cereals ready-to-eat, KASHI, HEART TO HEART, Oat Flakes & Blueberry Clusters	HIGH	80.3
Cereals ready-to-eat, KASHI, ORGANIC PROMISE Autumn Wheat",	HIGH	79
Cereals ready-to-eat, KELLOGG RAISIN BRAN with Omega-3 from flaxseed",	HIGH	82.69
Cereals ready-to-eat, KELLOGG SCOOBY-DOO! cereal",	HIGH	84
Cereals ready-to-eat, KELLOGG, KELLOGG'S ALL-BRAN BRAN BUDS",	HIGH	81
Cereals ready-to-eat, KELLOGG, KELLOGG'S ALL-BRAN COMPLETE Wheat Flak	HIGH	81.6
Cereals ready-to-eat, KELLOGG, KELLOGG'S ALL-BRAN Original",	HIGH	74.24
Cereals ready-to-eat, KELLOGG, KELLOGG'S APPLE JACKS",	HIGH	88.2
Cereals ready-to-eat, KELLOGG, KELLOGG'S CINNABON cereal",	HIGH	83.3
Cereals ready-to-eat, KELLOGG, KELLOGG'S COCOA KRISPIES",	HIGH	87.9
Cereals ready-to-eat, KELLOGG, KELLOGG'S Corn Flakes",	HIGH	84.1
Cereals ready-to-eat, KELLOGG, KELLOGG'S CORN POPS",	HIGH	89.7
Cereals ready-to-eat, KELLOGG, KELLOGG'S CRACKLIN' OAT BRAN",	HIGH	70.3
Cereals ready-to-eat, KELLOGG, KELLOGG'S CRISPIX",	HIGH	87.19
Cereals ready-to-eat, KELLOGG, KELLOGG'S FROOT LOOPS",	HIGH	88
Cereals ready-to-eat, KELLOGG, KELLOGG'S FROSTED FLAKES",	HIGH	89.2
Cereals ready-to-eat, KELLOGG, KELLOGG'S FROSTED MINI-WHEATS, bite size	HIGH	83.4
Cereals ready-to-eat, KELLOGG, KELLOGG'S FROSTED MINI-WHEATS, little bite	HIGH	83.4
Cereals ready-to-eat, KELLOGG, KELLOGG'S FROSTED RICE KRISPIES",	HIGH	91.3

Food name/ Category (100 g)	Status	Carbs content in g
Cereals ready-to-eat, KELLOGG, KELLOGG'S HONEY CRUNCH CORN FLAKES",	HIGH	87
Cereals ready-to-eat, KELLOGG, KELLOGG'S HONEY SMACKS",	HIGH	88.5
Cereals ready-to-eat, KELLOGG, KELLOGG'S Low Fat Granola with Raisins",	HIGH	80.1
Cereals ready-to-eat, KELLOGG, KELLOGG'S Low Fat Granola without Raisins",	HIGH	80.9
Cereals ready-to-eat, KELLOGG, KELLOGG'S MARSHMALLOW FROOT LOOPS",	HIGH	89.3
Cereals ready-to-eat, KELLOGG, KELLOGG'S MINI-WHEATS, unfrosted bite size"	HIGH	81
Cereals ready-to-eat, KELLOGG, KELLOGG'S MUESLIX",	HIGH	74.9
Cereals ready-to-eat, KELLOGG, KELLOGG'S PRODUCT 19",	HIGH	84.3
Cereals ready-to-eat, KELLOGG, KELLOGG'S RAISIN BRAN with cranberries",	HIGH	84.19
Cereals ready-to-eat, KELLOGG, KELLOGG'S RAISIN BRAN, Cinnamon Almond",	HIGH	81.19
Cereals ready-to-eat, KELLOGG, KELLOGG'S RAISIN BRAN",	HIGH	77.29
Cereals ready-to-eat, KELLOGG, KELLOGG'S RICE KRISPIES TREATS Cereal",	HIGH	85.59
Cereals ready-to-eat, KELLOGG, KELLOGG'S RICE KRISPIES",	HIGH	85.05
Cereals ready-to-eat, KELLOGG, KELLOGG'S SMART START Strong Heart Antiox	HIGH	86.8
Cereals ready-to-eat, KELLOGG, KELLOGG'S SPECIAL K Blueberry",	HIGH	86.3
Cereals ready-to-eat, KELLOGG, KELLOGG'S SPECIAL K Chocolatey Strawberry"	HIGH	83.3
Cereals ready-to-eat, KELLOGG, KELLOGG'S SPECIAL K Low Fat Granola",	HIGH	74.8
Cereals ready-to-eat, KELLOGG, KELLOGG'S SPECIAL K Multi-grain",	HIGH	86.59
Cereals ready-to-eat, KELLOGG, KELLOGG'S SPECIAL K Red Berries",	HIGH	87.09
Cereals ready-to-eat, KELLOGG, KELLOGG'S SPECIAL K, Cinnamon Pecan",	HIGH	81.2
Cereals ready-to-eat, KELLOGG, KELLOGG'S SPECIAL K",	HIGH	73.4
Cereals ready-to-eat, KELLOGG, KELLOGG'S, RAISIN BRAN CRUNCH",	HIGH	84.9
Cereals ready-to-eat, KELLOGG, SPECIAL K, Fruit & Yogurt",	HIGH	85.3
Cereals ready-to-eat, KELLOGG'S APPLE JACKS with marshmallows",	HIGH	89.6
Cereals ready-to-eat, KELLOGG'S CINNAMON JACKS",	HIGH	83
Cereals ready-to-eat, KELLOGG'S CRUNCHY NUT Golden Honey Nut flakes",	HIGH	83.3
Cereals ready-to-eat, KELLOGG'S FROSTED FLAKES, CHOCO ZUCARITAS",	HIGH	85.1
Cereals ready-to-eat, KELLOGG's FROSTED MINI-WHEATS Bite Size Blueberry M	HIGH	84.8
Cereals ready-to-eat, KELLOGG'S FROSTED MINI-WHEATS LITTLE BITES, choc	HIGH	81.4
Cereals ready-to-eat, KELLOGG'S FROSTED MINI-WHEATS Touch of Fruit in the l	HIGH	82.1
Cereals ready-to-eat, KELLOGG'S FROSTED MINI-WHEATS, Big Bite",	HIGH	83.4
Cereals ready-to-eat, KELLOGG'S KRAVE chocolate cereal",	HIGH	76.1
Cereals ready-to-eat, KELLOGG'S KRAVE double chocolate cereal",	HIGH	75.9
Cereals ready-to-eat, KELLOGG'S KRAVE Smores",	HIGH	76.4
Cereals ready-to-eat, KELLOGG'S RICE KRISPIES, Gluten Free",	HIGH	82.4
Cereals ready-to-eat, KELLOGG'S SPECIAL K Chocolate Almond",	HIGH	81.5
Cereals ready-to-eat, KELLOGG'S SPECIAL K Chocolatey Delight",	HIGH	81.2
Cereals ready-to-eat, KELLOGG'S SPECIAL K Multigrain Oats and Honey",	HIGH	85
Cereals ready-to-eat, KELLOGG'S, FROSTED MINI-WHEATS Bite Size Strawberry	HIGH	84.6
Cereals ready-to-eat, KELLOGG'S, Reduced Sugar Frosted Flakes Cereal",	HIGH	87.3
Cereals ready-to-eat, KELLOGG'S, SPECIAL K gluten free, touch of brown sugar",	HIGH	86.5
Cereals ready-to-eat, KELLOGG'S, SPECIAL K Protein Plus",	HIGH	60.6
Cereals ready-to-eat, KELLOGG'S, SPECIAL K protein, cinnamon brown sugar crur	HIGH	69.8
Cereals ready-to-eat, KELLOGG'S, SPECIAL K Vanilla Almond",	HIGH	83
Cereals ready-to-eat, MALT-O-MEAL, Apple ZINGS",	HIGH	87.3
Cereals ready-to-eat, MALT-O-MEAL, BERRY COLOSSAL CRUNCH",	HIGH	86.55
Cereals ready-to-eat, MALT-O-MEAL, Blueberry MUFFIN TOPS Cereal",	HIGH	79.91
Cereals ready-to-eat, MALT-O-MEAL, CHOCOLATE MARSHMALLOW MATEYS",	HIGH	88.18
Cereals ready-to-eat, MALT-O-MEAL, CINNAMON TOASTERS",	HIGH	78.33
Cereals ready-to-eat, MALT-O-MEAL, COCO-ROOS",	HIGH	86.75
Cereals ready-to-eat, MALT-O-MEAL, Cocoa DYNO-BITES",	HIGH	87.93
Cereals ready-to-eat, MALT-O-MEAL, COLOSSAL CRUNCH",	HIGH	81.59
Cereals ready-to-eat, MALT-O-MEAL, CORN BURSTS",	HIGH	90.59
Cereals ready-to-eat, MALT-O-MEAL, Crispy Rice",	HIGH	86.4
Cereals ready-to-eat, MALT-O-MEAL, Frosted Flakes",	HIGH	90.2
Cereals ready-to-eat, MALT-O-MEAL, Fruity DYNO-BITES",	HIGH	90.1
Cereals ready-to-eat, MALT-O-MEAL, GOLDEN PUFFS",	HIGH	89.72

Food name/ Category (100 g)	Status	Carbs content in g
Cereals ready-to-eat, MALT-O-MEAL, Honey BUZZERS",	HIGH	89.66
Cereals ready-to-eat, MALT-O-MEAL, Honey Nut SCOOTERS",	HIGH	79.62
Cereals ready-to-eat, MALT-O-MEAL, MARSHMALLOW MATEYS",	HIGH	82.77
Cereals ready-to-eat, MALT-O-MEAL, OAT BLENDERS with honey & almonds",	HIGH	77.26
Cereals ready-to-eat, MALT-O-MEAL, OAT BLENDERS with honey",	HIGH	84.94
Cereals ready-to-eat, MALT-O-MEAL, Raisin Bran Cereal",	HIGH	80.37
Cereals ready-to-eat, MALT-O-MEAL, TOOTIE FRUITIES",	HIGH	85.94
Cereals ready-to-eat, MOM'S BEST, Honey Nut TOASTY O'S",	HIGH	79.84
Cereals ready-to-eat, NATURE'S PATH, Organic FLAX PLUS flakes",	HIGH	75.27
Cereals ready-to-eat, NATURE'S PATH, Organic FLAX PLUS, Pumpkin Granola",	HIGH	66.1
Cereals ready-to-eat, OAT BRAN FLAKES, HEALTH VALLEY",	HIGH	78
Cereals ready-to-eat, POST Bran Flakes",	HIGH	80.5
Cereals ready-to-eat, POST GREAT GRAINS Banana Nut Crunch",	HIGH	70.9
Cereals ready-to-eat, POST GREAT GRAINS Cranberry Almond Crunch",	HIGH	76.6
Cereals ready-to-eat, POST HONEY BUNCHES OF OATS with cinnamon bunches'	HIGH	82.8
Cereals ready-to-eat, POST Raisin Bran Cereal",	HIGH	78.9
Cereals ready-to-eat, POST SELECTS Blueberry Morning",	HIGH	81.6
Cereals ready-to-eat, POST SELECTS Maple Pecan Crunch",	HIGH	77.4
Cereals ready-to-eat, POST, ALPHA-BITS",	HIGH	80.3
Cereals ready-to-eat, POST, COCOA PEBBLES",	HIGH	85.7
Cereals ready-to-eat, POST, FRUITY PEBBLES",	HIGH	86.1
Cereals ready-to-eat, POST, GOLDEN CRISP",	HIGH	90.1
Cereals ready-to-eat, POST, GRAPE-NUTS Cereal",	HIGH	80.49
Cereals ready-to-eat, POST, GRAPE-NUTS Flakes",	HIGH	82
Cereals ready-to-eat, POST, GREAT GRAINS Crunchy Pecan Cereal",	HIGH	73
Cereals ready-to-eat, POST, GREAT GRAINS, Raisin, Date & Pecan",	HIGH	74.3
Cereals ready-to-eat, POST, HONEY BUNCHES OF OATS with vanilla bunches",	HIGH	81.8
Cereals ready-to-eat, POST, HONEY BUNCHES OF OATS, honey roasted",	HIGH	81.19
Cereals ready-to-eat, POST, HONEY BUNCHES OF OATS, pecan bunches",	HIGH	82
Cereals ready-to-eat, POST, HONEY BUNCHES OF OATS, with almonds",	HIGH	79.6
Cereals ready-to-eat, POST, HONEY BUNCHES OF OATS, with real strawberries",	HIGH	83.3
Cereals ready-to-eat, POST, Honey Nut Shredded Wheat",	HIGH	83.6
Cereals ready-to-eat, POST, Honeycomb Cereal",	HIGH	86.63
Cereals ready-to-eat, POST, Shredded Wheat n' Bran, spoon-size",	HIGH	80.65
Cereals ready-to-eat, POST, Shredded Wheat, original big biscuit",	HIGH	78.96
Cereals ready-to-eat, POST, Shredded Wheat, original spoon-size",	HIGH	81.4
Cereals ready-to-eat, Post, Waffle Crisp",	HIGH	83
Cereals ready-to-eat, QUAKER Oatmeal Squares, Golden Maple",	HIGH	78.04
Cereals ready-to-eat, QUAKER WHOLE HEARTS oat cereal",	HIGH	80.1
Cereals ready-to-eat, QUAKER, 100% Natural Granola, Oats, Wheat and Honey",	HIGH	73.65
Cereals ready-to-eat, QUAKER, CAP'N CRUNCH with CRUNCHBERRIES",	HIGH	85.93
Cereals ready-to-eat, QUAKER, CAP'N CRUNCH'S Halloween Crunch",	HIGH	85.14
Cereals ready-to-eat, QUAKER, Cap'n Crunch's OOPS! All Berries Cereal",	HIGH	87.1
Cereals ready-to-eat, QUAKER, CAP'N CRUNCH'S PEANUT BUTTER CRUNCH",	HIGH	78.65
Cereals ready-to-eat, QUAKER, CAP'N CRUNCH",	HIGH	85.51
Cereals ready-to-eat, QUAKER, Christmas Crunch",	HIGH	85.92
Cereals ready-to-eat, QUAKER, KING VITAMAN",	HIGH	83.85
Cereals ready-to-eat, QUAKER, Low Fat 100% Natural Granola with Raisins",	HIGH	80.57
Cereals ready-to-eat, QUAKER, Maple Brown Sugar LIFE Cereal",	HIGH	78.86
Cereals ready-to-eat, QUAKER, MOTHER'S Cinnamon Oat Crunch",	HIGH	79.79
Cereals ready-to-eat, QUAKER, MOTHER'S COCOA BUMPERS",	HIGH	89.91
Cereals ready-to-eat, QUAKER, MOTHER'S PEANUT BUTTER BUMPERS Cereal"	HIGH	79.68
Cereals ready-to-eat, QUAKER, MOTHER'S Toasted Oat Bran cereal",	HIGH	75.41
Cereals ready-to-eat, QUAKER, Natural Granola Apple Cranberry Almond",	HIGH	74.73
Cereals ready-to-eat, QUAKER, Oatmeal Squares, cinnamon",	HIGH	78.09
Cereals ready-to-eat, QUAKER, Oatmeal Squares",	HIGH	77.77
Cereals ready-to-eat, QUAKER, QUAKER 100% Natural Granola with Oats, Wheat,	HIGH	74.67

Food name/ Category (100 g)	Status	Carbs content in g
Cereals ready-to-eat, QUAKER, QUAKER CRUNCHY BRAN",	HIGH	83.68
Cereals ready-to-eat, QUAKER, QUAKER OAT CINNAMON LIFE",	HIGH	79.02
Cereals ready-to-eat, QUAKER, QUAKER OAT LIFE, plain",	HIGH	77.74
Cereals ready-to-eat, QUAKER, QUAKER Puffed Rice",	HIGH	87.78
Cereals ready-to-eat, QUAKER, QUAKER Puffed Wheat",	HIGH	76.39
Cereals ready-to-eat, QUAKER, Shredded Wheat, bagged cereal",	HIGH	81.01
Cereals ready-to-eat, QUAKER, SWEET CRUNCH\/QUISP",	HIGH	85.03
Cereals ready-to-eat, QUAKER, Toasted Multigrain Crisps",	HIGH	74.9
Cereals ready-to-eat, RALSTON Corn Biscuits",	HIGH	85.79
Cereals ready-to-eat, RALSTON Corn Flakes",	HIGH	88.01
Cereals ready-to-eat, RALSTON CRISP RICE",	HIGH	86.22
Cereals ready-to-eat, RALSTON Crispy Hexagons",	HIGH	86.78
Cereals ready-to-eat, RALSTON Enriched Wheat Bran flakes",	HIGH	79.77
Cereals ready-to-eat, RALSTON TASTEEOS",	HIGH	75.5
Cereals ready-to-eat, rice, puffed, fortified",	HIGH	89.8
Cereals ready-to-eat, UNCLE SAM CEREAL",	HIGH	65.78
Cereals ready-to-eat, USDA Commodity Corn and Rice (includes all commodity bra	HIGH	86.85
Cereals ready-to-eat, USDA Commodity Rice Crisps (includes all commodity brand	HIGH	86.04
Cereals ready-to-eat, WEETABIX whole grain cereal",	HIGH	81.5
Cereals ready-to-eat, wheat and bran, presweetened with nuts and fruits",	HIGH	76.2
Cereals ready-to-eat, wheat germ, toasted, plain",	MEDIUM	49.6
Cereals ready-to-eat, wheat, puffed, fortified",	HIGH	79.6
Cereals, corn grits, white, regular and quick, enriched, cooked with water, with salt",	LOW	14.76
Cereals, corn grits, white, regular and quick, enriched, cooked with water, without salt",	LOW	14.76
Cereals, corn grits, white, regular and quick, enriched, dry",	HIGH	79.09
Cereals, corn grits, yellow, regular and quick, enriched, cooked with water, without salt",	LOW	13.86
Cereals, corn grits, yellow, regular and quick, enriched, dry",	HIGH	79.91
Cereals, corn grits, yellow, regular and quick, unenriched, dry",	HIGH	79.6
Cereals, corn grits, yellow, regular, quick, enriched, cooked with water, with salt",	LOW	13.86
Cereals, CREAM OF RICE, cooked with water, with salt",	LOW	11.5
Cereals, CREAM OF RICE, cooked with water, without salt",	LOW	11.4
Cereals, CREAM OF WHEAT, 1 minute cook time, cooked with water, microwaved, without salt",	LOW	10.67
Cereals, CREAM OF WHEAT, 1 minute cook time, cooked with water, stove-top, without salt",	LOW	11.16
Cereals, CREAM OF WHEAT, 2 1\/2 minute cook time, cooked with water, microwaved, without salt",	LOW	10.1
Cereals, CREAM OF WHEAT, 2 1\/2 minute cook time, dry",	HIGH	71.79
Cereals, CREAM OF WHEAT, instant, dry",	HIGH	75.5
Cereals, CREAM OF WHEAT, instant, prepared with water, without salt",	LOW	13.08
Cereals, CREAM OF WHEAT, regular (10 minute), cooked with water, with salt",	LOW	10.66
Cereals, farina, enriched, assorted brands including CREAM OF WHEAT, quick (1-	HIGH	73.19
Cereals, farina, enriched, cooked with water, with salt",	LOW	10.92
Cereals, farina, unenriched, dry",	HIGH	78
Cereals, KASHI GO LEAN Hot Cereal, Creamy TRULY VANILLA, dry",	HIGH	61.09
Cereals, KASHI GO LEAN Hot Cereal, Hearty Honey & Cinnamon, dry",	HIGH	68
Cereals, KASHI HEART TO HEART, Instant Oatmeal, Apple Cinnamon, dry",	HIGH	73.8
Cereals, KASHI HEART TO HEART, Instant Oatmeal, golden brown maple, dry",	HIGH	73.59

Food name/ Category (100 g)	Status	Carbs content in g
Cereals, KELLOGG'S SPECIAL K NOURISH, Cinnamon Raisin Pecan, dry",	HIGH	61.9
Cereals, KELLOGG'S SPECIAL K NOURISH, Cranberry Almond, dry",	HIGH	63.29
Cereals, KELLOGG'S SPECIAL K NOURISH, Maple Brown Sugar Crunch, dry",	HIGH	62.09
Cereals, MALT-O-MEAL, chocolate, prepared with water, without salt",	LOW	9.22
Cereals, MALT-O-MEAL, Farina Hot Wheat Cereal, dry",	HIGH	77.2
Cereals, MALT-O-MEAL, Maple & Brown Sugar Hot Wheat Cereal, dry",	HIGH	80.52
Cereals, MALT-O-MEAL, original, plain, dry",	HIGH	77.25
Cereals, MALT-O-MEAL, original, plain, prepared with water, without salt",	LOW	10.09
Cereals, oats, instant, fortified, maple and brown sugar, dry",	HIGH	76.67
Cereals, oats, instant, fortified, plain, dry",	HIGH	69.52
Cereals, oats, instant, fortified, plain, prepared with water (boiling water added or microwaved)",	LOW	11.67
Cereals, oats, instant, fortified, with cinnamon and spice, dry",	HIGH	76.08
Cereals, oats, instant, fortified, with cinnamon and spice, prepared with water",	LOW	18.95
Cereals, oats, instant, fortified, with raisins and spice, dry",	HIGH	76.33
Cereals, oats, instant, fortified, with raisins and spice, prepared with water",	LOW	17.91
Cereals, oats, regular and quick and instant, unenriched, cooked with water (includes boiling and microwaving), with salt",	LOW	12
Cereals, oats, regular and quick, unenriched, cooked with water (includes boiling and microwaving), without salt",	LOW	12
Cereals, QUAKER, corn grits, instant, cheddar cheese flavor, dry",	HIGH	72.96
Cereals, QUAKER, corn grits, instant, plain, dry",	HIGH	78.42
Cereals, QUAKER, corn grits, instant, plain, prepared (microwaved or boiling water added), without salt",	LOW	15.95
Cereals, QUAKER, hominy grits, white, quick, dry",	HIGH	79.6
Cereals, QUAKER, hominy grits, white, regular, dry",	HIGH	79.2
Cereals, QUAKER, Instant Grits Product with American Cheese Flavor, dry",	HIGH	74.18
Cereals, QUAKER, Instant Grits, Butter flavor, dry",	HIGH	74.83
Cereals, QUAKER, Instant Oatmeal Organic, Regular",	HIGH	67
Cereals, QUAKER, Instant Oatmeal, Apple and Cinnamon, reduced sugar",	HIGH	72.17
Cereals, QUAKER, Instant Oatmeal, apples and cinnamon, dry",	HIGH	76.74
Cereals, QUAKER, Instant Oatmeal, Banana Bread, dry",	HIGH	75.7
Cereals, QUAKER, Instant Oatmeal, Cinnamon Spice, reduced sugar",	HIGH	69.45
Cereals, QUAKER, Instant Oatmeal, Cinnamon Swirl, high fiber",	HIGH	75.67
Cereals, QUAKER, Instant Oatmeal, Cinnamon-Spice, dry",	HIGH	74.52
Cereals, QUAKER, Instant Oatmeal, DINOSAUR EGGS, Brown Sugar, dry",	HIGH	73.68
Cereals, QUAKER, Instant Oatmeal, fruit and cream variety, dry",	HIGH	75.42
Cereals, QUAKER, Instant Oatmeal, fruit and cream, variety of flavors, reduced su	HIGH	71.57
Cereals, QUAKER, Instant Oatmeal, maple and brown sugar, dry",	HIGH	76.91
Cereals, QUAKER, Instant Oatmeal, Raisin and Spice, dry",	HIGH	75.68
Cereals, QUAKER, Instant Oatmeal, raisins, dates and walnuts, dry",	HIGH	72.41
Cereals, QUAKER, Instant Oatmeal, weight control, cinnamon",	HIGH	64.21
Cereals, QUAKER, Oat Bran, QUAKER\/MOTHER'S Oat Bran, dry",	HIGH	62.94
Cereals, QUAKER, oatmeal, REAL MEDLEYS, apple walnut, dry",	HIGH	70.53
Cereals, QUAKER, oatmeal, REAL MEDLEYS, blueberry hazelnut, dry",	HIGH	69.47
Cereals, QUAKER, oatmeal, REAL MEDLEYS, cherry pistachio, dry",	HIGH	66.73
Cereals, QUAKER, oatmeal, REAL MEDLEYS, peach almond, dry",	HIGH	68.61
Cereals, QUAKER, oatmeal, REAL MEDLEYS, summer berry, dry",	HIGH	72.58
Cereals, QUAKER, Quick Oats with Iron, Dry",	HIGH	68.18
Cereals, QUAKER, Quick Oats, Dry",	HIGH	68.18
Cereals, QUAKER, Weight Control Instant Oatmeal, banana bread",	HIGH	64.42
Cereals, QUAKER, Weight Control Instant Oatmeal, maple and brown sugar",	HIGH	64.25
Cereals, ready-to-eat, MALT-O-MEAL, Blueberry Mini SPOONERS",	HIGH	79.4

Food name/ Category (100 g)	Status	Carbs content in g
Cereals, WHEATENA, cooked with water, with salt",	LOW	11.74
Cereals, WHEATENA, cooked with water",	LOW	11.8
Cereals, whole wheat hot natural cereal, cooked with water, with salt",	LOW	13.7
Cereals, whole wheat hot natural cereal, cooked with water, without salt",	LOW	13.7
Cereals, whole wheat hot natural cereal, dry",	HIGH	75.2
Chard, swiss, cooked, boiled, drained, with salt",	LOW	4.13
Chard, swiss, cooked, boiled, drained, without salt",	LOW	4.13
Chard, swiss, raw",	LOW	3.74
Chayote, fruit, cooked, boiled, drained, with salt",	LOW	4.5
Chayote, fruit, cooked, boiled, drained, without salt",	LOW	5.09
Chayote, fruit, raw",	LOW	4.51
Cheese food, cold pack, American",	LOW	8.32
Cheese food, pasteurized process, American, imitation, without added vitamin D",	LOW	16.18
Cheese food, pasteurized process, American, vitamin D fortified",	LOW	8.56
Cheese food, pasteurized process, American, without added vitamin D",	LOW	8.56
Cheese food, pasteurized process, swiss",	LOW	4.5
Cheese product, pasteurized process, American, reduced fat, fortified with vitamin D",	LOW	10.6
Cheese product, pasteurized process, American, vitamin D fortified",	LOW	8.8
Cheese product, pasteurized process, cheddar, reduced fat",	LOW	10.6
Cheese puffs and twists, corn based, baked, low fat",	HIGH	72.35
Cheese sauce, prepared from recipe",	LOW	5.48
Cheese spread, American or Cheddar cheese base, reduced fat",	LOW	10.71
Cheese spread, cream cheese base",	LOW	3.5
Cheese spread, pasteurized process, American",	LOW	8.73
Cheese substitute, mozzarella",	LOW	23.67
Cheese, american cheddar, imitation",	LOW	11.6
Cheese, American, nonfat or fat free",	LOW	10.53
Cheese, blue",	LOW	2.34
Cheese, brick",	LOW	2.79

Food name/ Category (100 g)	Status	Carbs content in g
Cheese, brie",	LOW	0.45
Cheese, camembert",	LOW	0.46
Cheese, caraway",	LOW	3.06
Cheese, cheddar, nonfat or fat free",	LOW	7.14
Cheese, cheddar, reduced fat",	LOW	4.06
Cheese, cheddar, sharp, sliced",	LOW	2.13
Cheese, cheddar",	LOW	3.09
Cheese, cheshire",	LOW	4.78
Cheese, colby",	LOW	2.57
Cheese, cottage, creamed, large or small curd",	LOW	3.38
Cheese, cottage, creamed, with fruit",	LOW	4.61
Cheese, cottage, lowfat, 1% milkfat, lactose reduced",	LOW	3.2
Cheese, cottage, lowfat, 1% milkfat, with vegetables",	LOW	3
Cheese, cottage, lowfat, 1% milkfat",	LOW	2.72
Cheese, cottage, lowfat, 2% milkfat",	LOW	4.76
Cheese, cottage, nonfat, uncreamed, dry, large or small curd",	LOW	6.66
Cheese, cottage, with vegetables",	LOW	3
Cheese, cream, fat free",	LOW	7.66
Cheese, cream, low fat",	LOW	8.13
Cheese, cream",	LOW	5.52
Cheese, dry white, queso seco",	LOW	2.04
Cheese, edam",	LOW	1.43
Cheese, feta",	LOW	4.09
Cheese, fontina",	LOW	1.55
Cheese, fresh, queso fresco",	LOW	2.98
Cheese, gjetost",	MEDIUM	42.65
Cheese, goat, hard type",	LOW	2.17
Cheese, goat, semisoft type",	LOW	0.12

Food name/ Category (100 g)	Status	Carbs content in g
Cheese, goat, soft type",	LOW	0
Cheese, gouda",	LOW	2.22
Cheese, gruyere",	LOW	0.36
Cheese, limburger",	LOW	0.49
Cheese, low fat, cheddar or colby",	LOW	1.91
Cheese, Mexican blend",	LOW	1.75
Cheese, Mexican, blend, reduced fat",	LOW	3.41
Cheese, mexican, queso anejo",	LOW	4.63
Cheese, mexican, queso asadero",	LOW	2.87
Cheese, mexican, queso chihuahua",	LOW	5.56
Cheese, mexican, queso cotija",	LOW	3.97
Cheese, monterey, low fat",	LOW	0.7
Cheese, monterey",	LOW	0.68
Cheese, mozzarella, low moisture, part-skim, shredded",	LOW	8.06
Cheese, mozzarella, low moisture, part-skim",	LOW	5.58
Cheese, mozzarella, nonfat",	LOW	3.5
Cheese, mozzarella, part skim milk",	LOW	2.77
Cheese, mozzarella, whole milk, low moisture",	LOW	2.47
Cheese, mozzarella, whole milk",	LOW	2.19
Cheese, muenster, low fat",	LOW	3.5
Cheese, muenster",	LOW	1.12
Cheese, neufchatel",	LOW	3.59
Cheese, parmesan, dry grated, reduced fat",	LOW	1.37
Cheese, parmesan, grated",	LOW	13.91
Cheese, parmesan, hard",	LOW	3.22
Cheese, parmesan, low sodium",	LOW	3.7
Cheese, parmesan, shredded",	LOW	3.41
Cheese, pasteurized process, American, fortified with vitamin D",	LOW	4.78

Food name/ Category (100 g)	Status	Carbs content in g
Cheese, pasteurized process, American, low fat",	LOW	3.5
Cheese, pasteurized process, American, without added vitamin D",	LOW	3.7
Cheese, pasteurized process, cheddar or American, fat-free",	LOW	13.4
Cheese, pasteurized process, pimento",	LOW	1.73
Cheese, pasteurized process, swiss, low fat",	LOW	4.3
Cheese, pasteurized process, swiss",	LOW	2.1
Cheese, port de salut",	LOW	0.57
Cheese, provolone, reduced fat",	LOW	3.5
Cheese, provolone",	LOW	2.14
Cheese, ricotta, part skim milk",	LOW	5.14
Cheese, ricotta, whole milk",	LOW	3.04
Cheese, romano",	LOW	3.63
Cheese, roquefort",	LOW	2
Cheese, swiss, low fat",	LOW	3.4
Cheese, Swiss, nonfat or fat free",	LOW	3.4
Cheese, swiss",	LOW	1.44
Cheese, tilsit",	LOW	1.88
Cheese, white, queso blanco",	LOW	2.53
Cheesecake commercially prepared",	LOW	25.5
Cheesecake prepared from mix, no-bake type",	LOW	35.5
Cherries, sour, canned, water pack, drained",	LOW	10.45
Cherries, sour, red, frozen, unsweetened",	LOW	11.02
Cherries, sour, red, raw",	LOW	12.18
Cherries, sweet, canned, extra heavy syrup pack, solids and liquids",	LOW	26.23
Cherries, sweet, canned, juice pack, solids and liquids",	LOW	13.81
Cherries, sweet, canned, light syrup pack, solids and liquids",	LOW	17.29
Cherries, sweet, canned, pitted, heavy syrup pack, solids and liquids",	LOW	21.27
Cherries, sweet, canned, pitted, heavy syrup, drained",	LOW	21.07

Food name/ Category (100 g)	Status	Carbs content in g
Cherries, sweet, canned, water pack, solids and liquids",	LOW	11.76
Cherries, sweet, frozen, sweetened",	LOW	22.36
Cherries, sweet, raw",	LOW	16.01
Chewing gum",	HIGH	96.7
CHICK-FIL-A, Chick-n-Strips",	LOW	10.39
CHICK-FIL-A, chicken sandwich",	LOW	20.89
CHICK-FIL-A, hash browns",	LOW	30.51
Chicken breast tenders, breaded, cooked, microwaved",	LOW	17.56
Chicken breast tenders, breaded, uncooked",	LOW	15.01
Chicken breast, deli, rotisserie seasoned, sliced, prepackaged",	LOW	2.92
Chicken breast, fat-free, mesquite flavor, sliced",	LOW	2.25
Chicken breast, oven-roasted, fat-free, sliced",	LOW	2.17
Chicken patty, frozen, cooked",	LOW	12.84
Chicken patty, frozen, uncooked",	LOW	13.61
Chicken pot pie, frozen entree, prepared",	LOW	19.21
Chicken spread",	LOW	4.05
Chicken tenders, breaded, frozen, prepared",	LOW	14.86
Chicken, broiler or fryers, breast, skinless, boneless, meat only, cooked, braised",	LOW	0
Chicken, broiler or fryers, breast, skinless, boneless, meat only, cooked, grilled",	LOW	0
Chicken, broiler or fryers, breast, skinless, boneless, meat only, raw",	LOW	0
Chicken, broiler or fryers, breast, skinless, boneless, meat only, with added solution, cooked, braised",	LOW	0
Chicken, broiler or fryers, breast, skinless, boneless, meat only, with added solution, cooked, grilled",	LOW	0
Chicken, broiler, rotisserie, BBQ, back meat and skin",	LOW	0.4
Chicken, broiler, rotisserie, BBQ, back meat only",	LOW	0.31
Chicken, broiler, rotisserie, BBQ, breast meat and skin",	LOW	0.09
Chicken, broiler, rotisserie, BBQ, breast meat only",	LOW	0
Chicken, broiler, rotisserie, BBQ, drumstick meat and skin",	LOW	0.12
Chicken, broiler, rotisserie, BBQ, drumstick, meat only",	LOW	0

Food name/ Category (100 g)	Status	Carbs content in g
Chicken, broiler, rotisserie, BBQ, skin",	LOW	0.7
Chicken, broiler, rotisserie, BBQ, thigh meat and skin",	LOW	0.12
Chicken, broiler, rotisserie, BBQ, thigh, meat only",	LOW	0
Chicken, broiler, rotisserie, BBQ, wing meat and skin",	LOW	0.6
Chicken, broiler, rotisserie, BBQ, wing, meat only",	LOW	0.54
Chicken, broilers or fryers, back, meat and skin, cooked, fried, batter",	LOW	10.25
Chicken, broilers or fryers, back, meat and skin, cooked, fried, flour",	LOW	6.5
Chicken, broilers or fryers, back, meat and skin, cooked, roasted",	LOW	0
Chicken, broilers or fryers, back, meat and skin, cooked, rotisserie, original seasoning",	LOW	0.03
Chicken, broilers or fryers, back, meat and skin, cooked, stewed",	LOW	0
Chicken, broilers or fryers, back, meat and skin, raw",	LOW	0
Chicken, broilers or fryers, back, meat only, cooked, fried",	LOW	5.68
Chicken, broilers or fryers, back, meat only, cooked, roasted",	LOW	0
Chicken, broilers or fryers, back, meat only, cooked, rotisserie, original seasoning",	LOW	0
Chicken, broilers or fryers, back, meat only, cooked, stewed",	LOW	0
Chicken, broilers or fryers, back, meat only, raw",	LOW	0
Chicken, broilers or fryers, breast, meat and skin, cooked, fried, batter",	LOW	8.99
Chicken, broilers or fryers, breast, meat and skin, cooked, fried, flour",	LOW	1.64
Chicken, broilers or fryers, breast, meat and skin, cooked, roasted",	LOW	0
Chicken, broilers or fryers, breast, meat and skin, cooked, rotisserie, original seasoning",	LOW	0.02
Chicken, broilers or fryers, breast, meat and skin, cooked, stewed",	LOW	0
Chicken, broilers or fryers, breast, meat and skin, raw",	LOW	0
Chicken, broilers or fryers, breast, meat only, cooked, fried",	LOW	0.51
Chicken, broilers or fryers, breast, meat only, cooked, roasted",	LOW	0
Chicken, broilers or fryers, breast, meat only, cooked, rotisserie, original seasoning",	LOW	0
Chicken, broilers or fryers, breast, meat only, cooked, stewed",	LOW	0
Chicken, broilers or fryers, breast, skinless, boneless, meat only, with added solution, raw",	LOW	0
Chicken, broilers or fryers, dark meat, drumstick, meat and skin, cooked, braised",	LOW	0

Food name/ Category (100 g)	Status	Carbs content in g
Chicken, broilers or fryers, dark meat, drumstick, meat only, cooked, braised",	LOW	0
Chicken, broilers or fryers, dark meat, drumstick, meat only, cooked, roasted",	LOW	0
Chicken, broilers or fryers, dark meat, drumstick, meat only, raw",	LOW	0
Chicken, broilers or fryers, dark meat, meat and skin, cooked, fried, batter",	LOW	9.38
Chicken, broilers or fryers, dark meat, meat and skin, cooked, fried, flour",	LOW	4.08
Chicken, broilers or fryers, dark meat, meat and skin, cooked, roasted",	LOW	0
Chicken, broilers or fryers, dark meat, meat and skin, cooked, stewed",	LOW	0
Chicken, broilers or fryers, dark meat, meat and skin, raw",	LOW	0
Chicken, broilers or fryers, dark meat, meat only, cooked, fried",	LOW	2.59
Chicken, broilers or fryers, dark meat, meat only, cooked, roasted",	LOW	0
Chicken, broilers or fryers, dark meat, meat only, cooked, stewed",	LOW	0
Chicken, broilers or fryers, dark meat, meat only, raw",	LOW	0
Chicken, broilers or fryers, dark meat, thigh, meat and skin, cooked, braised",	LOW	0
Chicken, broilers or fryers, dark meat, thigh, meat only, cooked, braised",	LOW	0
Chicken, broilers or fryers, dark meat, thigh, meat only, raw",	LOW	0
Chicken, broilers or fryers, drumstick, meat and skin, cooked, fried, batter",	LOW	8.28
Chicken, broilers or fryers, drumstick, meat and skin, cooked, fried, flour",	LOW	1.63
Chicken, broilers or fryers, drumstick, meat and skin, cooked, roasted",	LOW	0
Chicken, broilers or fryers, drumstick, meat and skin, cooked, rotisserie, original seasoning",	LOW	0.02
Chicken, broilers or fryers, drumstick, meat and skin, cooked, stewed",	LOW	0
Chicken, broilers or fryers, drumstick, meat and skin, raw",	LOW	0.11
Chicken, broilers or fryers, drumstick, meat only, cooked, fried",	LOW	0
Chicken, broilers or fryers, drumstick, meat only, cooked, rotisserie, original seasoning",	LOW	0
Chicken, broilers or fryers, drumstick, meat only, cooked, stewed",	LOW	0
Chicken, broilers or fryers, giblets, cooked, fried",	LOW	4.35
Chicken, broilers or fryers, giblets, cooked, simmered",	LOW	0
Chicken, broilers or fryers, giblets, raw",	LOW	1.8
Chicken, broilers or fryers, leg, meat and skin, cooked, fried, batter",	LOW	8.72

Food name/ Category (100 g)	Status	Carbs content in g
Chicken, broilers or fryers, leg, meat and skin, cooked, fried, flour",	LOW	2.5
Chicken, broilers or fryers, leg, meat and skin, cooked, roasted",	LOW	0
Chicken, broilers or fryers, leg, meat and skin, cooked, stewed",	LOW	0
Chicken, broilers or fryers, leg, meat and skin, raw",	LOW	0.17
Chicken, broilers or fryers, leg, meat only, cooked, fried",	LOW	0.65
Chicken, broilers or fryers, leg, meat only, cooked, roasted",	LOW	0
Chicken, broilers or fryers, leg, meat only, cooked, stewed",	LOW	0
Chicken, broilers or fryers, leg, meat only, raw",	LOW	0
Chicken, broilers or fryers, light meat, meat and skin, cooked, fried, batter",	LOW	9.5
Chicken, broilers or fryers, light meat, meat and skin, cooked, fried, flour",	LOW	1.82
Chicken, broilers or fryers, light meat, meat and skin, cooked, roasted",	LOW	0
Chicken, broilers or fryers, light meat, meat and skin, cooked, stewed",	LOW	0
Chicken, broilers or fryers, light meat, meat and skin, raw",	LOW	0
Chicken, broilers or fryers, light meat, meat only, cooked, fried",	LOW	0.42
Chicken, broilers or fryers, light meat, meat only, cooked, roasted",	LOW	0
Chicken, broilers or fryers, light meat, meat only, cooked, stewed",	LOW	0
Chicken, broilers or fryers, light meat, meat only, raw",	LOW	0
Chicken, broilers or fryers, meat and skin and giblets and neck, cooked, fried, batter",	LOW	9.03
Chicken, broilers or fryers, meat and skin and giblets and neck, cooked, fried, flour",	LOW	3.27
Chicken, broilers or fryers, meat and skin and giblets and neck, raw",	LOW	0.13
Chicken, broilers or fryers, meat and skin and giblets and neck, roasted",	LOW	0.06
Chicken, broilers or fryers, meat and skin and giblets and neck, stewed",	LOW	0.06
Chicken, broilers or fryers, meat and skin, cooked, fried, batter",	LOW	9.42
Chicken, broilers or fryers, meat and skin, cooked, fried, flour",	LOW	3.15
Chicken, broilers or fryers, meat and skin, cooked, roasted",	LOW	0
Chicken, broilers or fryers, meat and skin, cooked, stewed",	LOW	0
Chicken, broilers or fryers, meat and skin, raw",	LOW	0
Chicken, broilers or fryers, meat only, cooked, fried",	LOW	1.69

Food name/ Category (100 g)	Status	Carbs content in g
Chicken, broilers or fryers, meat only, raw",	LOW	0
Chicken, broilers or fryers, meat only, roasted",	LOW	0
Chicken, broilers or fryers, meat only, stewed",	LOW	0
Chicken, broilers or fryers, neck, meat and skin, cooked simmered",	LOW	0
Chicken, broilers or fryers, neck, meat and skin, cooked, fried, batter",	LOW	8.7
Chicken, broilers or fryers, neck, meat and skin, cooked, fried, flour",	LOW	4.24
Chicken, broilers or fryers, neck, meat and skin, raw",	LOW	0
Chicken, broilers or fryers, neck, meat only, cooked, fried",	LOW	1.77
Chicken, broilers or fryers, neck, meat only, cooked, simmered",	LOW	0
Chicken, broilers or fryers, neck, meat only, raw",	LOW	0
Chicken, broilers or fryers, skin only, cooked, fried, batter",	LOW	23.15
Chicken, broilers or fryers, skin only, cooked, fried, flour",	LOW	9.34
Chicken, broilers or fryers, skin only, cooked, roasted",	LOW	0
Chicken, broilers or fryers, skin only, cooked, rotisserie, original seasoning",	LOW	0.11
Chicken, broilers or fryers, skin only, cooked, stewed",	LOW	0
Chicken, broilers or fryers, skin only, raw",	LOW	0
Chicken, broilers or fryers, thigh, meat and skin, cooked, fried, batter",	LOW	9.08
Chicken, broilers or fryers, thigh, meat and skin, cooked, fried, flour",	LOW	3.18
Chicken, broilers or fryers, thigh, meat and skin, cooked, roasted",	LOW	0
Chicken, broilers or fryers, thigh, meat and skin, cooked, rotisserie, original seasoning",	LOW	0.02
Chicken, broilers or fryers, thigh, meat and skin, cooked, stewed",	LOW	0
Chicken, broilers or fryers, thigh, meat and skin, raw",	LOW	0.25
Chicken, broilers or fryers, thigh, meat only, cooked, fried",	LOW	1.18
Chicken, broilers or fryers, thigh, meat only, cooked, roasted",	LOW	0
Chicken, broilers or fryers, thigh, meat only, cooked, rotisserie, original seasoning",	LOW	0
Chicken, broilers or fryers, thigh, meat only, cooked, stewed",	LOW	0
Chicken, broilers or fryers, wing, meat and skin, cooked, fried, batter",	LOW	10.94
Chicken, broilers or fryers, wing, meat and skin, cooked, fried, flour",	LOW	2.39

Food name/ Category (100 g)	Status	Carbs content in g
Chicken, broilers or fryers, wing, meat and skin, cooked, roasted",	LOW	0
Chicken, broilers or fryers, wing, meat and skin, cooked, rotisserie, original seasoning",	LOW	0.04
Chicken, broilers or fryers, wing, meat and skin, cooked, stewed",	LOW	0
Chicken, broilers or fryers, wing, meat and skin, raw",	LOW	0
Chicken, broilers or fryers, wing, meat only, cooked, fried",	LOW	0
Chicken, broilers or fryers, wing, meat only, cooked, roasted",	LOW	0
Chicken, broilers or fryers, wing, meat only, cooked, rotisserie, original seasoning",	LOW	0
Chicken, broilers or fryers, wing, meat only, cooked, stewed",	LOW	0
Chicken, broilers or fryers, wing, meat only, raw",	LOW	0
Chicken, canned, meat only, with broth",	LOW	0
Chicken, canned, no broth",	LOW	0.9
Chicken, capons, giblets, cooked, simmered",	LOW	0.76
Chicken, capons, giblets, raw",	LOW	1.42
Chicken, capons, meat and skin and giblets and neck, cooked, roasted",	LOW	0.04
Chicken, capons, meat and skin and giblets and neck, raw",	LOW	0.08
Chicken, capons, meat and skin, cooked, roasted",	LOW	0
Chicken, capons, meat and skin, raw",	LOW	0
Chicken, cornish game hens, meat and skin, cooked, roasted",	LOW	0
Chicken, cornish game hens, meat and skin, raw",	LOW	0
Chicken, cornish game hens, meat only, cooked, roasted",	LOW	0
Chicken, cornish game hens, meat only, raw",	LOW	0
Chicken, dark meat, drumstick, meat and skin, with added solution, cooked, braised",	LOW	0.13
Chicken, dark meat, drumstick, meat and skin, with added solution, cooked, roasted",	LOW	0.05
Chicken, dark meat, drumstick, meat and skin, with added solution, raw",	LOW	0
Chicken, dark meat, drumstick, meat only, with added solution, cooked, braised",	LOW	0
Chicken, dark meat, drumstick, meat only, with added solution, cooked, roasted",	LOW	0
Chicken, dark meat, drumstick, meat only, with added solution, raw",	LOW	0
Chicken, dark meat, thigh, meat and skin, with added solution, cooked, braised",	LOW	0.21

Food name/ Category (100 g)	Status	Carbs content in g
Chicken, dark meat, thigh, meat and skin, with added solution, cooked, roasted",	LOW	0.09
Chicken, dark meat, thigh, meat and skin, with added solution, raw",	LOW	0
Chicken, dark meat, thigh, meat only, with added solution, cooked, braised",	LOW	0
Chicken, dark meat, thigh, meat only, with added solution, cooked, roasted",	LOW	0
Chicken, dark meat, thigh, meat only, with added solution, raw",	LOW	0
Chicken, feet, boiled",	LOW	0.2
Chicken, gizzard, all classes, cooked, simmered",	LOW	0
Chicken, gizzard, all classes, raw",	LOW	0
Chicken, ground, crumbles, cooked, pan-browned",	LOW	0
Chicken, ground, raw",	LOW	0.04
Chicken, heart, all classes, cooked, simmered",	LOW	0.1
Chicken, heart, all classes, raw",	LOW	0.71
Chicken, liver, all classes, cooked, pan-fried",	LOW	1.11
Chicken, liver, all classes, cooked, simmered",	LOW	0.87
Chicken, liver, all classes, raw",	LOW	0.73
Chicken, meatless, breaded, fried",	LOW	8.51
Chicken, meatless",	LOW	3.64
Chicken, nuggets, dark and white meat, precooked, frozen, not reheated",	LOW	16.32
Chicken, nuggets, white meat, precooked, frozen, not reheated",	LOW	16.24
Chicken, roasting, dark meat, meat only, cooked, roasted",	LOW	0
Chicken, roasting, dark meat, meat only, raw",	LOW	0
Chicken, roasting, giblets, cooked, simmered",	LOW	0.86
Chicken, roasting, giblets, raw",	LOW	1.14
Chicken, roasting, light meat, meat only, cooked, roasted",	LOW	0
Chicken, roasting, light meat, meat only, raw",	LOW	0
Chicken, roasting, meat and skin and giblets and neck, cooked, roasted",	LOW	0.05
Chicken, roasting, meat and skin and giblets and neck, raw",	LOW	0.09
Chicken, roasting, meat and skin, cooked, roasted",	LOW	0

Food name/ Category (100 g)	Status	Carbs content in g
Chicken, roasting, meat only, cooked, roasted",	LOW	0
Chicken, roasting, meat only, raw",	LOW	0
Chicken, skin (drumsticks and thighs), cooked, braised",	LOW	0
Chicken, skin (drumsticks and thighs), cooked, roasted",	LOW	0
Chicken, skin (drumsticks and thighs), raw",	LOW	0.79
Chicken, skin (drumsticks and thighs), with added solution, cooked, braised",	LOW	1
Chicken, skin (drumsticks and thighs), with added solution, cooked, roasted",	LOW	0.44
Chicken, skin (drumsticks and thighs), with added solution, raw",	LOW	0.01
Chicken, stewing, dark meat, meat only, cooked, stewed",	LOW	0
Chicken, stewing, dark meat, meat only, raw",	LOW	0
Chicken, stewing, giblets, cooked, simmered",	LOW	0.11
Chicken, stewing, giblets, raw",	LOW	2.13
Chicken, stewing, light meat, meat only, cooked, stewed",	LOW	0
Chicken, stewing, light meat, meat only, raw",	LOW	0
Chicken, stewing, meat and skin, and giblets and neck, cooked, stewed",	LOW	0
Chicken, stewing, meat and skin, and giblets and neck, raw",	LOW	0.19
Chicken, stewing, meat and skin, cooked, stewed",	LOW	0
Chicken, stewing, meat and skin, raw",	LOW	0
Chicken, stewing, meat only, cooked, stewed",	LOW	0
Chicken, stewing, meat only, raw",	LOW	0
Chicken, thighs, frozen, breaded, reheated",	LOW	14.23
Chicken, wing, frozen, glazed, barbecue flavored, heated (conventional oven)",	LOW	3.36
Chicken, wing, frozen, glazed, barbecue flavored, heated (microwave)",	LOW	3.84
Chicken, wing, frozen, glazed, barbecue flavored",	LOW	3.34
Chickpea flour (besan)",	HIGH	57.82
Chickpeas (garbanzo beans, bengal gram), mature seeds, canned, drained solids",	LOW	22.53
Chickpeas (garbanzo beans, bengal gram), mature seeds, canned, drained, rinsed in tap water",	LOW	22.87
Chickpeas (garbanzo beans, bengal gram), mature seeds, canned, solids and liquids, low sodium",	LOW	13.49

Food name/ Category (100 g)	Status	Carbs content in g
Chickpeas (garbanzo beans, bengal gram), mature seeds, canned, solids and liquids",	LOW	13.49
Chickpeas (garbanzo beans, bengal gram), mature seeds, cooked, boiled, with salt",	LOW	27.42
Chicory greens, raw",	LOW	4.7
Chicory roots, raw",	LOW	17.51
Chicory, witloof, raw",	LOW	4
Child formula, ABBOTT NUTRITION, PEDIASURE, ready-to-feed, with iron and fiber",	LOW	11.28
Child formula, ABBOTT NUTRITION, PEDIASURE, ready-to-feed",	LOW	11.15
Child formula, MEAD JOHNSON, PORTAGEN, with iron, powder, not reconstituted	MEDIUM	54.8
Child formula, MEAD JOHNSON, PORTAGEN, with iron, prepared from powder",	LOW	8.57
Chili con carne with beans, canned entree",	LOW	13.1
Chili with beans, canned",	LOW	13.24
Chili with beans, microwavable bowls",	LOW	10.88
Chili, no beans, canned entree",	LOW	6.1
Chives, freeze-dried",	HIGH	64.29
Chives, raw",	LOW	4.35
Chocolate-flavored hazelnut spread",	HIGH	62.16
Chokecherries, raw, pitted (Northern Plains Indians)",	LOW	33.62
Chrysanthemum leaves, raw",	LOW	3.01
Chrysanthemum, garland, cooked, boiled, drained, with salt",	LOW	4.31
Chrysanthemum, garland, cooked, boiled, drained, without salt",	LOW	4.31
Chrysanthemum, garland, raw",	LOW	3.02
Cinnamon buns, frosted (includes honey buns)",	MEDIUM	48.6
Clementines, raw",	LOW	12.02
Cocoa mix, NESTLE, Rich Chocolate Hot Cocoa Mix",	HIGH	75
Cocoa, dry powder, unsweetened, HERSHEY'S European Style Cocoa",	HIGH	60
Coffeecake, cheese",	MEDIUM	44.3
Coffeecake, cinnamon with crumb topping, commercially prepared, enriched",	MEDIUM	46.7
Coffeecake, cinnamon with crumb topping, commercially prepared, unenriched",	MEDIUM	46.7
Coffeecake, cinnamon with crumb topping, dry mix, prepared",	MEDIUM	52.8
Coffeecake, cinnamon with crumb topping, dry mix",	HIGH	77.7
Coffeecake, creme-filled with chocolate frosting",	MEDIUM	53.8
Coffeecake, fruit",	MEDIUM	51.5
Collards, cooked, boiled, drained, with salt",	LOW	5.65
Collards, frozen, chopped, cooked, boiled, drained, with salt",	LOW	7.1

Food name/ Category (100 g)	Status	Carbs content in g
Collards, frozen, chopped, cooked, boiled, drained, without salt",	LOW	7.1
Collards, frozen, chopped, unprepared",	LOW	6.46
CONTINENTAL MILLS, KRUSTEAZ Almond Poppyseed Muffin Mix, Artificially Fla	HIGH	75.6
Cookie, butter or sugar, with chocolate icing or filling",	HIGH	68.83
Cookie, chocolate, with icing or coating",	HIGH	67.87
Cookie, vanilla with caramel, coconut, and chocolate coating",	HIGH	64.1
Cookie, with peanut butter filling, chocolate-coated",	MEDIUM	52.9
Cookies, animal crackers (includes arrowroot, tea biscuits)",	HIGH	74.1
Cookies, animal, with frosting or icing",	HIGH	70.09
Cookies, brownies, commercially prepared, reduced fat, with added fiber",	HIGH	61.58
Cookies, brownies, commercially prepared",	HIGH	63.9
Cookies, brownies, dry mix, regular",	HIGH	76.6
Cookies, brownies, dry mix, sugar free",	HIGH	80.4
Cookies, brownies, prepared from recipe",	MEDIUM	50.2
Cookies, butter, commercially prepared, enriched",	HIGH	68.9
Cookies, butter, commercially prepared, unenriched",	HIGH	68.9
Cookies, chocolate chip sandwich, with creme filling",	HIGH	63.52
Cookies, chocolate chip, commercially prepared, regular, higher fat, enriched",	HIGH	65.36
Cookies, chocolate chip, commercially prepared, regular, higher fat, unenriched",	HIGH	66.8
Cookies, chocolate chip, commercially prepared, regular, lower fat",	HIGH	67.49
Cookies, chocolate chip, commercially prepared, soft-type",	HIGH	65.75
Cookies, chocolate chip, commercially prepared, special dietary",	HIGH	73.4
Cookies, chocolate chip, dry mix",	HIGH	66.1
Cookies, chocolate chip, prepared from recipe, made with butter",	HIGH	58.2
Cookies, chocolate chip, prepared from recipe, made with margarine",	HIGH	58.4
Cookies, chocolate chip, refrigerated dough, baked",	HIGH	68.2
Cookies, chocolate chip, refrigerated dough",	HIGH	61.02
Cookies, chocolate cream covered biscuit sticks",	MEDIUM	51.08
Cookies, chocolate sandwich, with creme filling, reduced fat",	HIGH	76.17
Cookies, chocolate sandwich, with creme filling, regular, chocolate-coated",	HIGH	66.4
Cookies, chocolate sandwich, with creme filling, regular",	HIGH	71
Cookies, chocolate sandwich, with creme filling, special dietary",	HIGH	68
Cookies, chocolate sandwich, with extra creme filling",	HIGH	68.2
Cookies, chocolate wafers",	HIGH	72.7
Cookies, chocolate, made with rice cereal",	HIGH	63.26
Cookies, coconut macaroon",	HIGH	61.22
Cookies, fig bars",	HIGH	70.9
Cookies, fudge, cake-type (includes trolley cakes)",	HIGH	78.3
Cookies, gingersnaps",	HIGH	76.9
Cookies, gluten-free, chocolate sandwich, with creme filling",	HIGH	76.03
Cookies, gluten-free, chocolate wafer",	HIGH	62.82
Cookies, gluten-free, lemon wafer",	HIGH	74.39
Cookies, gluten-free, vanilla sandwich, with creme filling",	HIGH	74.61
Cookies, ladyfingers, with lemon juice and rind",	HIGH	59.7
Cookies, ladyfingers, without lemon juice and rind",	HIGH	59.7
Cookies, Marie biscuit",	HIGH	70.54
Cookies, marshmallow, chocolate-coated (includes marshmallow pies)",	HIGH	67.7
Cookies, marshmallow, with rice cereal and chocolate chips",	HIGH	63.26
Cookies, molasses",	HIGH	73.8
Cookies, oatmeal sandwich, with creme filling",	MEDIUM	55.62
Cookies, oatmeal, commercially prepared, regular",	HIGH	68.7
Cookies, oatmeal, commercially prepared, soft-type",	HIGH	65.7
Cookies, oatmeal, commercially prepared, special dietary",	HIGH	69.9
Cookies, oatmeal, dry mix",	HIGH	67.3
Cookies, oatmeal, prepared from recipe, with raisins",	HIGH	68.4

Food name/ Category (100 g)	Status	Carbs content in g
Cookies, oatmeal, prepared from recipe, without raisins",	HIGH	66.4
Cookies, oatmeal, reduced fat",	HIGH	64.62
Cookies, oatmeal, refrigerated dough, baked",	HIGH	65.7
Cookies, oatmeal, refrigerated dough",	HIGH	59.1
Cookies, peanut butter sandwich, regular",	HIGH	65.6
Cookies, peanut butter sandwich, special dietary",	MEDIUM	50.8
Cookies, peanut butter, commercially prepared, regular",	HIGH	58.15
Cookies, peanut butter, commercially prepared, soft-type",	HIGH	57.7
Cookies, peanut butter, commercially prepared, sugar free",	MEDIUM	50.52
Cookies, peanut butter, prepared from recipe",	HIGH	58.9
Cookies, peanut butter, refrigerated dough, baked",	HIGH	57.3
Cookies, peanut butter, refrigerated dough",	MEDIUM	52.1
Cookies, raisin, soft-type",	HIGH	68
Cookies, shortbread, commercially prepared, pecan",	HIGH	58.3
Cookies, shortbread, commercially prepared, plain",	HIGH	63.78
Cookies, shortbread, reduced fat",	HIGH	75.99
Cookies, sugar wafer, chocolate-covered",	HIGH	65.99
Cookies, sugar wafer, with creme filling, sugar free",	HIGH	66.26
Cookies, sugar wafers with creme filling, regular",	HIGH	70.64
Cookies, sugar, commercially prepared, regular (includes vanilla)",	HIGH	67.34
Cookies, sugar, prepared from recipe, made with margarine",	HIGH	60
Cookies, sugar, refrigerated dough, baked",	HIGH	65.6
Cookies, sugar, refrigerated dough",	HIGH	61.22
Cookies, vanilla sandwich with creme filling, reduced fat",	HIGH	78.16
Cookies, vanilla sandwich with creme filling",	HIGH	72.1
Cookies, vanilla wafers, higher fat",	HIGH	72.6
Cookies, vanilla wafers, lower fat",	HIGH	73.6
Coriander (cilantro) leaves, raw",	LOW	3.67
Corn dogs, frozen, prepared",	LOW	26.96
Corn flour, masa, enriched, white",	HIGH	76.59
Corn flour, masa, unenriched, white",	HIGH	76.59
Corn flour, whole-grain, blue (harina de maiz morado)",	HIGH	73.89
Corn flour, whole-grain, white",	HIGH	76.85
Corn flour, whole-grain, yellow",	HIGH	76.85
Corn flour, yellow, degermed, unenriched",	HIGH	82.75
Corn flour, yellow, masa, enriched",	HIGH	76.59
Corn pudding, home prepared",	LOW	16.97
Corn with red and green peppers, canned, solids and liquids",	LOW	18.17
Corn, dried, yellow (Northern Plains Indians)",	HIGH	66.27
Corn, sweet, white, canned, cream style, no salt added",	LOW	18.13
Corn, sweet, white, canned, cream style, regular pack",	LOW	18.62
Corn, sweet, white, canned, vacuum pack, no salt added",	LOW	19.44
Corn, sweet, white, canned, vacuum pack, regular pack",	LOW	19.44
Corn, sweet, white, canned, whole kernel, drained solids",	LOW	15.06
Corn, sweet, white, canned, whole kernel, regular pack, solids and liquids",	LOW	15.41
Corn, sweet, white, cooked, boiled, drained, with salt",	LOW	21.71

Food name/ Category (100 g)	Status	Carbs content in g
Corn, sweet, white, cooked, boiled, drained, without salt",	LOW	21.71
Corn, sweet, white, frozen, kernels cut off cob, boiled, drained, with salt",	LOW	19.56
Corn, sweet, white, frozen, kernels cut off cob, boiled, drained, without salt",	LOW	19.56
Corn, sweet, white, frozen, kernels cut off cob, unprepared",	LOW	20.73
Corn, sweet, white, frozen, kernels on cob, cooked, boiled, drained, with salt",	LOW	22.33
Corn, sweet, white, frozen, kernels on cob, cooked, boiled, drained, without salt",	LOW	22.33
Corn, sweet, white, frozen, kernels on cob, unprepared",	LOW	23.5
Corn, sweet, yellow, canned, brine pack, regular pack, solids and liquids",	LOW	13.86
Corn, sweet, yellow, canned, cream style, no salt added",	LOW	18.13
Corn, sweet, yellow, canned, cream style, regular pack",	LOW	18.13
Corn, sweet, yellow, canned, drained solids, rinsed with tap water",	LOW	13.02
Corn, sweet, yellow, canned, vacuum pack, no salt added",	LOW	19.44
Corn, sweet, yellow, canned, vacuum pack, regular pack",	LOW	19.44
Corn, sweet, yellow, canned, whole kernel, drained solids",	LOW	14.34
Corn, sweet, yellow, cooked, boiled, drained, with salt",	LOW	20.98
Corn, sweet, yellow, cooked, boiled, drained, without salt",	LOW	20.98
Corn, sweet, yellow, frozen, kernels cut off cob, boiled, drained, without salt",	LOW	19.3
Corn, sweet, yellow, frozen, kernels cut off cob, unprepared",	LOW	20.71
Corn, sweet, yellow, frozen, kernels on cob, cooked, boiled, drained, with salt",	LOW	22.33
Corn, sweet, yellow, frozen, kernels on cob, cooked, boiled, drained, without salt",	LOW	22.33
Corn, sweet, yellow, frozen, kernels on cob, unprepared",	LOW	23.5
Corn, sweet, yellow, frozen, kernels, cut off cob, boiled, drained, with salt",	LOW	18.71
Corn, yellow, whole kernel, frozen, microwaved",	LOW	25.87
Corned beef loaf, jellied",	LOW	0
Cornmeal, white, self-rising, bolted, plain, enriched",	HIGH	70.28
Cornmeal, white, self-rising, bolted, with wheat flour added, enriched",	HIGH	73.43
Cornmeal, white, self-rising, degermed, enriched",	HIGH	74.79
Cornmeal, yellow, self-rising, bolted, plain, enriched",	HIGH	70.28
Cornmeal, yellow, self-rising, bolted, with wheat flour added, enriched",	HIGH	73.43
Cornmeal, yellow, self-rising, degermed, enriched",	HIGH	74.79
Cornsalad, raw",	LOW	3.6

Food name/ Category (100 g)	Status	Carbs content in g
Couscous, cooked",	LOW	23.22
Cowpeas (blackeyes), immature seeds, cooked, boiled, drained, with salt",	LOW	19.73
Cowpeas (blackeyes), immature seeds, cooked, boiled, drained, without salt",	LOW	20.32
Cowpeas (blackeyes), immature seeds, frozen, cooked, boiled, drained, with salt",	LOW	23.5
Cowpeas (blackeyes), immature seeds, frozen, cooked, boiled, drained, without salt",	LOW	23.76
Cowpeas (blackeyes), immature seeds, raw",	LOW	18.83
Cowpeas, catjang, mature seeds, cooked, boiled, with salt",	LOW	20.32
Cowpeas, catjang, mature seeds, raw",	HIGH	59.64
Cowpeas, common (blackeyes, crowder, southern), mature seeds, canned, plain",	LOW	13.63
Cowpeas, common (blackeyes, crowder, southern), mature seeds, cooked, boiled, with salt",	LOW	20.76
Cowpeas, common (blackeyes, crowder, southern), mature seeds, cooked, boiled, without salt",	LOW	20.76
Cowpeas, leafy tips, cooked, boiled, drained, with salt",	LOW	2.8
Cowpeas, young pods with seeds, cooked, boiled, drained, with salt",	LOW	7
Cowpeas, young pods with seeds, cooked, boiled, drained, without salt",	LOW	7
Cowpeas, young pods with seeds, raw",	LOW	9.5
Crabapples, raw",	LOW	19.95
CRACKER BARREL, chicken tenderloin platter, fried, from kid's menu",	LOW	20.24
CRACKER BARREL, chicken tenderloin platter, fried",	LOW	20.29
CRACKER BARREL, coleslaw",	LOW	13.01
CRACKER BARREL, country fried shrimp platter",	LOW	21.4
CRACKER BARREL, farm raised catfish platter",	LOW	5.31
CRACKER BARREL, grilled sirloin steak",	LOW	0
CRACKER BARREL, macaroni n' cheese plate, from kid's menu",	LOW	15.58
CRACKER BARREL, macaroni n' cheese",	LOW	15.61
CRACKER BARREL, onion rings, thick-cut",	MEDIUM	40.95
CRACKER BARREL, steak fries",	LOW	30.87
Crackers, cheese, low sodium",	HIGH	58.2
Crackers, cheese, reduced fat",	HIGH	68.19
Crackers, cheese, regular",	HIGH	59.42
Crackers, cheese, sandwich-type with cheese filling",	HIGH	58.76
Crackers, cheese, sandwich-type with peanut butter filling",	MEDIUM	56.74
Crackers, cheese, whole grain",	HIGH	57.29

Food name/ Category (100 g)	Status	Carbs content in g
Crackers, cream, GAMESA SABROSAS",	HIGH	64.55
Crackers, cream, LA MODERNA RIKIS CREAM CRACKERS",	HIGH	64.88
Crackers, crispbread, rye",	HIGH	82.2
Crackers, flavored, fish-shaped",	HIGH	65.67
Crackers, gluten-free, multi-seeded and multigrain",	HIGH	66.3
Crackers, gluten-free, multigrain and vegetable, made with corn starch and white ric	HIGH	76.94
Crackers, matzo, egg and onion",	HIGH	77.1
Crackers, matzo, plain",	HIGH	83.7
Crackers, matzo, whole-wheat",	HIGH	78.9
Crackers, melba toast, plain",	HIGH	76.6
Crackers, melba toast, rye (includes pumpernickel)",	HIGH	77.3
Crackers, melba toast, wheat",	HIGH	76.4
Crackers, milk",	HIGH	71.73
Crackers, multigrain",	HIGH	67.6
Crackers, rusk toast",	HIGH	72.3
Crackers, rye, sandwich-type with cheese filling",	HIGH	60.8
Crackers, rye, wafers, plain",	HIGH	80.4
Crackers, rye, wafers, seasoned",	HIGH	73.8
Crackers, saltines (includes oyster, soda, soup)",	HIGH	74.05
Crackers, saltines, fat-free, low-sodium",	HIGH	82.3
Crackers, saltines, low salt (includes oyster, soda, soup)",	HIGH	74.34
Crackers, saltines, unsalted tops (includes oyster, soda, soup)",	HIGH	71.5
Crackers, saltines, whole wheat (includes multi-grain)",	HIGH	68.25
Crackers, sandwich-type, peanut butter filled, reduced fat",	HIGH	63.49
Crackers, snack, GOYA CRACKERS",	HIGH	64.35
Crackers, standard snack-type, regular, low salt",	HIGH	61
Crackers, standard snack-type, regular",	HIGH	61.3
Crackers, standard snack-type, sandwich, with cheese filling",	HIGH	61.7
Crackers, standard snack-type, sandwich, with peanut butter filling",	HIGH	58.38
Crackers, standard snack-type, with whole wheat",	HIGH	68.37
Crackers, toast thins, low sodium",	HIGH	67.66
Crackers, water biscuits",	HIGH	72.81
Crackers, wheat, low salt",	HIGH	64.9
Crackers, wheat, reduced fat",	HIGH	71.52
Crackers, wheat, regular",	HIGH	70.73
Crackers, wheat, sandwich, with cheese filling",	HIGH	58.2
Crackers, wheat, sandwich, with peanut butter filling",	MEDIUM	53.8
Crackers, whole grain, sandwich-type, with peanut butter filling",	MEDIUM	54.59
Crackers, whole-wheat, low salt",	HIGH	68.6
Crackers, whole-wheat, reduced fat",	HIGH	75.52
Crackers, whole-wheat",	HIGH	69.55
Cranberries, dried, sweetened",	HIGH	82.8
Cranberries, raw",	LOW	11.97
Cranberry juice cocktail, bottled, low calorie, with calcium, saccharin and corn sweetener",	LOW	4.6
Cranberry juice cocktail, bottled",	LOW	13.52
Cranberry juice cocktail, frozen concentrate, prepared with water",	LOW	11.81
Cranberry juice cocktail, frozen concentrate",	MEDIUM	51.45
Cranberry juice, unsweetened",	LOW	12.2
Cranberry sauce, canned, sweetened",	MEDIUM	40.4
Cranberry sauce, jellied, canned, OCEAN SPRAY",	MEDIUM	40.61
Cranberry sauce, whole, canned, OCEAN SPRAY",	MEDIUM	40.4

Food name/ Category (100 g)	Status	Carbs content in g
Cream puff shell, prepared from recipe",	LOW	22.8
Cream puff, eclair, custard or cream filled, iced",	LOW	37.43
Cream substitute, flavored, liquid",	LOW	35.07
Cream substitute, flavored, powdered",	HIGH	75.42
Cream substitute, liquid, light",	LOW	9.1
Cream substitute, liquid, with hydrogenated vegetable oil and soy protein",	LOW	11.38
Cream substitute, liquid, with lauric acid oil and sodium caseinate",	LOW	11.38
Cream substitute, powdered, light",	HIGH	73.4
Cream substitute, powdered",	HIGH	59.29
Cream, fluid, half and half",	LOW	4.73
Cream, fluid, light (coffee cream or table cream)",	LOW	2.82
Cream, half and half, fat free",	LOW	9
Cream, sour, reduced fat, cultured",	LOW	4.26
Creamy dressing, made with sour cream and\/or buttermilk and oil, reduced calorie, cholesterol-free",	LOW	16
Creamy dressing, made with sour cream and\/or buttermilk and oil, reduced calorie, fat-free",	LOW	20
Creamy dressing, made with sour cream and\/or buttermilk and oil, reduced calorie",	LOW	7
Cress, garden, cooked, boiled, drained, with salt",	LOW	3.8
Croissants, apple",	LOW	37.1
Croissants, butter",	MEDIUM	45.8
Croissants, cheese",	MEDIUM	47
Croutons, plain",	HIGH	73.5
Croutons, seasoned",	HIGH	63.5
CRUNCHMASTER, Multi-Grain Crisps, Snack Crackers, Gluten-Free",	HIGH	67.18
Crustaceans, crab, alaska king, cooked, moist heat",	LOW	0
Crustaceans, crab, alaska king, imitation, made from surimi",	LOW	15
Crustaceans, crab, alaska king, raw",	LOW	0
Crustaceans, crab, blue, canned",	LOW	0
Crustaceans, crab, blue, cooked, moist heat",	LOW	0
Crustaceans, crab, blue, crab cakes, home recipe",	LOW	0.48
Crustaceans, crab, blue, raw",	LOW	0.04
Crustaceans, crab, dungeness, cooked, moist heat",	LOW	0.95
Crustaceans, crab, dungeness, raw",	LOW	0.74

Food name/ Category (100 g)	Status	Carbs content in g
Crustaceans, crab, queen, cooked, moist heat",	LOW	0
Crustaceans, crab, queen, raw",	LOW	0
Crustaceans, crayfish, mixed species, farmed, cooked, moist heat",	LOW	0
Crustaceans, crayfish, mixed species, farmed, raw",	LOW	0
Crustaceans, crayfish, mixed species, wild, cooked, moist heat",	LOW	0
Crustaceans, crayfish, mixed species, wild, raw",	LOW	0
Crustaceans, lobster, northern, cooked, moist heat",	LOW	0
Crustaceans, lobster, northern, raw",	LOW	0
Crustaceans, shrimp, cooked (not previously frozen)",	LOW	0.2
Crustaceans, shrimp, mixed species, canned",	LOW	0
Crustaceans, shrimp, mixed species, cooked, breaded and fried",	LOW	11.47
Crustaceans, shrimp, mixed species, cooked, moist heat (may have been previously frozen)",	LOW	1.52
Crustaceans, shrimp, mixed species, imitation, made from surimi",	LOW	9.13
Crustaceans, shrimp, mixed species, raw (may have been previously frozen)",	LOW	0.91
Crustaceans, shrimp, raw (not previously frozen)",	LOW	0
Crustaceans, spiny lobster, mixed species, cooked, moist heat",	LOW	3.12
Crustaceans, spiny lobster, mixed species, raw",	LOW	2.43
Cucumber, peeled, raw",	LOW	2.16
Cucumber, with peel, raw",	LOW	3.63
Currants, european black, raw",	LOW	15.38
Currants, red and white, raw",	LOW	13.8
Dandelion greens, cooked, boiled, drained, with salt",	LOW	6.4
Dandelion greens, cooked, boiled, drained, without salt",	LOW	6.4
Dandelion greens, raw",	LOW	9.2
Danish pastry, cheese",	LOW	37.2
Danish pastry, cinnamon, enriched",	MEDIUM	44.6
Danish pastry, cinnamon, unenriched",	MEDIUM	44.6
Danish pastry, fruit, enriched (includes apple, cinnamon, raisin, lemon, raspberry, s	MEDIUM	47.8
Danish pastry, fruit, unenriched (includes apple, cinnamon, raisin, strawberry)",	MEDIUM	47.8
Danish pastry, lemon, unenriched",	MEDIUM	47.8
Danish pastry, nut (includes almond, raisin nut, cinnamon nut)",	MEDIUM	45.7

Food name/ Category (100 g)	Status	Carbs content in g
Danish pastry, raspberry, unenriched",	MEDIUM	47.8
Dates, deglet noor",	HIGH	75.03
Dates, medjool",	HIGH	74.97
DENNY'S, chicken nuggets, star shaped, from kid's menu",	LOW	13.59
DENNY'S, chicken strips",	LOW	22.03
DENNY'S, coleslaw",	LOW	10.88
DENNY'S, fish fillet, battered or breaded, fried",	LOW	17.41
DENNY'S, french fries",	LOW	35.2
DENNY'S, golden fried shrimp",	LOW	20.93
DENNY'S, hash browns",	LOW	26.59
DENNY'S, macaroni & cheese, from kid's menu",	LOW	21.16
DENNY'S, mozzarella cheese sticks",	LOW	27.22
DENNY'S, onion rings",	MEDIUM	41.05
DENNY'S, spaghetti and meatballs",	LOW	15.51
DENNY'S, top sirloin steak",	LOW	0.14
Dessert topping, powdered, 1.5 ounce prepared with 1V2 cup milk",	LOW	17.13
Dessert topping, powdered",	MEDIUM	52.54
Dessert topping, pressurized",	LOW	16.07
Desserts, apple crisp, prepared-from-recipe",	LOW	30.84
Desserts, egg custard, baked, prepared-from-recipe",	LOW	11
Desserts, flan, caramel custard, prepared-from-recipe",	LOW	22.78
Desserts, mousse, chocolate, prepared-from-recipe",	LOW	16.07
Desserts, rennin, chocolate, dry mix",	HIGH	91.5
Desserts, rennin, tablets, unsweetened",	LOW	19.8
DIGIORNO Pizza, cheese topping, cheese stuffed crust, frozen, baked",	LOW	29.86
DIGIORNO Pizza, cheese topping, rising crust, frozen, baked",	LOW	31.78
DIGIORNO Pizza, cheese topping, thin crispy crust, frozen, baked",	LOW	26.47
DIGIORNO Pizza, pepperoni topping, cheese stuffed crust, frozen, baked",	LOW	29.46
DIGIORNO Pizza, pepperoni topping, rising crust, frozen, baked",	LOW	31.15
DIGIORNO Pizza, pepperoni topping, thin crispy crust, frozen, baked",	LOW	28.67
DIGIORNO Pizza, supreme topping, rising crust, frozen, baked",	LOW	27.93

Food name/ Category (100 g)	Status	Carbs content in g
DIGIORNO Pizza, supreme topping, thin crispy crust, frozen, baked",	LOW	28.05
Dill weed, fresh",	LOW	7.02
Dip, bean, original flavor",	LOW	15.89
Dip, FRITO'S, bean, original flavor",	LOW	15.89
Dip, OLD EL PASO, Cheese 'n Salsa, medium",	LOW	10.65
Dip, salsa con queso, cheese and salsa- medium",	LOW	11.14
Dip, TOSTITOS, salsa con queso, medium",	LOW	11.72
Dock, raw",	LOW	3.2
DOMINO'S 14\" Cheese Pizza, Classic Hand-Tossed Crust",	LOW	33.24
DOMINO'S 14\" Cheese Pizza, Crunchy Thin Crust",	LOW	28.18
DOMINO'S 14\" Cheese Pizza, Ultimate Deep Dish Crust",	LOW	33.48
DOMINO'S 14\" EXTRAVAGANZZA FEAST Pizza, Classic Hand-Tossed Crust",	LOW	25.72
DOMINO'S 14\" Pepperoni Pizza, Classic Hand-Tossed Crust",	LOW	31.86
DOMINO'S 14\" Pepperoni Pizza, Crunchy Thin Crust",	LOW	25.35
DOMINO'S 14\" Pepperoni Pizza, Ultimate Deep Dish Crust",	LOW	31.89
DOMINO'S 14\" Sausage Pizza, Classic Hand-Tossed Crust",	LOW	31.84
DOMINO'S 14\" Sausage Pizza, Crunchy Thin Crust",	LOW	25.3
DOMINO'S 14\" Sausage Pizza, Ultimate Deep Dish Crust",	LOW	31.17
Doughnuts, cake-type, chocolate, sugared or glazed",	HIGH	57.4
Doughnuts, cake-type, plain (includes unsugared, old-fashioned)",	MEDIUM	47.06
Doughnuts, cake-type, plain, chocolate-coated or frosted",	MEDIUM	51.33
Doughnuts, cake-type, plain, sugared or glazed",	MEDIUM	50.8
Doughnuts, french crullers, glazed",	HIGH	59.5
Doughnuts, yeast-leavened, glazed, enriched (includes honey buns)",	MEDIUM	47.93
Doughnuts, yeast-leavened, glazed, unenriched (includes honey buns)",	MEDIUM	44.3
Doughnuts, yeast-leavened, with creme filling",	LOW	30
Doughnuts, yeast-leavened, with jelly filling",	LOW	39
Dove, cooked (includes squab)",	LOW	0
Dressing, honey mustard, fat-free",	LOW	38.43
Drumstick leaves, cooked, boiled, drained, with salt",	LOW	11.15
Drumstick pods, cooked, boiled, drained, with salt",	LOW	8.18

Food name/ Category (100 g)	Status	Carbs content in g
Drumstick pods, cooked, boiled, drained, without salt",	LOW	8.18
Drumstick pods, raw",	LOW	8.53
Duck, domesticated, liver, raw",	LOW	3.53
Duck, domesticated, meat and skin, cooked, roasted",	LOW	0
Duck, domesticated, meat and skin, raw",	LOW	0
Duck, domesticated, meat only, cooked, roasted",	LOW	0
Duck, domesticated, meat only, raw",	LOW	0.94
Duck, wild, breast, meat only, raw",	LOW	0
Duck, wild, meat and skin, raw",	LOW	0
Duck, young duckling, domesticated, White Pekin, breast, meat and skin, boneless, cooked, roasted",	LOW	0
Duck, young duckling, domesticated, White Pekin, breast, meat only, boneless, cooked without skin, broiled",	LOW	0
Duck, young duckling, domesticated, White Pekin, leg, meat and skin, bone in, cooked, roasted",	LOW	0
Duck, young duckling, domesticated, White Pekin, leg, meat only, bone in, cooked without skin, braised",	LOW	0
Dulce de Leche",	MEDIUM	55.35
Dumpling, potato- or cheese-filled, frozen",	LOW	29.64
Durian, raw or frozen",	LOW	27.09
Egg custards, dry mix, prepared with 2% milk",	LOW	17.61
Egg custards, dry mix, prepared with whole milk",	LOW	17.6
Egg custards, dry mix",	HIGH	82.8
Egg Mix, USDA Commodity",	LOW	23.97
Egg rolls, chicken, refrigerated, heated",	LOW	28.54
Egg rolls, vegetable, frozen, prepared",	LOW	31.77
Egg substitute, liquid or frozen, fat free",	LOW	2
Egg substitute, powder",	LOW	21.8
Egg, duck, whole, fresh, raw",	LOW	1.45
Egg, goose, whole, fresh, raw",	LOW	1.35
Egg, quail, whole, fresh, raw",	LOW	0.41
Egg, turkey, whole, fresh, raw",	LOW	1.15
Egg, white, dried, flakes, stabilized, glucose reduced",	LOW	4.17

Food name/ Category (100 g)	Status	Carbs content in g
Egg, white, dried, powder, stabilized, glucose reduced",	LOW	4.47
Egg, white, dried, stabilized, glucose reduced",	LOW	4.51
Egg, white, dried",	LOW	7.8
Egg, white, raw, fresh",	LOW	0.73
Egg, white, raw, frozen, pasteurized",	LOW	1.04
Egg, whole, cooked, fried",	LOW	0.83
Egg, whole, cooked, hard-boiled",	LOW	1.12
Egg, whole, cooked, omelet",	LOW	0.64
Egg, whole, cooked, poached",	LOW	0.71
Egg, whole, cooked, scrambled",	LOW	1.61
Egg, whole, dried, stabilized, glucose reduced",	LOW	2.38
Egg, whole, dried",	LOW	1.13
Egg, whole, raw, fresh",	LOW	0.72
Egg, whole, raw, frozen, pasteurized",	LOW	1.01
Egg, whole, raw, frozen, salted, pasteurized",	LOW	0.83
Egg, yolk, dried",	LOW	0.66
Egg, yolk, raw, fresh",	LOW	3.59
Egg, yolk, raw, frozen, pasteurized",	LOW	0.81
Egg, yolk, raw, frozen, salted, pasteurized",	LOW	1.77
Egg, yolk, raw, frozen, sugared, pasteurized",	LOW	10.95
Eggnog",	LOW	8.05
Eggplant, cooked, boiled, drained, with salt",	LOW	8.14
Eggplant, cooked, boiled, drained, without salt",	LOW	8.73
Eggplant, pickled",	LOW	9.77
Eggplant, raw",	LOW	5.88
Eggs, scrambled, frozen mixture",	LOW	7.5
Emu, fan fillet, cooked, broiled",	LOW	0
Emu, fan fillet, raw",	LOW	0

Food name/ Category (100 g)	Status	Carbs content in g
Emu, flat fillet, raw",	LOW	0
Emu, full rump, cooked, broiled",	LOW	0
Emu, full rump, raw",	LOW	0
Emu, ground, cooked, pan-broiled",	LOW	0
Emu, ground, raw",	LOW	0
Emu, inside drum, raw",	LOW	0
Emu, inside drums, cooked, broiled",	LOW	0
Emu, outside drum, raw",	LOW	0
Emu, oyster, raw",	LOW	0
Emu, top loin, cooked, broiled",	LOW	0
English muffins, mixed-grain (includes granola)",	MEDIUM	46.3
English muffins, mixed-grain, toasted (includes granola)",	MEDIUM	50.3
English muffins, plain, enriched, with ca prop (includes sourdough)",	MEDIUM	44.17
English muffins, plain, enriched, without calcium propionate(includes sourdough)",	MEDIUM	46
English muffins, plain, toasted, enriched, with calcium propionate (includes sourdou	MEDIUM	52.65
English muffins, plain, unenriched, with calcium propionate (includes sourdough)",	MEDIUM	46
English muffins, plain, unenriched, without calcium propionate (includes sourdough)	MEDIUM	46
English muffins, raisin-cinnamon (includes apple-cinnamon)",	MEDIUM	48.1
English muffins, raisin-cinnamon, toasted (includes apple-cinnamon)",	MEDIUM	55.04
English muffins, wheat, toasted",	MEDIUM	48.7
English muffins, wheat",	MEDIUM	44.8
English muffins, whole grain white",	MEDIUM	50.17
English muffins, whole-wheat, toasted",	MEDIUM	44.1
English muffins, whole-wheat",	MEDIUM	40.4
Epazote, raw",	LOW	7.44
Falafel, home-prepared",	LOW	31.84
FAMOUS AMOS, Chocolate Chip Cookies",	HIGH	67.7
FAMOUS AMOS, Chocolate Chip Pecan Cookies",	HIGH	63.8
FAMOUS AMOS, Chocolate Sandwich Creme Cookies",	HIGH	72.3
FAMOUS AMOS, Vanilla Sandwich Creme Cookies",	HIGH	73.8
Fast food, biscuit",	MEDIUM	42.82
Fast Food, Pizza Chain, 14\" pizza, cheese topping, regular crust",	LOW	33.33
Fast Food, Pizza Chain, 14\" pizza, cheese topping, stuffed crust",	LOW	30
Fast Food, Pizza Chain, 14\" pizza, cheese topping, thick crust",	LOW	33.17
Fast Food, Pizza Chain, 14\" pizza, cheese topping, thin crust",	LOW	31.2
Fast Food, Pizza Chain, 14\" pizza, meat and vegetable topping, regular crust",	LOW	25.38
Fast Food, Pizza Chain, 14\" pizza, pepperoni topping, regular crust",	LOW	31.98

Food name/ Category (100 g)	Status	Carbs content in g
Fast Food, Pizza Chain, 14\" pizza, pepperoni topping, thick crust",	LOW	31.84
Fast Food, Pizza Chain, 14\" pizza, pepperoni topping, thin crust",	LOW	29
Fast Food, Pizza Chain, 14\" pizza, sausage topping, regular crust",	LOW	30.62
Fast Food, Pizza Chain, 14\" pizza, sausage topping, thick crust",	LOW	30.36
Fast Food, Pizza Chain, 14\" pizza, sausage topping, thin crust",	LOW	27
Fast foods, bagel, with breakfast steak, egg, cheese, and condiments",	LOW	22.99
Fast foods, bagel, with egg, sausage patty, cheese, and condiments",	LOW	22.64
Fast foods, biscuit with egg and steak",	LOW	14.37
Fast foods, biscuit, with crispy chicken fillet",	LOW	30.56
Fast Foods, biscuit, with egg and sausage",	LOW	21.05
Fast foods, biscuit, with egg",	LOW	23.46
Fast foods, biscuit, with sausage",	LOW	29.99
Fast foods, breadstick, soft, prepared with garlic and parmesan cheese",	MEDIUM	44.48
Fast foods, breakfast burrito, with egg, cheese, and sausage",	LOW	22.97
Fast foods, burrito, with beans and beef",	LOW	19.52
Fast foods, burrito, with beans and cheese",	LOW	31.23
Fast foods, burrito, with beans, cheese, and beef",	LOW	23.37
Fast foods, burrito, with beans",	LOW	32.92
Fast foods, cheeseburger, double, regular patty and bun, with condiments",	LOW	17.97
Fast foods, cheeseburger; double, large patty, with condiments and vegetables",	LOW	15.37
Fast Foods, cheeseburger; double, large patty; with condiments, vegetables and mayonnaise",	LOW	12.62
Fast foods, cheeseburger; double, large patty; with condiments",	LOW	14.43
Fast foods, cheeseburger; double, regular patty, with condiments and vegetables",	LOW	21.2
Fast foods, cheeseburger; double, regular patty; double decker bun with condiments and special sauce",	LOW	21.53
Fast foods, cheeseburger; double, regular patty; plain",	LOW	20.8
Fast foods, cheeseburger; double, regular patty; with condiments",	LOW	17.97
Fast foods, cheeseburger; double, regular, patty and bun; with condiments and vegetables",	LOW	23.3
Fast foods, cheeseburger; single, large patty; plain",	LOW	24.07

Food name/ Category (100 g)	Status	Carbs content in g
Fast foods, cheeseburger; single, large patty; with condiments and vegetables",	LOW	16.81
Fast foods, cheeseburger; single, large patty; with condiments, vegetables and mayonnaise",	LOW	17.73
Fast foods, cheeseburger; single, large patty; with condiments",	LOW	19.72
Fast foods, cheeseburger; single, regular patty, with condiments and vegetables",	LOW	24.97
Fast foods, cheeseburger; single, regular patty, with condiments",	LOW	25.46
Fast foods, cheeseburger; single, regular patty; plain",	LOW	28.03
Fast foods, cheeseburger; triple, regular patty; plain",	LOW	16.16
Fast foods, chicken fillet sandwich, plain with pickles",	LOW	20.89
Fast foods, chicken tenders",	LOW	17.25
Fast foods, chicken, breaded and fried, boneless pieces, plain",	LOW	14.93
Fast foods, coleslaw",	LOW	14.89
Fast Foods, crispy chicken filet sandwich, with lettuce and mayonnaise",	LOW	27.4
Fast foods, crispy chicken in tortilla, with lettuce, cheese, and ranch sauce",	LOW	23.22
Fast foods, croissant, with egg and cheese",	LOW	22.45
Fast foods, croissant, with egg, cheese, and sausage",	LOW	15.9
Fast foods, egg, scrambled",	LOW	2.08
Fast foods, english muffin, with cheese and sausage",	LOW	25.28
Fast foods, english muffin, with egg, cheese, and sausage",	LOW	17.44
Fast foods, fish sandwich, with tartar sauce and cheese",	LOW	26.39
Fast foods, fish sandwich, with tartar sauce",	LOW	26.69
Fast foods, french toast sticks",	MEDIUM	41.21
Fast foods, french toast with butter",	LOW	26.7
Fast Foods, Fried Chicken, Breast, meat and skin and breading",	LOW	6.03
Fast Foods, Fried Chicken, Breast, meat only, skin and breading removed",	LOW	0
Fast Foods, Fried Chicken, Drumstick, meat and skin with breading",	LOW	7.59
Fast Foods, Fried Chicken, Drumstick, meat only, skin and breading removed",	LOW	0
Fast Foods, Fried Chicken, Thigh, meat and skin and breading",	LOW	8.68
Fast Foods, Fried Chicken, Thigh, meat only, skin and breading removed",	LOW	0.24

Food name/ Category (100 g)	Status	Carbs content in g
Fast Foods, Fried Chicken, Wing, meat and skin and breading",	LOW	11.19
Fast Foods, Fried Chicken, Wing, meat only, skin and breading removed",	LOW	2.13
Fast foods, griddle cake sandwich, egg, cheese, and sausage",	LOW	22.04
Fast foods, griddle cake sandwich, sausage",	LOW	31.25
Fast Foods, grilled chicken filet sandwich, with lettuce, tomato and spread",	LOW	16.78
Fast foods, grilled chicken in tortilla, with lettuce, cheese, and ranch sauce",	LOW	18.43
Fast foods, hotdog, plain",	LOW	18.4
Fast foods, hotdog, with chili",	LOW	27.45
Fast foods, hotdog, with corn flour coating (corndog)",	LOW	31.88
Fast foods, hush puppies",	MEDIUM	40.21
Fast foods, miniature cinnamon rolls",	MEDIUM	53.38
Fast foods, nachos, with cheese, beans, ground beef, and tomatoes",	LOW	21.39
Fast foods, nachos, with cheese",	LOW	34.91
Fast foods, onion rings, breaded and fried",	MEDIUM	43.58
Fast foods, potato, french fried in vegetable oil",	MEDIUM	41.44
Fast foods, potato, mashed",	LOW	14.65
Fast foods, potatoes, hash browns, round pieces or patty",	LOW	28.88
Fast foods, quesadilla, with chicken",	LOW	24.04
Fast foods, roast beef sandwich, plain",	LOW	22.21
Fast foods, shrimp, breaded and fried",	LOW	27.99
Fast foods, submarine sandwich, cold cut on white bread with lettuce and tomato",	LOW	20.43
Fast foods, submarine sandwich, meatball marinara on white bread",	LOW	26.01
Fast foods, submarine sandwich, oven roasted chicken on white bread with lettuce and tomato",	LOW	21.35
Fast foods, submarine sandwich, roast beef on white bread with lettuce and tomato",	LOW	20.34
Fast foods, submarine sandwich, steak and cheese on white bread with cheese, lettuce and tomato",	LOW	21.49
Fast foods, submarine sandwich, sweet onion chicken teriyaki on white bread with lettuce, tomato and sweet onion sauce",	LOW	22.54
Fast foods, submarine sandwich, tuna on white bread with lettuce and tomato",	LOW	15.95
Fast foods, submarine sandwich, turkey breast on white bread with lettuce and tomato",	LOW	22.42
Fast foods, sundae, caramel",	LOW	31.81
Fast foods, sundae, hot fudge",	LOW	30.17

Food name/ Category (100 g)	Status	Carbs content in g
Fast foods, sundae, strawberry",	LOW	29.18
Fast foods, taco salad",	LOW	11.91
Fast foods, taco with beef, cheese and lettuce, hard shell",	LOW	19.85
Fast foods, taco with beef, cheese and lettuce, soft",	LOW	20.23
Fast foods, taco with chicken, lettuce and cheese, soft",	LOW	19.69
Fast foods, vanilla, light, soft-serve ice cream, with cone",	LOW	26.36
Fat free ice cream, no sugar added, flavors other than chocolate",	LOW	27.94
Fat, beef tallow",	LOW	0
Fat, chicken",	LOW	0
Fat, duck",	LOW	0
Fat, goose",	LOW	0
Fat, mutton tallow",	LOW	0
Fat, turkey",	LOW	0
Feijoa, raw",	LOW	15.21
Fennel, bulb, raw",	LOW	7.3
Figs, canned, extra heavy syrup pack, solids and liquids",	LOW	27.86
Figs, canned, heavy syrup pack, solids and liquids",	LOW	22.9
Figs, canned, light syrup pack, solids and liquids",	LOW	17.95
Figs, canned, water pack, solids and liquids",	LOW	13.99
Figs, dried, stewed",	LOW	27.57
Figs, raw",	LOW	19.18
Fish broth",	LOW	0.4
Fish oil, cod liver",	LOW	0
Fish oil, herring",	LOW	0
Fish oil, menhaden, fully hydrogenated",	LOW	0
Fish oil, menhaden",	LOW	0
Fish oil, salmon",	LOW	0
Fish oil, sardine",	LOW	0

Food name/ Category (100 g)	Status	Carbs content in g
Fish, anchovy, european, canned in oil, drained solids",	LOW	0
Fish, anchovy, european, raw",	LOW	0
Fish, bass, fresh water, mixed species, raw",	LOW	0
Fish, bass, freshwater, mixed species, cooked, dry heat",	LOW	0
Fish, bass, striped, cooked, dry heat",	LOW	0
Fish, bass, striped, raw",	LOW	0
Fish, bluefish, cooked, dry heat",	LOW	0
Fish, bluefish, raw",	LOW	0
Fish, burbot, cooked, dry heat",	LOW	0
Fish, burbot, raw",	LOW	0
Fish, butterfish, cooked, dry heat",	LOW	0
Fish, butterfish, raw",	LOW	0
Fish, carp, cooked, dry heat",	LOW	0
Fish, carp, raw",	LOW	0
Fish, catfish, channel, cooked, breaded and fried",	LOW	8.04
Fish, catfish, channel, farmed, cooked, dry heat",	LOW	0
Fish, catfish, channel, farmed, raw",	LOW	0
Fish, catfish, channel, wild, cooked, dry heat",	LOW	0
Fish, catfish, channel, wild, raw",	LOW	0
Fish, caviar, black and red, granular",	LOW	4
Fish, cisco, raw",	LOW	0
Fish, cisco, smoked",	LOW	0
Fish, cod, Atlantic, canned, solids and liquid",	LOW	0
Fish, cod, Atlantic, cooked, dry heat",	LOW	0
Fish, cod, Atlantic, dried and salted",	LOW	0
Fish, cod, Atlantic, raw",	LOW	0
Fish, cod, Pacific, cooked (not previously frozen)",	LOW	0
Fish, cod, Pacific, cooked, dry heat (may have been previously frozen)",	LOW	0

Food name/ Category (100 g)	Status	Carbs content in g
Fish, cod, Pacific, raw (may have been previously frozen)",	LOW	0
Fish, cod, Pacific, raw (not previously frozen)",	LOW	0
Fish, croaker, Atlantic, cooked, breaded and fried",	LOW	7.54
Fish, croaker, Atlantic, raw",	LOW	0
Fish, cusk, cooked, dry heat",	LOW	0
Fish, drum, freshwater, cooked, dry heat",	LOW	0
Fish, drum, freshwater, raw",	LOW	0
Fish, eel, mixed species, cooked, dry heat",	LOW	0
Fish, eel, mixed species, raw",	LOW	0
Fish, fish sticks, frozen, prepared",	LOW	21.66
Fish, flatfish (flounder and sole species), cooked, dry heat",	LOW	0
Fish, flatfish (flounder and sole species), raw",	LOW	0
Fish, gefiltefish, commercial, sweet recipe",	LOW	7.41
Fish, grouper, mixed species, cooked, dry heat",	LOW	0
Fish, grouper, mixed species, raw",	LOW	0
Fish, haddock, cooked, dry heat",	LOW	0
Fish, haddock, raw",	LOW	0
Fish, haddock, smoked",	LOW	0
Fish, halibut, Atlantic and Pacific, cooked, dry heat",	LOW	0
Fish, halibut, Atlantic and Pacific, raw",	LOW	0
Fish, halibut, greenland, cooked, dry heat",	LOW	0
Fish, halibut, Greenland, raw",	LOW	0
Fish, herring, Atlantic, cooked, dry heat",	LOW	0
Fish, herring, Atlantic, kippered",	LOW	0
Fish, herring, Atlantic, pickled",	LOW	9.64
Fish, herring, Atlantic, raw",	LOW	0
Fish, herring, Pacific, cooked, dry heat",	LOW	0
Fish, herring, Pacific, raw",	LOW	0

Food name/ Category (100 g)	Status	Carbs content in g
Fish, ling, cooked, dry heat",	LOW	0
Fish, ling, raw",	LOW	0
Fish, lingcod, cooked, dry heat",	LOW	0
Fish, lingcod, raw",	LOW	0
Fish, mackerel, Atlantic, cooked, dry heat",	LOW	0
Fish, mackerel, Atlantic, raw",	LOW	0
Fish, mackerel, jack, canned, drained solids",	LOW	0
Fish, mackerel, king, cooked, dry heat",	LOW	0
Fish, mackerel, king, raw",	LOW	0
Fish, mackerel, Pacific and jack, mixed species, cooked, dry heat",	LOW	0
Fish, mackerel, Pacific and jack, mixed species, raw",	LOW	0
Fish, mackerel, salted",	LOW	0
Fish, mackerel, spanish, cooked, dry heat",	LOW	0
Fish, mackerel, spanish, raw",	LOW	0
Fish, mahimahi, cooked, dry heat",	LOW	0
Fish, mahimahi, raw",	LOW	0
Fish, milkfish, cooked, dry heat",	LOW	0
Fish, milkfish, raw",	LOW	0
Fish, mullet, striped, cooked, dry heat",	LOW	0
Fish, mullet, striped, raw",	LOW	0
Fish, ocean perch, Atlantic, cooked, dry heat",	LOW	0
Fish, ocean perch, Atlantic, raw",	LOW	0
Fish, perch, mixed species, cooked, dry heat",	LOW	0
Fish, perch, mixed species, raw",	LOW	0
Fish, pike, northern, cooked, dry heat",	LOW	0
Fish, pike, northern, raw",	LOW	0
Fish, pike, walleye, cooked, dry heat",	LOW	0
Fish, pike, walleye, raw",	LOW	0

Food name/ Category (100 g)	Status	Carbs content in g
Fish, pollock, Alaska, cooked (not previously frozen)",	LOW	0
Fish, pollock, Alaska, cooked, dry heat (may have been previously frozen)",	LOW	0
Fish, pollock, Alaska, raw (may have been previously frozen)",	LOW	0
Fish, pollock, Alaska, raw (not previously frozen)",	LOW	0
Fish, pollock, Atlantic, cooked, dry heat",	LOW	0
Fish, pollock, Atlantic, raw",	LOW	0
Fish, pompano, florida, cooked, dry heat",	LOW	0
Fish, pompano, florida, raw",	LOW	0
Fish, pout, ocean, cooked, dry heat",	LOW	0
Fish, pout, ocean, raw",	LOW	0
Fish, rockfish, Pacific, mixed species, cooked, dry heat",	LOW	0
Fish, rockfish, Pacific, mixed species, raw",	LOW	0
Fish, roe, mixed species, cooked, dry heat",	LOW	1.92
Fish, roe, mixed species, raw",	LOW	1.5
Fish, roughy, orange, cooked, dry heat",	LOW	0
Fish, roughy, orange, raw",	LOW	0
Fish, sablefish, cooked, dry heat",	LOW	0
Fish, sablefish, raw",	LOW	0
Fish, sablefish, smoked",	LOW	0
Fish, salmon, Atlantic, farmed, cooked, dry heat",	LOW	0
Fish, salmon, Atlantic, farmed, raw",	LOW	0
Fish, salmon, Atlantic, wild, cooked, dry heat",	LOW	0
Fish, salmon, Atlantic, wild, raw",	LOW	0
Fish, salmon, chinook, cooked, dry heat",	LOW	0
Fish, salmon, chinook, raw",	LOW	0
Fish, salmon, chinook, smoked, (lox), regular",	LOW	0
Fish, salmon, chinook, smoked",	LOW	0
Fish, salmon, chum, canned, drained solids with bone",	LOW	0

Food name/ Category (100 g)	Status	Carbs content in g
Fish, salmon, chum, canned, without salt, drained solids with bone",	LOW	0
Fish, salmon, chum, cooked, dry heat",	LOW	0
Fish, salmon, chum, raw",	LOW	0
Fish, salmon, coho, farmed, cooked, dry heat",	LOW	0
Fish, salmon, coho, farmed, raw",	LOW	0
Fish, salmon, coho, wild, cooked, dry heat",	LOW	0
Fish, salmon, coho, wild, cooked, moist heat",	LOW	0
Fish, salmon, coho, wild, raw",	LOW	0
Fish, Salmon, pink, canned, drained solids, without skin and bones",	LOW	0
Fish, salmon, pink, canned, drained solids",	LOW	0
Fish, salmon, pink, canned, total can contents",	LOW	0
Fish, salmon, pink, canned, without salt, solids with bone and liquid",	LOW	0
Fish, salmon, pink, cooked, dry heat",	LOW	0
Fish, salmon, pink, raw",	LOW	0
Fish, salmon, sockeye, canned, drained solids",	LOW	0
Fish, salmon, sockeye, canned, without salt, drained solids with bone",	LOW	0
Fish, salmon, sockeye, cooked, dry heat",	LOW	0
Fish, salmon, sockeye, raw",	LOW	0
Fish, sardine, Atlantic, canned in oil, drained solids with bone",	LOW	0
Fish, sardine, Pacific, canned in tomato sauce, drained solids with bone",	LOW	0.54
Fish, scup, cooked, dry heat",	LOW	0
Fish, scup, raw",	LOW	0
Fish, sea bass, mixed species, cooked, dry heat",	LOW	0
Fish, sea bass, mixed species, raw",	LOW	0
Fish, seatrout, mixed species, cooked, dry heat",	LOW	0
Fish, seatrout, mixed species, raw",	LOW	0
Fish, shad, american, cooked, dry heat",	LOW	0
Fish, shad, american, raw",	LOW	0

Food name/ Category (100 g)	Status	Carbs content in g
Fish, shark, mixed species, cooked, batter-dipped and fried",	LOW	6.39
Fish, shark, mixed species, raw",	LOW	0
Fish, sheepshead, cooked, dry heat",	LOW	0
Fish, sheepshead, raw",	LOW	0
Fish, smelt, rainbow, cooked, dry heat",	LOW	0
Fish, smelt, rainbow, raw",	LOW	0
Fish, snapper, mixed species, cooked, dry heat",	LOW	0
Fish, snapper, mixed species, raw",	LOW	0
Fish, spot, cooked, dry heat",	LOW	0
Fish, sturgeon, mixed species, cooked, dry heat",	LOW	0
Fish, sturgeon, mixed species, raw",	LOW	0
Fish, sturgeon, mixed species, smoked",	LOW	0
Fish, sucker, white, cooked, dry heat",	LOW	0
Fish, sucker, white, raw",	LOW	0
Fish, sunfish, pumpkin seed, cooked, dry heat",	LOW	0
Fish, sunfish, pumpkin seed, raw",	LOW	0
Fish, surimi",	LOW	6.85
Fish, swordfish, cooked, dry heat",	LOW	0
Fish, swordfish, raw",	LOW	0
Fish, tilapia, cooked, dry heat",	LOW	0
Fish, tilapia, raw",	LOW	0
Fish, tilefish, cooked, dry heat",	LOW	0
Fish, tilefish, raw",	LOW	0
Fish, trout, brook, raw, New York State",	LOW	0
Fish, trout, mixed species, cooked, dry heat",	LOW	0
Fish, trout, mixed species, raw",	LOW	0
Fish, trout, rainbow, farmed, cooked, dry heat",	LOW	0
Fish, trout, rainbow, farmed, raw",	LOW	0

Food name/ Category (100 g)	Status	Carbs content in g
Fish, trout, rainbow, wild, cooked, dry heat",	LOW	0
Fish, tuna salad",	LOW	9.41
Fish, tuna, fresh, bluefin, cooked, dry heat",	LOW	0
Fish, tuna, fresh, bluefin, raw",	LOW	0
Fish, tuna, fresh, skipjack, raw",	LOW	0
Fish, tuna, fresh, yellowfin, raw",	LOW	0
Fish, tuna, light, canned in oil, drained solids",	LOW	0
Fish, tuna, light, canned in oil, without salt, drained solids",	LOW	0
Fish, tuna, light, canned in water, drained solids",	LOW	0
Fish, tuna, light, canned in water, without salt, drained solids",	LOW	0
Fish, tuna, skipjack, fresh, cooked, dry heat",	LOW	0
Fish, tuna, white, canned in oil, drained solids",	LOW	0
Fish, tuna, white, canned in oil, without salt, drained solids",	LOW	0
Fish, tuna, white, canned in water, drained solids",	LOW	0
Fish, tuna, white, canned in water, without salt, drained solids",	LOW	0
Fish, tuna, yellowfin, fresh, cooked, dry heat",	LOW	0
Fish, turbot, european, cooked, dry heat",	LOW	0
Fish, turbot, european, raw",	LOW	0
Fish, whitefish, mixed species, cooked, dry heat",	LOW	0
Fish, whitefish, mixed species, raw",	LOW	0
Fish, whitefish, mixed species, smoked",	LOW	0
Fish, whiting, mixed species, cooked, dry heat",	LOW	0
Fish, whiting, mixed species, raw",	LOW	0
Fish, wolffish, Atlantic, cooked, dry heat",	LOW	0
Fish, wolffish, Atlantic, raw",	LOW	0
Fish, yellowtail, mixed species, cooked, dry heat",	LOW	0
Fish, yellowtail, mixed species, raw",	LOW	0
Flan, caramel custard, dry mix",	HIGH	91.6

Food name/ Category (100 g)	Status	Carbs content in g
Fluid replacement, electrolyte solution (include PEDIALYTE)",	LOW	2.45
Focaccia, Italian flatbread, plain",	LOW	35.82
Formulated bar, high fiber, chewy, oats and chocolate",	HIGH	69.78
Fomulated bar, LUNA BAR, NUTZ OVER CHOCOLATE",	MEDIUM	52.49
Formulated bar, MARS SNACKFOOD US, COCOAVIA, Chocolate Almond Snack E	MEDIUM	51.68
Formulated bar, MARS SNACKFOOD US, COCOAVIA, Chocolate Blueberry Snack	HIGH	57.87
Formulated bar, MARS SNACKFOOD US, SNICKERS MARATHON Chewy Chocol	MEDIUM	47.24
Formulated bar, MARS SNACKFOOD US, SNICKERS MARATHON Double Chocol	MEDIUM	52.47
Formulated bar, MARS SNACKFOOD US, SNICKERS MARATHON Energy Bar, al	MEDIUM	50.3
Formulated bar, MARS SNACKFOOD US, SNICKERS MARATHON Honey Nut Oa	MEDIUM	54.3
Formulated bar, MARS SNACKFOOD US, SNICKERS MARATHON MULTIGRAIN	HIGH	57.27
Formulated bar, MARS SNACKFOOD US, SNICKERS MARATHON Protein Perforr	MEDIUM	50.5
Formulated bar, POWER BAR, chocolate",	HIGH	69.63
Formulated bar, SLIM-FAST OPTIMA meal bar, milk chocolate peanut",	HIGH	60.21
Formulated bar, ZONE PERFECT CLASSIC CRUNCH BAR, mixed flavors",	MEDIUM	45
Frankfurter, beef, heated",	LOW	2.66
Frankfurter, beef, low fat",	LOW	1.6
Frankfurter, beef, unheated",	LOW	3.36
Frankfurter, chicken",	LOW	2.74
Frankfurter, low sodium",	LOW	1.8
Frankfurter, meat and poultry, cooked, boiled",	LOW	4.96
Frankfurter, meat and poultry, cooked, grilled",	LOW	5.24
Frankfurter, meat and poultry, low fat",	LOW	8.4
Frankfurter, meat and poultry, unheated",	LOW	5.02
Frankfurter, meat, heated",	LOW	4.9
Frankfurter, meat",	LOW	4.17
Frankfurter, meatless",	LOW	7.7
Frankfurter, turkey",	LOW	3.81
French toast, frozen, ready-to-heat",	LOW	32.1
French toast, prepared from recipe, made with low fat (2%) milk",	LOW	25
Frijoles rojos volteados (Refried beans, red, canned)",	LOW	15.47
Frog legs, raw",	LOW	0
Frostings, chocolate, creamy, dry mix, prepared with butter",	HIGH	71.8
Frostings, chocolate, creamy, dry mix, prepared with margarine",	HIGH	71.02
Frostings, chocolate, creamy, dry mix",	HIGH	92
Frostings, chocolate, creamy, ready-to-eat",	HIGH	63.2
Frostings, coconut-nut, ready-to-eat",	MEDIUM	52.7

Food name/ Category (100 g)	Status	Carbs content in g
Frostings, cream cheese-flavor, ready-to-eat",	HIGH	67.32
Frostings, glaze, chocolate, prepared-from-recipe, with butter, NFSMI Recipe No. C	HIGH	72.18
Frostings, vanilla, creamy, dry mix, prepared with margarine",	HIGH	74.28
Frostings, vanilla, creamy, ready-to-eat",	HIGH	67.89
Frostings, white, fluffy, dry mix, prepared with water",	HIGH	62.6
Frostings, white, fluffy, dry mix",	HIGH	94.9
Frozen novelties, fruit and juice bars",	LOW	20.2
Frozen novelties, ice cream type, chocolate or caramel covered, with nuts",	LOW	30.9
Frozen novelties, ice cream type, vanilla ice cream, light, no sugar added, chocolate coated",	LOW	26.11
Frozen novelties, ice type, fruit, no sugar added",	LOW	6.2
Frozen novelties, ice type, italian, restaurant-prepared",	LOW	13.5
Frozen novelties, juice type, juice with cream",	LOW	24.11
Frozen novelties, KLONDIKE, SLIM-A-BEAR Chocolate Cone",	MEDIUM	45.32
Frozen novelties, KLONDIKE, SLIM-A-BEAR Fudge Bar, 98% fat free, no sugar added",	LOW	30.07
Frozen novelties, KLONDIKE, SLIM-A-BEAR Vanilla Sandwich",	MEDIUM	42.75
Frozen novelties, KLONDIKE, SLIM-A-BEAR, No Sugar Added, Stickless Bar",	LOW	25.98
Frozen novelties, No Sugar Added CREAMSICLE Pops",	LOW	12.88
Frozen novelties, No Sugar Added, FUDGSICLE pops",	LOW	23.11
Frozen yogurts, chocolate, nonfat milk, sweetened without sugar",	LOW	19.7
Frozen yogurts, chocolate, soft-serve",	LOW	24.9
Frozen yogurts, chocolate",	LOW	21.6
Frozen yogurts, flavors other than chocolate",	LOW	21.6
Frozen yogurts, vanilla, soft-serve",	LOW	24.2
Fruit cocktail, (peach and pineapple and pear and grape and cherry), canned, extra light syrup, solids and liquids",	LOW	11.63
Fruit cocktail, (peach and pineapple and pear and grape and cherry), canned, juice pack, solids and liquids",	LOW	11.86
Fruit cocktail, (peach and pineapple and pear and grape and cherry), canned, water pack, solids and liquids",	LOW	8.51
Fruit juice smoothie, BOLTHOUSE FARMS, BERRY BOOST",	LOW	10.9
Fruit juice smoothie, BOLTHOUSE FARMS, strawberry banana",	LOW	12.37
Fruit juice smoothie, NAKED JUICE, BLUE MACHINE",	LOW	16.67
Fruit juice smoothie, NAKED JUICE, MIGHTY MANGO",	LOW	15
Fruit juice smoothie, NAKED JUICE, strawberry banana",	LOW	11.66
Fruit juice smoothie, ODWALLA, ORIGINAL SUPERFOOD",	LOW	11.51

Food name/ Category (100 g)	Status	Carbs content in g
Fruit juice smoothie, ODWALLA, strawberry banana",	LOW	11.05
Fruit salad, (peach and pear and apricot and pineapple and cherry), canned, extra heavy syrup, solids and liquids",	LOW	22.77
Fruit salad, (peach and pear and apricot and pineapple and cherry), canned, juice pack, solids and liquids",	LOW	13.05
Fruit salad, (peach and pear and apricot and pineapple and cherry), canned, water pack, solids and liquids",	LOW	7.87
Fruit salad, (pineapple and papaya and banana and guava), tropical, canned, heavy syrup, solids and liquids",	LOW	22.36
Fruit syrup",	HIGH	85.13
Frybread, made with lard (Navajo)",	MEDIUM	48.26
Game meat , bison, ground, raw",	LOW	0
Game meat , bison, top sirloin, separable lean only, 1\" steak, cooked, broiled",	LOW	0
Game meat, antelope, cooked, roasted",	LOW	0
Game meat, antelope, raw",	LOW	0
Game meat, bear, cooked, simmered",	LOW	0
Game meat, beaver, cooked, roasted",	LOW	0
Game meat, beaver, raw",	LOW	0
Game meat, beefalo, composite of cuts, cooked, roasted",	LOW	0
Game meat, beefalo, composite of cuts, raw",	LOW	0
Game meat, bison, chuck, shoulder clod, separable lean only, cooked, braised",	LOW	0
Game meat, bison, chuck, shoulder clod, separable lean only, raw",	LOW	0
Game meat, bison, ground, cooked, pan-broiled",	LOW	0
Game meat, bison, ribeye, separable lean only, 1\" steak, cooked, broiled",	LOW	0
Game meat, bison, ribeye, separable lean only, trimmed to 0\" fat, raw",	LOW	0
Game meat, bison, separable lean only, cooked, roasted",	LOW	0
Game meat, bison, separable lean only, raw",	LOW	0
Game meat, bison, shoulder clod, separable lean only, trimmed to 0\" fat, raw",	LOW	0
Game meat, bison, top round, separable lean only, 1\" steak, cooked, broiled",	LOW	0
Game meat, bison, top round, separable lean only, 1\" steak, raw",	LOW	0
Game meat, bison, top sirloin, separable lean only, trimmed to 0\" fat, raw",	LOW	0
Game meat, boar, wild, cooked, roasted",	LOW	0
Game meat, buffalo, water, cooked, roasted",	LOW	0

Food name/ Category (100 g)	Status	Carbs content in g
Game meat, buffalo, water, raw",	LOW	0
Game meat, caribou, cooked, roasted",	LOW	0
Game meat, caribou, raw",	LOW	0
Game meat, deer, cooked, roasted",	LOW	0
Game meat, deer, ground, cooked, pan-broiled",	LOW	0
Game meat, deer, ground, raw",	LOW	0
Game meat, deer, loin, separable lean only, 1\" steak, cooked, broiled",	LOW	0
Game meat, deer, raw",	LOW	0
Game meat, deer, shoulder clod, separable lean only, cooked, braised",	LOW	0
Game meat, deer, tenderloin, separable lean only, cooked, broiled",	LOW	0
Game meat, deer, top round, separable lean only, 1\" steak, cooked, broiled",	LOW	0
Game meat, elk, cooked, roasted",	LOW	0
Game meat, elk, ground, cooked, pan-broiled",	LOW	0
Game meat, elk, ground, raw",	LOW	0
Game meat, elk, loin, separable lean only, cooked, broiled",	LOW	0
Game meat, elk, raw",	LOW	0
Game meat, elk, round, separable lean only, cooked, broiled",	LOW	0
Game meat, elk, tenderloin, separable lean only, cooked, broiled",	LOW	0
Game meat, goat, cooked, roasted",	LOW	0
Game meat, horse, cooked, roasted",	LOW	0
Game meat, horse, raw",	LOW	0
Game meat, moose, cooked, roasted",	LOW	0
Game meat, moose, raw",	LOW	0
Game meat, muskrat, cooked, roasted",	LOW	0
Game meat, muskrat, raw",	LOW	0
Game meat, opossum, cooked, roasted",	LOW	0
Game meat, rabbit, domesticated, composite of cuts, cooked, roasted",	LOW	0
Game meat, rabbit, domesticated, composite of cuts, cooked, stewed",	LOW	0

Food name/ Category (100 g)	Status	Carbs content in g
Game meat, rabbit, domesticated, composite of cuts, raw",	LOW	0
Game meat, rabbit, wild, cooked, stewed",	LOW	0
Game meat, rabbit, wild, raw",	LOW	0
Game meat, raccoon, cooked, roasted",	LOW	0
Game meat, squirrel, cooked, roasted",	LOW	0
Game meat, squirrel, raw",	LOW	0
GARDENBURGER Black Bean Chipotle Burger, frozen, unprepared",	LOW	22
GARDENBURGER Flame Grilled Burger, frozen, unprepared",	LOW	6.8
GARDENBURGER Original, frozen, unprepared",	LOW	22.1
GARDENBURGER Savory Portabella Veggie Burger, frozen, unprepared",	LOW	22.1
GARDENBURGER Sun-Dried Tomato Basil Burger, frozen, unprepared",	LOW	23.7
GARDENBURGER Veggie Medley Burger, frozen, unprepared",	LOW	24
Garlic bread, frozen",	MEDIUM	41.72
Gelatin desserts, dry mix, prepared with water",	LOW	14.19
Gelatin desserts, dry mix, reduced calorie, with aspartame, added phosphorus, potassium, sodium, vitamin C",	LOW	33.3
Gelatin desserts, dry mix, reduced calorie, with aspartame, no added sodium",	LOW	33.3
Gelatin desserts, dry mix, reduced calorie, with aspartame, prepared with water",	LOW	4.22
Gelatin desserts, dry mix, reduced calorie, with aspartame",	HIGH	80.21
Gelatin desserts, dry mix, with added ascorbic acid, sodium-citrate and salt",	HIGH	90.5
Gelatin desserts, dry mix",	HIGH	90.5
Gelatins, dry powder, unsweetened",	LOW	0
GENERAL MILLS, BETTY CROCKER SUPERMOIST Yellow Cake Mix, dry",	HIGH	81.3
GEORGE WESTON BAKERIES, Brownberry Sage and Onion Stuffing Mix, dry",	HIGH	72.7
GEORGE WESTON BAKERIES, Thomas English Muffins",	MEDIUM	46
Ginger root, pickled, canned, with artificial sweetener",	LOW	4.83
GIRL SCOUTS, Caramel Dulce De Leche Cookies",	HIGH	64.8
GIRL SCOUTS, Chalet Cookies",	HIGH	72.3
GIRL SCOUTS, Do-si-dos Cookies",	HIGH	66
GIRL SCOUTS, Samoas Cookies",	HIGH	64.1
GIRL SCOUTS, Tagalongs Cookies",	MEDIUM	52.2
GIRL SCOUTS, Thank U Berry Munch Cookies",	HIGH	70
GIRL SCOUTS, Thin Mints Cookies",	HIGH	67.3
GIRL SCOUTS, Trefoils Cookies",	HIGH	68
GLUTINO, Gluten Free Cookies, Chocolate Vanilla Creme",	HIGH	76.03
GLUTINO, Gluten Free Cookies, Vanilla Creme",	HIGH	77.34
GLUTINO, Gluten Free Wafers, Lemon Flavored",	HIGH	74.39
GLUTINO, Gluten Free Wafers, Milk Chocolate",	HIGH	62.82

Food name/ Category (100 g)	Status	Carbs content in g
Goat, raw",	LOW	0
Goji berries, dried",	HIGH	77.06
Goose, domesticated, meat and skin, cooked, roasted",	LOW	0
Goose, domesticated, meat and skin, raw",	LOW	0
Goose, domesticated, meat only, cooked, roasted",	LOW	0
Goose, domesticated, meat only, raw",	LOW	0
Goose, liver, raw",	LOW	6.32
Gooseberries, canned, light syrup pack, solids and liquids",	LOW	18.75
Gooseberries, raw",	LOW	10.18
Gourd, dishcloth (towelgourd), cooked, boiled, drained, with salt",	LOW	13.75
Gourd, dishcloth (towelgourd), raw",	LOW	4.35
Gourd, white-flowered (calabash), cooked, boiled, drained, with salt",	LOW	3.1
Gourd, white-flowered (calabash), cooked, boiled, drained, without salt",	LOW	3.69
Gourd, white-flowered (calabash), raw",	LOW	3.39
Granola bar, soft, milk chocolate coated, peanut butter",	MEDIUM	54.1
Grape juice, canned or bottled, unsweetened, with added ascorbic acid and calcium",	LOW	14.77
Grape juice, canned or bottled, unsweetened, with added ascorbic acid",	LOW	14.77
Grape juice, canned or bottled, unsweetened, without added ascorbic acid",	LOW	14.77
Grape leaves, canned",	LOW	11.71
Grapefruit juice, pink or red, with added calcium",	LOW	8.69
Grapefruit juice, pink, raw",	LOW	9.2
Grapefruit juice, white, bottled, unsweetened, OCEAN SPRAY",	LOW	7.93
Grapefruit juice, white, canned or bottled, unsweetened",	LOW	7.93
Grapefruit juice, white, canned, sweetened",	LOW	11.13
Grapefruit juice, white, frozen concentrate, unsweetened, diluted with 3 volume water",	LOW	9.73
Grapefruit juice, white, frozen concentrate, unsweetened, undiluted",	LOW	34.56
Grapefruit juice, white, raw",	LOW	9.2
Grapefruit, raw, pink and red and white, all areas",	LOW	8.08
Grapefruit, raw, pink and red, all areas",	LOW	10.66

Food name/ Category (100 g)	Status	Carbs content in g
Grapefruit, raw, pink and red, California and Arizona",	LOW	9.69
Grapefruit, raw, pink and red, Florida",	LOW	7.5
Grapefruit, raw, white, all areas",	LOW	8.41
Grapefruit, raw, white, California",	LOW	9.09
Grapefruit, raw, white, Florida",	LOW	8.19
Grapefruit, sections, canned, light syrup pack, solids and liquids",	LOW	15.44
Grapefruit, sections, canned, water pack, solids and liquids",	LOW	9.15
Grapes, american type (slip skin), raw",	LOW	17.15
Grapes, canned, thompson seedless, heavy syrup pack, solids and liquids",	LOW	19.65
Grapes, muscadine, raw",	LOW	13.93
Grapes, red or green (European type, such as Thompson seedless), raw",	LOW	18.1
Gravy, au jus, canned",	LOW	2.5
Gravy, au jus, dry",	MEDIUM	47.49
Gravy, beef, canned, ready-to-serve",	LOW	4.81
Gravy, brown instant, dry",	HIGH	59.78
Gravy, brown, dry",	HIGH	59.38
Gravy, CAMPBELL'S, au jus",	LOW	0
Gravy, CAMPBELL'S, beef, fat free",	LOW	5.08
Gravy, CAMPBELL'S, beef, microwavable",	LOW	5.08
Gravy, CAMPBELL'S, beef",	LOW	5.08
Gravy, CAMPBELL'S, brown with onions",	LOW	6.78
Gravy, CAMPBELL'S, chicken, fat free",	LOW	5.08
Gravy, CAMPBELL'S, chicken, microwavable",	LOW	5
Gravy, CAMPBELL'S, chicken",	LOW	5.87
Gravy, CAMPBELL'S, country style cream",	LOW	5.08
Gravy, CAMPBELL'S, country style sausage",	LOW	5.08
Gravy, CAMPBELL'S, mushroom",	LOW	5.08
Gravy, CAMPBELL'S, turkey, fat free",	LOW	6.67
Gravy, CAMPBELL'S, turkey, microwavable",	LOW	5

Food name/ Category (100 g)	Status	Carbs content in g
Gravy, CAMPBELL'S, turkey",	LOW	5.08
Gravy, chicken, canned or bottled, ready-to-serve",	LOW	5.29
Gravy, chicken, dry",	HIGH	62.09
Gravy, FRANCO-AMERICAN, beef, slow roast, fat free",	LOW	5.08
Gravy, FRANCO-AMERICAN, beef, slow roast",	LOW	5.08
Gravy, FRANCO-AMERICAN, chicken, slow roast, fat free",	LOW	6.78
Gravy, FRANCO-AMERICAN, chicken, slow roast",	LOW	5.08
Gravy, FRANCO-AMERICAN, turkey, slow roast",	LOW	6.78
Gravy, HEINZ Home Style, classic chicken",	LOW	5.01
Gravy, HEINZ Home Style, savory beef",	LOW	6.24
Gravy, instant beef, dry",	HIGH	61.1
Gravy, instant turkey, dry",	HIGH	57.56
Gravy, mushroom, canned",	LOW	5.47
Gravy, mushroom, dry, powder",	HIGH	64.66
Gravy, onion, dry, mix",	HIGH	67.64
Gravy, turkey, canned, ready-to-serve",	LOW	5.1
Gravy, turkey, dry",	HIGH	65.12
Gravy, unspecified type, dry",	HIGH	58
Ground turkey, 85% lean, 15% fat, pan-broiled crumbles",	LOW	0
Ground turkey, 85% lean, 15% fat, patties, broiled",	LOW	0
Ground turkey, 85% lean, 15% fat, raw",	LOW	0
Ground turkey, 93% lean, 7% fat, pan-broiled crumbles",	LOW	0
Ground turkey, 93% lean, 7% fat, patties, broiled",	LOW	0
Ground turkey, 93% lean, 7% fat, raw",	LOW	0
Ground turkey, cooked",	LOW	0
Ground turkey, fat free, pan-broiled crumbles",	LOW	0
Ground turkey, fat free, patties, broiled",	LOW	0
Ground turkey, fat free, raw",	LOW	0
Ground turkey, raw",	LOW	0
Guava sauce, cooked",	LOW	9.48
Guavas, common, raw",	LOW	14.32

Food name/ Category (100 g)	Status	Carbs content in g
Guavas, strawberry, raw",	LOW	17.36
Guinea hen, meat and skin, raw",	LOW	0
Guinea hen, meat only, raw",	LOW	0
Gums, seed gums (includes locust bean, guar)",	HIGH	77.3
Hazelnuts, beaked (Northern Plains Indians)",	LOW	22.98
HEALTHY REQUEST Tomato juice",	LOW	4.53
HEALTHY REQUEST, Cream of Celery Soup, condensed",	LOW	9.68
HEALTHY REQUEST, Minestrone Soup, condensed",	LOW	11.9
HEALTHY REQUEST, Tomato Soup, condensed",	LOW	13.71
HEALTHY REQUEST, Vegetable Soup, condensed",	LOW	15.87
Hearts of palm, canned",	LOW	4.62
HEINZ, WEIGHT WATCHER, Chocolate Eclair, frozen",	MEDIUM	40.3
Hominy, canned, white",	LOW	14.26
Hominy, canned, yellow",	LOW	14.26
Honey roll sausage, beef",	LOW	2.18
Honey",	HIGH	82.4
HORMEL Pillow Pak Sliced Turkey Pepperoni",	LOW	3.78
Horned melon (Kiwano)",	LOW	7.56
Horseradish, prepared",	LOW	11.29
HOT POCKETS, CROISSANT POCKETS Chicken, Broccoli, and Cheddar Stuffed Sandwich, frozen",	LOW	30.4
HOT POCKETS, meatballs & mozzarella stuffed sandwich, frozen",	LOW	30.45
Hummus, commercial",	LOW	14.29
Hummus, home prepared",	LOW	20.12
HUNGRY MAN, Salisbury Steak With Gravy, frozen, unprepared",	LOW	6.96
Hush puppies, prepared from recipe",	MEDIUM	46
Hyacinth beans, mature seeds, cooked, boiled, with salt",	LOW	20.7
Hyacinth-beans, immature seeds, cooked, boiled, drained, with salt",	LOW	9.2
Hyacinth-beans, immature seeds, cooked, boiled, drained, without salt",	LOW	9.2
Hyacinth-beans, immature seeds, raw",	LOW	9.19
Ice cream bar, stick or nugget, with crunch coating",	LOW	37.12

Food name/ Category (100 g)	Status	Carbs content in g
Ice cream cone, chocolate covered, with nuts, flavors other than chocolate",	LOW	34.38
Ice cream cones, cake or wafer-type",	HIGH	79
Ice cream cones, sugar, rolled-type",	HIGH	84.1
Ice cream cookie sandwich",	LOW	39.6
Ice cream sandwich, made with light ice cream, vanilla",	LOW	39.64
Ice cream sandwich, vanilla, light, no sugar added",	MEDIUM	42.86
Ice cream sandwich",	LOW	37.14
Ice cream, bar or stick, chocolate covered",	LOW	24.5
Ice cream, light, soft serve, chocolate",	LOW	23.15
Ice cream, soft serve, chocolate",	LOW	22.2
Ice creams, BREYERS, 98% Fat Free Chocolate",	LOW	30.18
Ice creams, BREYERS, 98% Fat Free Vanilla",	LOW	30.51
Ice creams, BREYERS, All Natural Light French Chocolate",	LOW	29.68
Ice creams, BREYERS, All Natural Light French Vanilla",	LOW	26.03
Ice creams, BREYERS, All Natural Light Mint Chocolate Chip",	LOW	28.39
Ice creams, BREYERS, All Natural Light Vanilla Chocolate Strawberry",	LOW	26.06
Ice creams, BREYERS, All Natural Light Vanilla",	LOW	25.3
Ice creams, BREYERS, No Sugar Added, Butter Pecan",	LOW	21.3
Ice creams, BREYERS, No Sugar Added, Chocolate Caramel",	LOW	25.17
Ice creams, BREYERS, No Sugar Added, French Vanilla",	LOW	20.75
Ice creams, BREYERS, No Sugar Added, Vanilla Chocolate Strawberry",	LOW	21.7
Ice creams, BREYERS, No Sugar Added, Vanilla Fudge Twirl",	LOW	25.63
Ice creams, BREYERS, No Sugar Added, Vanilla",	LOW	21.92
Ice creams, chocolate, light, no sugar added",	LOW	26.79
Ice creams, chocolate, light",	LOW	25.7
Ice creams, chocolate, rich",	LOW	19.78
Ice creams, chocolate",	LOW	28.2
Ice creams, french vanilla, soft-serve",	LOW	22.2
Ice creams, regular, low carbohydrate, chocolate",	LOW	26.8

Food name/ Category (100 g)	Status	Carbs content in g
Ice creams, regular, low carbohydrate, vanilla",	LOW	22.23
Ice creams, strawberry",	LOW	27.6
Ice creams, vanilla, fat free",	LOW	30.06
Ice creams, vanilla, light, no sugar added",	LOW	21.42
Ice creams, vanilla, light, soft-serve",	LOW	21.8
Ice creams, vanilla, light",	LOW	29.46
Ice creams, vanilla, rich",	LOW	22.29
Ice creams, vanilla",	LOW	23.6
Imitation cheese, american or cheddar, low cholesterol",	LOW	1
Incaparina, dry mix (corn and soy flours), unprepared",	HIGH	60.53
Infant formula, ABBOTT NUTRITION, ALIMENTUM ADVANCE, with iron, powder,	MEDIUM	51.91
Infant formula, ABBOTT NUTRITION, SIMILAC, ADVANCE, with iron, powder, not	MEDIUM	54.73
Infant formula, ABBOTT NUTRITION, SIMILAC, For Spit Up, powder, with ARA an	MEDIUM	55
Infant formula, ABBOTT NUTRITION, SIMILAC, GO AND GROW, powder, with AR	MEDIUM	52.2
Infant formula, ABBOTT NUTRITION, SIMILAC, ISOMIL, ADVANCE with iron, liquid concentrate",	LOW	13.21
Infant formula, ABBOTT NUTRITION, SIMILAC, ISOMIL, ADVANCE with iron, pow	MEDIUM	53.57
Infant formula, ABBOTT NUTRITION, SIMILAC, ISOMIL, with iron, liquid concentrate",	LOW	13.21
Infant formula, ABBOTT NUTRITION, SIMILAC, ISOMIL, with iron, powder, not rec	MEDIUM	53.57
Infant formula, ABBOTT NUTRITION, SIMILAC, low iron, powder, not reconstituted	MEDIUM	54.78
Infant formula, ABBOTT NUTRITION, SIMILAC, NEOSURE, powder, with ARA anc	MEDIUM	51.75
Infant formula, ABBOTT NUTRITION, SIMILAC, PM 60\/40, powder not reconstitut	MEDIUM	54.94
Infant formula, ABBOTT NUTRITION, SIMILAC, SENSITIVE, (LACTOSE FREE), liquid concentrate, with ARA and DHA",	LOW	13.64
Infant formula, ABBOTT NUTRITION, SIMILAC, SENSITIVE, (LACTOSE FREE), p	MEDIUM	55.67
Infant formula, ABBOTT NUTRITION, SIMILAC, with iron, powder, not reconstitutec	MEDIUM	54.73
Infant Formula, GERBER GOOD START 2, GENTLE PLUS, powder",	HIGH	57.1
Infant formula, GERBER, GOOD START 2 SOY, with iron, powder",	MEDIUM	55.6
Infant formula, GERBER, GOOD START 2, PROTECT PLUS, powder",	MEDIUM	56.3
Infant formula, GERBER, GOOD START, PROTECT PLUS, powder",	HIGH	57
Infant formula, MEAD JOHNSON, ENFAMIL, AR LIPIL, powder, with ARA and DH/	MEDIUM	56.03
Infant formula, MEAD JOHNSON, ENFAMIL, ENFACARE LIPIL, with iron, powder,	MEDIUM	56
Infant formula, MEAD JOHNSON, ENFAMIL, ENFAGROW, GENTLEASE, Toddler	MEDIUM	52
Infant formula, MEAD JOHNSON, ENFAMIL, ENFAGROW, Soy, Toddler, LIPIL, pc	MEDIUM	56
Infant Formula, MEAD JOHNSON, ENFAMIL, GENTLEASE, powder",	MEDIUM	56
Infant formula, MEAD JOHNSON, ENFAMIL, LACTOFREE LIPIL, with iron, powde	MEDIUM	56.3
Infant formula, MEAD JOHNSON, ENFAMIL, LACTOFREE, LIPIL, with iron, liquid concentrate, not reconstituted, with ARA and DHA",	LOW	14.42
Infant formula, MEAD JOHNSON, ENFAMIL, LACTOFREE, with iron, powder, not	HIGH	57
Infant formula, MEAD JOHNSON, ENFAMIL, LIPIL, low iron, liquid concentrate, with ARA and DHA",	LOW	14.24
Infant formula, MEAD JOHNSON, ENFAMIL, LIPIL, with iron, powder, with ARA an	MEDIUM	56.2
Infant formula, MEAD JOHNSON, ENFAMIL, low iron, powder, not reconstituted",	MEDIUM	56.2
Infant formula, MEAD JOHNSON, ENFAMIL, NUTRAMIGEN LIPIL, with iron, powd	MEDIUM	51
Infant formula, MEAD JOHNSON, ENFAMIL, NUTRAMIGEN, AA LIPIL, powder, no	MEDIUM	51
Infant formula, MEAD JOHNSON, ENFAMIL, NUTRAMIGEN, LIPIL, with iron, liquid concentrate not reconstituted, with ARA and DHA",	LOW	13.12

Food name/ Category (100 g)	Status	Carbs content in g
Infant formula, MEAD JOHNSON, ENFAMIL, NUTRAMIGEN, with iron, liquid concentrate, not reconstituted",	LOW	13.12
Infant formula, MEAD JOHNSON, ENFAMIL, NUTRAMIGEN, with iron, powder, no	MEDIUM	55
Infant formula, MEAD JOHNSON, ENFAMIL, Premature, 20 calories ready-to-feed Low iron",	LOW	7.21
Infant formula, MEAD JOHNSON, ENFAMIL, Premature, 20 calories ready-to-feed",	LOW	7.21
Infant formula, MEAD JOHNSON, ENFAMIL, Premature, 24 calo ready-to-feed",	LOW	7.19
Infant formula, MEAD JOHNSON, ENFAMIL, Premature, 24 calories ready-to-feed Low iron",	LOW	7.19
Infant Formula, MEAD JOHNSON, ENFAMIL, Premium LIPIL, Infant, powder",	HIGH	57
Infant formula, MEAD JOHNSON, ENFAMIL, Premium, Infant, powder",	HIGH	57
Infant Formula, MEAD JOHNSON, ENFAMIL, Premium, Newborn, powder",	HIGH	57
Infant formula, MEAD JOHNSON, ENFAMIL, PROSOBEE LIPIL, with iron, powder	MEDIUM	53
Infant formula, MEAD JOHNSON, ENFAMIL, PROSOBEE, LIPIL, liquid concentrate, not reconstituted, with ARA and DHA",	LOW	13.58
Infant formula, MEAD JOHNSON, ENFAMIL, PROSOBEE, with iron, powder, not r	MEDIUM	54.3
Infant formula, MEAD JOHNSON, ENFAMIL, with iron, powder",	MEDIUM	56.2
Infant formula, MEAD JOHNSON, NEXT STEP PROSOBEE, powder, not reconstit	HIGH	57.1
Infant formula, MEAD JOHNSON, NEXT STEP, PROSOBEE LIPIL, powder, with /	HIGH	57.1
Infant formula, MEAD JOHNSON, PREGESTIMIL, with iron, powder, not reconstitu	MEDIUM	52.8
Infant formula, MEAD JOHNSON, PROSOBEE, with iron, liquid concentrate, not reconstituted",	LOW	13.58
Infant formula, NESTLE, GOOD START 2 ESSENTIALS, with iron, liquid concentrate, not reconstituted",	LOW	16.5
Infant formula, NESTLE, GOOD START 2 ESSENTIALS, with iron, powder",	HIGH	62.23
Infant formula, NESTLE, GOOD START ESSENTIALS SOY, with iron, liquid concentrate, not reconstituted",	LOW	14.1
Infant formula, NESTLE, GOOD START ESSENTIALS SOY, with iron, powder",	MEDIUM	55.7
Infant formula, NESTLE, GOOD START SOY, with ARA and DHA, powder",	MEDIUM	55.6
Infant formula, NESTLE, GOOD START SOY, with DHA and ARA, liquid concentrate",	LOW	14.71
Infant formula, NESTLE, GOOD START SUPREME, with iron, powder",	HIGH	57.32
Infant formula, PBM PRODUCTS, store brand, powder",	MEDIUM	56
Infant formula, PBM PRODUCTS, store brand, soy, liquid concentrate, not reconstituted",	LOW	12.18
Infant formula, PBM PRODUCTS, store brand, soy, powder",	MEDIUM	52.2
Jackfruit, raw",	LOW	23.25
JACKSON'S, Old Fashioned Lemon Jumble Cookies",	HIGH	71.7
JACKSON'S, Old Fashioned Vanilla Wafers",	HIGH	74
Jams and preserves, apricot",	HIGH	64.4
Jams and preserves, no sugar (with sodium saccharin), any flavor",	MEDIUM	53.42
Jellies, no sugar (with sodium saccharin), any flavors",	LOW	29.6
Jellies, reduced sugar, home preserved",	MEDIUM	46.1
Jellyfish, dried, salted",	LOW	0
Jerusalem-artichokes, raw",	LOW	17.44
JIMMY DEAN, Sausage, Egg, and Cheese Breakfast Biscuit, frozen, unprepared",	LOW	21.07
Juice, apple, grape and pear blend, with added ascorbic acid and calcium",	LOW	12.96

Food name/ Category (100 g)	Status	Carbs content in g
Jute, potherb, cooked, boiled, drained, with salt",	LOW	7.29
Kale, cooked, boiled, drained, with salt",	LOW	5.63
Kale, frozen, cooked, boiled, drained, with salt",	LOW	5.23
Kale, raw",	LOW	8.75
Kale, scotch, cooked, boiled, drained, with salt",	LOW	5.62
Kale, scotch, cooked, boiled, drained, without salt",	LOW	5.63
Kale, scotch, raw",	LOW	8.32
KASHI Black Bean Mango, frozen, unprepared",	LOW	18
KASHI Italian Vegetable Medley Pasta, frozen, unprepared",	LOW	16.3
KASHI Mayan Harvest Bake, frozen, unprepared",	LOW	21
KASHI Mushroom & Asparagus Risotto, frozen, unprepared",	LOW	17
KASHI Pesto Pasta Primavera, frozen, unprepared",	LOW	13
KASHI Pizza, Greek Tzatziki, single serve, frozen, unprepared",	LOW	29.7
KASHI Pizza, Margherita, frozen, unprepared",	LOW	25.7
KASHI Pizza, Mediterranean, frozen, unprepared",	LOW	31
KASHI Pizza, Mushroom and Spinach, single serve, frozen, unprepared",	LOW	36.5
KASHI Pizza, Mushroom Trio & Spinach, frozen, unprepared",	LOW	24.6
KASHI Pizza, Roasted Vegetable, frozen, unprepared",	LOW	24.5
KASHI Pizza, Tikka Masala, single serve, frozen, unprepared",	LOW	29.5
KASHI Spicy Black Bean Enchilada, frozen, unprepared",	LOW	17.7
KASHI Spinach Artichoke Pasta, frozen, unprepared",	LOW	15.1
KASHI Three Cheese Penne, frozen, unprepared",	LOW	16.8
KASHI Three Cheese Ravioli with Mediterranean Tomato Sauce, frozen, unprepared",	LOW	19.7
KASHI, Blueberry Waffle",	LOW	34.6
KASHI, Chicken and Chipotle BBQ Sauce with Mango, Frozen Entree",	LOW	17.6
KASHI, Chicken Enchilada with Ancho Sauce, Frozen Entree",	LOW	14.9
KASHI, Chicken Florentine, Frozen Entree",	LOW	11
KASHI, Chicken Pasta Pomodoro, Frozen Entree",	LOW	13

Food name/ Category (100 g)	Status	Carbs content in g
KASHI, H2H Woven Wheat Cracker, Original",	HIGH	73.4
KASHI, H2H Woven Wheat Cracker, Roasted Garlic",	HIGH	73.2
KASHI, Lemongrass Coconut Chicken, Frozen Entree",	LOW	13.4
KASHI, Original Waffle",	LOW	35.4
KASHI, Pilaf, 7 Whole Grain, unprepared",	HIGH	71
KASHI, Red Curry Chicken, Frozen Entree",	LOW	15.6
KASHI, Southwest Style Chicken, Frozen Entree",	LOW	17.4
KASHI, STEAM MEAL, Chicken Fettuccine, Frozen Entree",	LOW	14
KASHI, STEAM MEAL, Roasted Garlic Chicken Farfalle, Frozen Entree",	LOW	14.6
KASHI, STEAM MEAL, Sesame Chicken, Frozen Entree",	LOW	15.7
KASHI, Sweet and Sour Chicken, Frozen Entree",	LOW	19
KASHI, TLC, Country Cheddar Crackers",	HIGH	68
KASHI, TLC, Fire Roasted Vegetable Crackers",	HIGH	64.6
KASHI, TLC, Happy Trail Mix Cookies",	HIGH	63.86
KASHI, TLC, Honey Sesame Crackers",	HIGH	72.2
KASHI, TLC, Oatmeal Dark Chocolate Cookies",	HIGH	67
KASHI, TLC, Oatmeal Raisin Flax Cookies",	HIGH	67
KASHI, TLC, Original 7-Grain Crackers",	HIGH	63.2
KASHI, TLC, Pita Crisps, Sea Salt",	HIGH	72.4
KASHI, TLC, Pita Crisps, Zesty Salsa",	HIGH	71.6
KASHI, TLC, Toasted Asiago Crackers",	HIGH	66.4
KASHI, Tuscan Veggie Bake, Frozen Entree",	LOW	15
KEEBLER, 100 Calorie RIGHT BITES, CHIPS DELUXE, Chocolate Chip Cookies",	HIGH	77.7
KEEBLER, 100 Calorie RIGHT BITES, FUDGE SHOPPE, Cookies 'N Creme",	HIGH	72.2
KEEBLER, 100 Calorie RIGHT BITES, FUDGE SHOPPE, Dark Chocolate Fudge S	HIGH	71.2
KEEBLER, 100 Calorie RIGHT BITES, FUDGE SHOPPE, Fudge Covered Pretzels	HIGH	71.3
KEEBLER, 100 Calorie RIGHT BITES, FUDGE SHOPPE, Mini Brownies",	HIGH	65.1
KEEBLER, 100 Calorie RIGHT BITES, FUDGE SHOPPE, Mini Fudge Stripes Cook	HIGH	74.3
KEEBLER, 100 Calorie RIGHT BITES, FUDGE SHOPPE, Mini Mints Grasshopper	HIGH	75
KEEBLER, 100 Calorie RIGHT BITES, Sandies Shortbread Cookies, Fudge Dipped	HIGH	72.4
KEEBLER, 100 Calorie RIGHT BITES, Sandies Shortbread Cookies",	HIGH	73.9
KEEBLER, 100 Calorie RIGHT BITES, White Fudge Dipped Pretzels",	HIGH	68.8
KEEBLER, Almond Crescents Cookies, Holiday",	HIGH	70.1
KEEBLER, ANIMALS, Cookies",	HIGH	75.3
KEEBLER, ANIMALS, Crackers",	HIGH	75.3
KEEBLER, ANIMALS, Frosted Cookies",	HIGH	70
KEEBLER, ANIMALS, Iced Cookies",	HIGH	74.2
KEEBLER, BAKER'S TREASURES, Chocolate Chip Cookie, soft",	HIGH	69.9
KEEBLER, BAKER'S TREASURES, Oatmeal Raisin Cookie, soft",	HIGH	69.1
KEEBLER, Cheese & Cheddar Sandwich Crackers",	HIGH	59.5
KEEBLER, Cheese & Peanut Butter Sandwich Crackers",	HIGH	59
KEEBLER, Cheese on Wheat Sandwich Crackers",	HIGH	59.8
KEEBLER, CHIPS DELUXE, Chocolate Lovers Cookies",	HIGH	63
KEEBLER, CHIPS DELUXE, Chocolate Malt Chunk Cookies",	HIGH	61.8
KEEBLER, CHIPS DELUXE, Coconut Cookies",	HIGH	61.5
KEEBLER, CHIPS DELUXE, Dark Chocolate Chunk Cookies",	HIGH	64
KEEBLER, CHIPS DELUXE, Mini Chocolate Chip Cookies",	HIGH	68
KEEBLER, CHIPS DELUXE, Oatmeal Chocolate Chip Cookies",	HIGH	65.3

Food name/ Category (100 g)	Status	Carbs content in g
KEEBLER, CHIPS DELUXE, Original Chocolate Chip Cookies",	HIGH	62.7
KEEBLER, CHIPS DELUXE, Peanut Butter Cups Cookies",	HIGH	60.8
KEEBLER, CHIPS DELUXE, Rainbow Chocolate Chip Cookies, bite size",	HIGH	68.55
KEEBLER, CHIPS DELUXE, Rainbow Chocolate Chip Cookies",	HIGH	65
KEEBLER, CHIPS DELUXE, Soft 'n Chewy Chocolate Chip Cookies",	HIGH	67.4
KEEBLER, Club & Cheddar Sandwich Crackers",	HIGH	61.3
KEEBLER, CLUB Crackers, Snack Sticks, Honey Wheat",	HIGH	66
KEEBLER, CLUB Crackers, Snack Sticks, Original",	HIGH	65
KEEBLER, CLUB, Dash of Salt Crackers",	HIGH	66.3
KEEBLER, CLUB, Minis Multigrain Crackers",	HIGH	67.4
KEEBLER, CLUB, Minis Original Crackers",	HIGH	66.4
KEEBLER, CLUB, Multigrain Crackers",	HIGH	65.9
KEEBLER, CLUB, Original Crackers",	HIGH	66.2
KEEBLER, CLUB, Reduced Fat Crackers",	HIGH	73.1
KEEBLER, Country Style Oatmeal Cookies with Raisins",	HIGH	67
KEEBLER, Danish Wedding Cookies",	HIGH	68.3
KEEBLER, E.L. FUDGE, Butter Flavored Cookies",	HIGH	70
KEEBLER, E.L. FUDGE, Double Stuffed Cookies",	HIGH	67.6
KEEBLER, FUDGE SHOPPE, Caramel Filled Cookies",	HIGH	66.7
KEEBLER, FUDGE SHOPPE, Cheesecake Middles, Dark Chocolate",	HIGH	64.7
KEEBLER, FUDGE SHOPPE, Coconut Dreams Cookies",	HIGH	61.4
KEEBLER, FUDGE SHOPPE, Fudge Sticks, Peanut Butter",	HIGH	60
KEEBLER, FUDGE SHOPPE, Fudge Sticks",	HIGH	68.8
KEEBLER, FUDGE SHOPPE, Fudge Stripes, Dark Chocolate",	HIGH	70.1
KEEBLER, FUDGE SHOPPE, Fudge Stripes, Holiday\/Spiderman",	HIGH	68.8
KEEBLER, FUDGE SHOPPE, Fudge Stripes, Mini",	HIGH	68.7
KEEBLER, FUDGE SHOPPE, Fudge Stripes, Oatmeal",	HIGH	66.4
KEEBLER, FUDGE SHOPPE, Fudge Stripes, Original",	HIGH	68.6
KEEBLER, FUDGE SHOPPE, Fudge-Dipped Ice Cream Cups",	HIGH	73.1
KEEBLER, FUDGE SHOPPE, Grasshopper Cookies, Fudge Mint",	HIGH	68.3
KEEBLER, FUDGE SHOPPE, Jumbo Fudge Sticks, Peanut Butter",	HIGH	60.6
KEEBLER, FUDGE SHOPPE, Jumbo Fudge Sticks, Vanilla",	HIGH	68.6
KEEBLER, FUDGE SHOPPE, Magic Middles Fudge Filled Cookies, Original",	HIGH	62.5
KEEBLER, FUDGE SHOPPE, Magic Middles Fudge Filled Cookies, Peanut Butter'	HIGH	59.2
KEEBLER, FUDGE SHOPPE, Merry Mint Patties, Holiday",	HIGH	66.7
KEEBLER, FUDGE SHOPPE, Peanut Creme Filled Cookies",	HIGH	57.6
KEEBLER, FUDGE SHOPPE, Triple Fudge Filled Cookies",	HIGH	64.2
KEEBLER, Gingerbread Men Cookies, Holiday",	HIGH	77.9
KEEBLER, GRIPZ, CHIPS DELUXE, Chocolate Chip Cookies, bite-size",	HIGH	71.3
KEEBLER, GRIPZ, CHIPS DELUXE, Rainbow Chocolate Chip Cookies, bite-size",	HIGH	74.3
KEEBLER, Holiday Jingles Cookies",	HIGH	73.9
KEEBLER, Iced Oatmeal Cookies",	HIGH	69.5
KEEBLER, Oatmeal Cookies",	HIGH	67.7
KEEBLER, READY CRUST, Chocolate Pie Crust",	HIGH	67.7
KEEBLER, READY CRUST, Shortbread Pie Crust",	HIGH	69.1
KEEBLER, SANDIES, Cashew Shortbread Cookies",	HIGH	59.3
KEEBLER, SANDIES, Chocolate Chip & Pecan Shortbread Cookies",	HIGH	59.2
KEEBLER, SANDIES, Dark Chocolate Almond Shortbread Cookies",	HIGH	59.9
KEEBLER, SANDIES, Pecan Shortbread Cookies, bite size",	HIGH	58.7
KEEBLER, SANDIES, Pecan Shortbread Cookies, Reduced Fat",	HIGH	67.1
KEEBLER, SANDIES, Pecan Shortbread Cookies",	HIGH	59
KEEBLER, SANDIES, Simply Shortbread Cookies",	HIGH	62.2
KEEBLER, SOFT BATCH, Chocolate Chip Cookies",	HIGH	66.2
KEEBLER, Sugar Cones",	HIGH	78
KEEBLER, Sweet Cremes Cookies",	HIGH	71
KEEBLER, Toast & Peanut Butter Sandwich Crackers",	HIGH	60.2
KEEBLER, Toasted Coconut Cookies",	HIGH	69.9

Food name/ Category (100 g)	Status	Carbs content in g
KEEBLER, TOASTEDS, Buttercrisps Crackers",	HIGH	65
KEEBLER, TOASTEDS, Onion Crackers",	HIGH	67.7
KEEBLER, TOASTEDS, Party Pack Cracker Assortment",	HIGH	64.4
KEEBLER, TOASTEDS, Sesame Crackers",	HIGH	62.6
KEEBLER, TOASTEDS, Wheat Crackers",	HIGH	66.1
KEEBLER, TOWN HOUSE, Bistro Multigrain Crackers",	HIGH	67
KEEBLER, TOWN HOUSE, FLATBREAD CRISPS, Sea Salt and Olive Oil Cracker	HIGH	72.8
KEEBLER, TOWN HOUSE, FLIPSIDES, Pretzel Crackers, Cheese",	HIGH	61.3
KEEBLER, TOWN HOUSE, FLIPSIDES, Pretzel Crackers, Garlic Herb",	HIGH	63
KEEBLER, TOWN HOUSE, FLIPSIDES, Pretzel Crackers, Original",	HIGH	64.3
KEEBLER, TOWN HOUSE, FLIPSIDES, Pretzel Crackers, Reduced Fat",	HIGH	70.4
KEEBLER, TOWN HOUSE, Original Crackers",	HIGH	59.8
KEEBLER, TOWN HOUSE, Reduced Fat Crackers",	HIGH	77.1
KEEBLER, TOWN HOUSE, TOPPERS, Garlic Herb Crackers",	HIGH	71.6
KEEBLER, TOWN HOUSE, TOPPERS, Multigrain Crackers",	HIGH	68.4
KEEBLER, TOWN HOUSE, TOPPERS, Original Crackers",	HIGH	66.8
KEEBLER, TOWN HOUSE, Wheat Crackers",	HIGH	63.2
KEEBLER, TRADITIONS, Iced Lemonade Cookies",	HIGH	66.3
KEEBLER, TRADITIONS, Iced Oatmeal Cookies",	HIGH	71
KEEBLER, Vanilla Wafers Minis, Rainbow",	HIGH	72.3
KEEBLER, Vanilla Wafers",	HIGH	73.1
KEEBLER, Vienna Fingers with Creme Filling, Reduced Fat",	HIGH	78.1
KEEBLER, Vienna Fingers with Creme Filling",	HIGH	73.2
KEEBLER, Waffle Bowls",	HIGH	87.7
KEEBLER, Waffle Cones",	HIGH	87.7
KEEBLER, WHEATABLES, Honey Wheat Crackers",	HIGH	67
KEEBLER, WHEATABLES, Nut Crisp Crackers, Roasted Almond",	HIGH	66.5
KEEBLER, WHEATABLES, Nut Crisp Crackers, Toasted Pecan",	HIGH	65.7
KEEBLER, ZESTA, Export Sodas Crackers",	HIGH	74
KEEBLER, ZESTA, Saltines with Whole Wheat",	HIGH	75.1
KEEBLER, ZESTA, Saltines, Original",	HIGH	76.1
Keikitos (muffins), Latino bakery item",	MEDIUM	53.16
KELLOGG, KELLOG'S NUTRI-GRAIN CEREAL BARS, Mixed Berry",	HIGH	72.8
KELLOGG, KELLOGG'S EGGO, Buttermilk Pancake",	LOW	38.6
KELLOGG'S EGGO Lowfat Blueberry Nutri-Grain Waffles",	MEDIUM	42.71
KELLOGG'S, ALL-BRAN, Garlic and Herb Crackers",	HIGH	63.5
KELLOGG'S, ALL-BRAN, Multigrain Crackers",	HIGH	65.7
KELLOGG'S, BEANATURAL, Original 3-Bean Chips",	MEDIUM	46.5
KELLOGG'S, CINNABON, Pancakes, Caramel",	MEDIUM	43.4
KELLOGG'S, CINNABON, Pancakes, Original",	MEDIUM	43.1
KELLOGG'S, Com Flakes Crumbs",	HIGH	84.4
KELLOGG'S, EGGO Minis, Pancakes, Buttermilk",	LOW	39.6
KELLOGG'S, EGGO Protein, Waffles, Homestyle",	LOW	37
KELLOGG'S, EGGO Seasons, Waffles, Pumpkin Spice",	MEDIUM	41.4
KELLOGG'S, EGGO, Biscuit Scramblers, Egg & Cheese",	LOW	38.3
KELLOGG'S, EGGO, FIBERPLUS Waffles, Buttermilk",	MEDIUM	41.8
KELLOGG'S, EGGO, FIBERPLUS Waffles, Chocolate Chip",	MEDIUM	44.4
KELLOGG'S, EGGO, French Toaster Sticks, Cinnamon",	MEDIUM	42.6
KELLOGG'S, EGGO, French Toaster Sticks, Original",	LOW	39.4
KELLOGG'S, EGGO, Mini Muffin Tops, Blueberry",	MEDIUM	45.8
KELLOGG'S, EGGO, Mini Muffin Tops, Chocolate Chip",	MEDIUM	45
KELLOGG'S, EGGO, NUTRI-GRAIN Frozen Fruit Pizza, Mixed Berry Granola",	MEDIUM	41.4

Food name/ Category (100 g)	Status	Carbs content in g
KELLOGG'S, EGGO, NUTRI-GRAIN Frozen Fruit Pizza, Strawberry Granola",	MEDIUM	43.7
KELLOGG'S, EGGO, NUTRI-GRAIN, Waffles, Blueberry",	MEDIUM	43.6
KELLOGG'S, EGGO, NUTRI-GRAIN, Waffles, Honey Oat",	MEDIUM	44.1
KELLOGG'S, EGGO, NUTRI-GRAIN, Waffles, Low Fat",	LOW	39
KELLOGG'S, EGGO, NUTRI-GRAIN, Waffles, Original",	LOW	37.6
KELLOGG'S, EGGO, Pancakes, Blueberry",	LOW	39.9
KELLOGG'S, EGGO, Pancakes, Chocolate Chip",	LOW	39.9
KELLOGG'S, EGGO, Thick & Fluffy, Waffles, Brown Sugar",	MEDIUM	44.5
KELLOGG'S, EGGO, Thick & Fluffy, Waffles, Original",	LOW	37.4
KELLOGG'S, EGGO, Wafflers, Brown Sugar Cinnamon Roll",	MEDIUM	52.2
KELLOGG'S, EGGO, Wafflers, Strawberry Strudel",	MEDIUM	50
KELLOGG'S, EGGO, Waffles, Blueberry",	MEDIUM	41.7
KELLOGG'S, EGGO, Waffles, Buttermilk",	LOW	39
KELLOGG'S, EGGO, Waffles, Chocolate Chip",	MEDIUM	44.8
KELLOGG'S, EGGO, Waffles, Cinnamon Toast",	MEDIUM	49.5
KELLOGG'S, EGGO, Waffles, French Toast",	MEDIUM	43.4
KELLOGG'S, EGGO, Waffles, Homestyle, Low Fat",	MEDIUM	44.9
KELLOGG'S, EGGO, Waffles, Homestyle",	LOW	39.8
KELLOGG'S, EGGO, Waffles, Strawberry",	MEDIUM	41.6
KELLOGG'S, POP-TARTS MINI CRISPS, Cinnamon Brown Sugar Baked Bites",	HIGH	79
KELLOGG'S, POP-TARTS MINI CRISPS, Frosted Chocolate Baked Bites",	HIGH	78.9
KELLOGG'S, POP-TARTS MINI CRISPS, Frosted Strawberry Baked Bites",	HIGH	79.1
KELLOGG'S, POP-TARTS, Chocolate Chip Cookie Dough Toaster Pastries",	HIGH	69.4
KELLOGG'S, POP-TARTS, Frosted Apple Strudel Toaster Pastries",	HIGH	70.5
KELLOGG'S, POP-TARTS, Frosted Blueberry Muffin Toaster Pastries",	HIGH	70.9
KELLOGG'S, POP-TARTS, Frosted Cinnamon Roll Toaster Pastries",	HIGH	67.8
KELLOGG'S, POP-TARTS, Frosted Confetti Cake Toaster Pastries",	HIGH	73
KELLOGG'S, POP-TARTS, Frosted Cookies & Creme Toaster Pastries",	HIGH	69.3
KELLOGG'S, POP-TARTS, Frosted Orange Cream Toaster Pastries",	HIGH	70.6
KELLOGG'S, POP-TARTS, Frosted Pumpkin Pie Toaster Pastries",	HIGH	70.6
KELLOGG'S, POP-TARTS, Frosted Spring Berry Toaster Pastries",	HIGH	72.3
KELLOGG'S, POP-TARTS, Frosted Sugar Cookie Toaster Pastries",	HIGH	70.2
KELLOGG'S, POP-TARTS, Frosted Waffle Cone Toaster Pastries",	HIGH	74.3
KELLOGG'S, POP-TARTS, Frosted Wild Fruit Fusion Toaster Pastries",	HIGH	72.3
KELLOGG'S, POP-TARTS, Frosted Wild Grape Toaster Pastries",	HIGH	71.8
KELLOGG'S, POP-TARTS, Frosted Wild Strawberry Toaster Pastries",	HIGH	72.1
KELLOGG'S, POP-TARTS, Gingerbread Toaster Pastries",	HIGH	70.8
KELLOGG'S, POP-TARTS, Ice Cream Shoppe Frosted Hot Fudge Sundae Toaster	HIGH	69.8
KELLOGG'S, POP-TARTS, Ice Cream Shoppe Frosted Ice Creme Sandwich Toast	HIGH	69.4
KELLOGG'S, POP-TARTS, Ice Cream Shoppe Frosted Rainbow Chip Toaster Past	HIGH	70.8
KELLOGG'S, POP-TARTS, Ice Cream Shoppe Frosted Strawberry Milkshake Toas	HIGH	70
KELLOGG'S, POP-TARTS, Ice Cream Shoppe Frosted Vanilla Milkshake Toaster F	HIGH	70.1
KELLOGG'S, POP-TARTS, Yum-azing Vanilla Milkshake Toaster Pastries",	HIGH	70.2
KELLOGG'S, SIMPLY EGGO, Original",	MEDIUM	43.3
KELLOGG'S, SPECIAL K, Cracker Chips, Cheddar",	HIGH	73.7
KELLOGG'S, SPECIAL K, Cracker Chips, Sea Salt",	HIGH	75.4
KELLOGG'S, SPECIAL K, Cracker Chips, Sour Cream & Onion",	HIGH	74.3
KELLOGG'S, SPECIAL K, Cracker Chips, Southwest Ranch",	HIGH	74.8
KELLOGG'S, SPECIAL K, Multigrain Crackers",	HIGH	75.4
KELLOGG'S, SPECIAL K, Savory Herb Crackers",	HIGH	73.8

Food name/ Category (100 g)	Status	Carbs content in g
KFC, biscuit",	MEDIUM	43.55
KFC, Coleslaw",	LOW	15.65
KFC, Crispy Chicken Strips",	LOW	13.66
KFC, Fried Chicken, EXTRA CRISPY, Breast, meat and skin with breading",	LOW	8.47
KFC, Fried Chicken, EXTRA CRISPY, Breast, meat only, skin and breading removed",	LOW	0.25
KFC, Fried Chicken, EXTRA CRISPY, Drumstick, meat and skin with breading",	LOW	7.96
KFC, Fried Chicken, EXTRA CRISPY, Drumstick, meat only, skin and breading removed",	LOW	0
KFC, Fried Chicken, EXTRA CRISPY, Thigh, meat and skin with breading",	LOW	10.3
KFC, Fried Chicken, EXTRA CRISPY, Thigh, meat only, skin and breading removed",	LOW	0
KFC, Fried Chicken, EXTRA CRISPY, Wing, meat and skin with breading",	LOW	11.66
KFC, Fried Chicken, EXTRA CRISPY, Wing, meat only, skin and breading removed",	LOW	2.97
KFC, Fried Chicken, ORIGINAL RECIPE, Breast, meat and skin with breading",	LOW	6.28
KFC, Fried Chicken, ORIGINAL RECIPE, Breast, meat only, skin and breading removed",	LOW	0
KFC, Fried Chicken, ORIGINAL RECIPE, Drumstick, meat and skin with breading",	LOW	5.39
KFC, Fried Chicken, ORIGINAL RECIPE, Drumstick, meat only, skin and breading removed",	LOW	0.11
KFC, Fried Chicken, ORIGINAL RECIPE, Thigh, meat and skin with breading",	LOW	8.46
KFC, Fried Chicken, ORIGINAL RECIPE, Thigh, meat only, skin and breading removed",	LOW	0.01
KFC, Fried Chicken, ORIGINAL RECIPE, Wing, meat and skin with breading",	LOW	9.93
KFC, Fried Chicken, ORIGINAL RECIPE, Wing, meat only, skin and breading removed",	LOW	1.76
KFC, Popcorn Chicken",	LOW	21.18
Kielbasa, fully cooked, grilled",	LOW	5.03
Kielbasa, fully cooked, pan-fried",	LOW	4.78
Kielbasa, fully cooked, unheated",	LOW	3.72
Kielbasa, Polish, turkey and beef, smoked",	LOW	3.9
Kiwifruit, green, raw",	LOW	14.66
Kiwifruit, ZESPRI SunGold, raw",	LOW	15.79
Kohlrabi, cooked, boiled, drained, with salt",	LOW	6.69
KRAFT BREAKSTONE'S FREE Fat Free Sour Cream",	LOW	15.1

Food name/ Category (100 g)	Status	Carbs content in g
KRAFT BREAKSTONE'S Reduced Fat Sour Cream",	LOW	6.5
KRAFT CHEEZ WHIZ LIGHT Pasteurized Process Cheese Product",	LOW	16.2
KRAFT CHEEZ WHIZ Pasteurized Process Cheese Sauce",	LOW	9.2
KRAFT FREE Singles American Nonfat Pasteurized Process Cheese Product",	LOW	11.7
KRAFT VELVEETA LIGHT Reduced Fat Pasteurized Process Cheese Product",	LOW	11.8
KRAFT VELVEETA Pasteurized Process Cheese Spread",	LOW	9.8
KRAFT, STOVE TOP Stuffing Mix Chicken Flavor",	HIGH	73.1
Lamb, Australian, ground, 85% lean \/ 15% fat, raw",	LOW	0
Lamb, Australian, imported, fresh, composite of trimmed retail cuts, separable lean and fat, trimmed to 1\/8\" fat, cooked",	LOW	0
Lamb, Australian, imported, fresh, composite of trimmed retail cuts, separable lean and fat, trimmed to 1\/8\" fat, raw",	LOW	0
Lamb, Australian, imported, fresh, composite of trimmed retail cuts, separable lean only, trimmed to 1\/8\" fat, cooked",	LOW	0
Lamb, Australian, imported, fresh, composite of trimmed retail cuts, separable lean only, trimmed to 1\/8\" fat, raw",	LOW	0
Lamb, Australian, imported, fresh, external fat, cooked",	LOW	0
Lamb, Australian, imported, fresh, foreshank, separable lean and fat, trimmed to 1\/8\" fat, cooked, braised",	LOW	0
Lamb, Australian, imported, fresh, foreshank, separable lean and fat, trimmed to 1\/8\" fat, raw",	LOW	0
Lamb, Australian, imported, fresh, foreshank, separable lean only, trimmed to 1\/8\" fat, cooked, braised",	LOW	0
Lamb, Australian, imported, fresh, foreshank, separable lean only, trimmed to 1\/8\" fat, raw",	LOW	0
Lamb, Australian, imported, fresh, leg, bottom, boneless, separable lean and fat, trimmed to 1\/8\" fat, cooked, roasted",	LOW	0
Lamb, Australian, imported, fresh, leg, bottom, boneless, separable lean and fat, trimmed to 1\/8\" fat, raw",	LOW	0
Lamb, Australian, imported, fresh, leg, bottom, boneless, separable lean only, trimmed to 1\/8\" fat, cooked, roasted",	LOW	0
Lamb, Australian, imported, fresh, leg, bottom, boneless, separable lean only, trimmed to 1\/8\" fat, raw",	LOW	0
Lamb, Australian, imported, fresh, leg, center slice, bone-in, separable lean and fat, trimmed to 1\/8\" fat, cooked, broiled",	LOW	0
Lamb, Australian, imported, fresh, leg, center slice, bone-in, separable lean and fat, trimmed to 1\/8\" fat, raw",	LOW	0
Lamb, Australian, imported, fresh, leg, center slice, bone-in, separable lean only, trimmed to 1\/8\" fat, cooked, broiled",	LOW	0
Lamb, Australian, imported, fresh, leg, center slice, bone-in, separable lean only, trimmed to 1\/8\" fat, raw",	LOW	0
Lamb, Australian, imported, fresh, leg, hindshank, heel on, bone-in, separable lean and fat, trimmed to 1\/8\" fat, cooked, braised",	LOW	0
Lamb, Australian, imported, fresh, leg, hindshank, heel on, bone-in, separable lean and fat, trimmed to 1\/8\" fat, raw",	LOW	0
Lamb, Australian, imported, fresh, leg, hindshank, heel on, bone-in, separable lean only, trimmed to 1\/8\" fat, cooked, braised",	LOW	0

Food name/ Category (100 g)	Status	Carbs content in g
Lamb, Australian, imported, fresh, leg, hindshank, heel on, bone-in, separable lean only, trimmed to 1\/8\" fat, raw",	LOW	0
Lamb, Australian, imported, fresh, leg, shank half, separable lean and fat, trimmed to 1\/8\" fat, cooked, roasted",	LOW	0
Lamb, Australian, imported, fresh, leg, shank half, separable lean and fat, trimmed to 1\/8\" fat, raw",	LOW	0
Lamb, Australian, imported, fresh, leg, shank half, separable lean only, trimmed to 1\/8\" fat, cooked, roasted",	LOW	0
Lamb, Australian, imported, fresh, leg, shank half, separable lean only, trimmed to 1\/8\" fat, raw",	LOW	0
Lamb, Australian, imported, fresh, leg, sirloin chops, boneless, separable lean and fat, trimmed to 1\/8\" fat, cooked, broiled",	LOW	0
Lamb, Australian, imported, fresh, leg, sirloin chops, boneless, separable lean and fat, trimmed to 1\/8\" fat, raw",	LOW	0
Lamb, Australian, imported, fresh, leg, sirloin chops, boneless, separable lean only, trimmed to 1\/8\" fat, cooked, broiled",	LOW	0
Lamb, Australian, imported, fresh, leg, sirloin chops, boneless, separable lean only, trimmed to 1\/8\" fat, raw",	LOW	0
Lamb, Australian, imported, fresh, leg, sirloin half, boneless, separable lean and fat, trimmed to 1\/8\" fat, cooked, roasted",	LOW	0
Lamb, Australian, imported, fresh, leg, sirloin half, boneless, separable lean and fat, trimmed to 1\/8\" fat, raw",	LOW	0
Lamb, Australian, imported, fresh, leg, sirloin half, boneless, separable lean only, trimmed to 1\/8\" fat, cooked, roasted",	LOW	0
Lamb, Australian, imported, fresh, leg, sirloin half, boneless, separable lean only, trimmed to 1\/8\" fat, raw",	LOW	0
Lamb, Australian, imported, fresh, leg, trotter off, bone-in, separable lean and fat, trimmed to 1\/8\" fat, cooked, roasted",	LOW	**0.08**
Lamb, Australian, imported, fresh, leg, trotter off, bone-in, separable lean and fat, trimmed to 1\/8\" fat, raw",	LOW	0
Lamb, Australian, imported, fresh, leg, trotter off, bone-in, separable lean only, trimmed to 1\/8\" fat, cooked, roasted",	LOW	0
Lamb, Australian, imported, fresh, leg, trotter off, bone-in, separable lean only, trimmed to 1\/8\" fat, raw",	LOW	0
Lamb, Australian, imported, fresh, leg, whole (shank and sirloin), separable lean and fat, trimmed to 1\/8\" fat, cooked, roasted",	LOW	0
Lamb, Australian, imported, fresh, leg, whole (shank and sirloin), separable lean and fat, trimmed to 1\/8\" fat, raw",	LOW	0
Lamb, Australian, imported, fresh, leg, whole (shank and sirloin), separable lean only, trimmed to 1\/8\" fat, cooked, roasted",	LOW	0
Lamb, Australian, imported, fresh, leg, whole (shank and sirloin), separable lean only, trimmed to 1\/8\" fat, raw",	LOW	0
Lamb, Australian, imported, fresh, loin, separable lean and fat, trimmed to 1\/8\" fat, cooked, broiled",	LOW	0
Lamb, Australian, imported, fresh, loin, separable lean and fat, trimmed to 1\/8\" fat, raw",	LOW	0
Lamb, Australian, imported, fresh, loin, separable lean only, trimmed to 1\/8\" fat, cooked, broiled",	LOW	0
Lamb, Australian, imported, fresh, loin, separable lean only, trimmed to 1\/8\" fat, raw",	LOW	0
Lamb, Australian, imported, fresh, rack, roast, frenched, bone-in, separable lean and fat, trimmed to 1\/8\" fat, cooked, roasted",	LOW	0
Lamb, Australian, imported, fresh, rack, roast, frenched, bone-in, separable lean only, trimmed to 1\/8\" fat, cooked, roasted",	LOW	0
Lamb, Australian, imported, fresh, rack, roast, frenched, denuded, bone-in, separable lean and fat, trimmed to 0\" fat, cooked, roasted",	LOW	0

Food name/ Category (100 g)	Status	Carbs content in g
Lamb, Australian, imported, fresh, rack, roast, frenched, denuded, bone-in, separable lean only, trimmed to 0\" fat, cooked, roasted",	LOW	0
Lamb, Australian, imported, fresh, rib chop, frenched, bone-in, separable lean and fat, trimmed to 1\/8\" fat, cooked, grilled",	LOW	0
Lamb, Australian, imported, fresh, rib chop, frenched, bone-in, separable lean only, trimmed to 1\/8\" fat, cooked, grilled",	LOW	0
Lamb, Australian, imported, fresh, rib chop, frenched, denuded, bone-in, separable lean and fat, trimmed to 0\" fat, cooked, grilled",	LOW	0
Lamb, Australian, imported, fresh, rib chop, frenched, denuded, bone-in, separable lean only, trimmed to 0\" fat, cooked, grilled",	LOW	0
Lamb, Australian, imported, fresh, rib chop\/rack roast, frenched, bone-in, separable lean and fat, trimmed to 1\/8\" fat, raw",	LOW	0
Lamb, Australian, imported, fresh, rib chop\/rack roast, frenched, bone-in, separable lean only, trimmed to 1\/8\" fat, raw",	LOW	0
Lamb, Australian, imported, fresh, separable fat, cooked",	LOW	0
Lamb, Australian, imported, fresh, shoulder ,blade, separable lean only, trimmed to 1\/8\" fat, cooked, broiled",	LOW	0
Lamb, Australian, imported, fresh, shoulder, arm, separable lean and fat, trimmed to 1\/8\" fat, cooked, braised",	LOW	0
Lamb, Australian, imported, fresh, shoulder, arm, separable lean and fat, trimmed to 1\/8\" fat, raw",	LOW	0
Lamb, Australian, imported, fresh, shoulder, arm, separable lean only, trimmed to 1\/8\" fat, cooked, braised",	LOW	0
Lamb, Australian, imported, fresh, shoulder, arm, separable lean only, trimmed to 1\/8\" fat, raw",	LOW	0
Lamb, Australian, imported, fresh, shoulder, blade, separable lean and fat, trimmed to 1\/8\" fat, cooked, broiled",	LOW	0
Lamb, Australian, imported, fresh, shoulder, blade, separable lean and fat, trimmed to 1\/8\" fat, raw",	LOW	0
Lamb, Australian, imported, fresh, shoulder, blade, separable lean only, trimmed to 1\/8\" fat, raw",	LOW	0
Lamb, Australian, imported, fresh, shoulder, whole (arm and blade), separable lean and fat, trimmed to 1\/8\" fat, cooked",	LOW	0
Lamb, Australian, imported, fresh, shoulder, whole (arm and blade), separable lean and fat, trimmed to 1\/8\" fat, raw",	LOW	0
Lamb, Australian, imported, fresh, shoulder, whole (arm and blade), separable lean only, trimmed to 1\/8\" fat, cooked",	LOW	0
Lamb, Australian, imported, fresh, shoulder, whole (arm and blade), separable lean only, trimmed to 1\/8\" fat, raw",	LOW	0
Lamb, Australian, imported, fresh, tenderloin, boneless, separable lean and fat, trimmed to 1\/8\" fat, cooked, roasted",	LOW	0
Lamb, Australian, imported, fresh, tenderloin, boneless, separable lean and fat, trimmed to 1\/8\" fat, raw",	LOW	0
Lamb, Australian, imported, fresh, tenderloin, boneless, separable lean only, trimmed to 1\/8\" fat, cooked, roasted",	LOW	0
Lamb, Australian, imported, fresh, tenderloin, boneless, separable lean only, trimmed to 1\/8\" fat, raw",	LOW	0
Lamb, domestic, composite of trimmed retail cuts, separable fat, trimmed to 1\/4\" fat, choice, cooked",	LOW	0
Lamb, domestic, composite of trimmed retail cuts, separable lean and fat, trimmed to 1\/4\" fat, choice, cooked",	LOW	0
Lamb, domestic, composite of trimmed retail cuts, separable lean and fat, trimmed to 1\/4\" fat, choice, raw",	LOW	0
Lamb, domestic, composite of trimmed retail cuts, separable lean and fat, trimmed to 1\/8\" fat, choice, cooked",	LOW	0

Food name/ Category (100 g)	Status	Carbs content in g
Lamb, domestic, composite of trimmed retail cuts, separable lean and fat, trimmed to 1\/8\" fat, choice, raw",	LOW	0
Lamb, domestic, composite of trimmed retail cuts, separable lean only, trimmed to 1\/4\" fat, choice, cooked",	LOW	0
Lamb, domestic, composite of trimmed retail cuts, separable lean only, trimmed to 1\/4\" fat, choice, raw",	LOW	0
Lamb, domestic, cubed for stew or kabob (leg and shoulder), separable lean only, trimmed to 1\/4\" fat, cooked, braised",	LOW	0
Lamb, domestic, cubed for stew or kabob (leg and shoulder), separable lean only, trimmed to 1\/4\" fat, cooked, broiled",	LOW	0
Lamb, domestic, cubed for stew or kabob (leg and shoulder), separable lean only, trimmed to 1\/4\" fat, raw",	LOW	0
Lamb, domestic, foreshank, separable lean and fat, trimmed to 1\/4\" fat, choice, cooked, braised",	LOW	0
Lamb, domestic, foreshank, separable lean and fat, trimmed to 1\/4\" fat, choice, raw",	LOW	0
Lamb, domestic, foreshank, separable lean and fat, trimmed to 1\/8\" fat, choice, raw",	LOW	0
Lamb, domestic, foreshank, separable lean and fat, trimmed to 1\/8\" fat, cooked, braised",	LOW	0
Lamb, domestic, foreshank, separable lean only, trimmed to 1\/4\" fat, choice, cooked, braised",	LOW	0
Lamb, domestic, foreshank, separable lean only, trimmed to 1\/4\" fat, choice, raw",	LOW	0
Lamb, domestic, leg, shank half, separable lean and fat, trimmed to 1\/4\" fat, choice, cooked, roasted",	LOW	0
Lamb, domestic, leg, shank half, separable lean and fat, trimmed to 1\/4\" fat, choice, raw",	LOW	0
Lamb, domestic, leg, shank half, separable lean and fat, trimmed to 1\/8\" fat, choice, cooked, roasted",	LOW	0
Lamb, domestic, leg, shank half, separable lean and fat, trimmed to 1\/8\" fat, choice, raw",	LOW	0
Lamb, domestic, leg, shank half, separable lean only, trimmed to 1\/4\" fat, choice, cooked, roasted",	LOW	0
Lamb, domestic, leg, shank half, separable lean only, trimmed to 1\/4\" fat, choice, raw",	LOW	0
Lamb, domestic, leg, sirloin half, separable lean and fat, trimmed to 1\/4\" fat, choice, cooked, roasted",	LOW	0
Lamb, domestic, leg, sirloin half, separable lean and fat, trimmed to 1\/4\" fat, choice, raw",	LOW	0
Lamb, domestic, leg, sirloin half, separable lean and fat, trimmed to 1\/8\" fat, choice, cooked, roasted",	LOW	0
Lamb, domestic, leg, sirloin half, separable lean and fat, trimmed to 1\/8\" fat, choice, raw",	LOW	0
Lamb, domestic, leg, sirloin half, separable lean only, trimmed to 1\/4\" fat, choice, cooked, roasted",	LOW	0
Lamb, domestic, leg, sirloin half, separable lean only, trimmed to 1\/4\" fat, choice, raw",	LOW	0
Lamb, domestic, leg, whole (shank and sirloin), separable lean and fat, trimmed to 1\/4\" fat, choice, cooked, roasted",	LOW	0
Lamb, domestic, leg, whole (shank and sirloin), separable lean and fat, trimmed to 1\/4\" fat, choice, raw",	LOW	0
Lamb, domestic, leg, whole (shank and sirloin), separable lean and fat, trimmed to 1\/8\" fat, choice, cooked, roasted",	LOW	0
Lamb, domestic, leg, whole (shank and sirloin), separable lean and fat, trimmed to 1\/8\" fat, choice, raw",	LOW	0

Food name/ Category (100 g)	Status	Carbs content in g
Lamb, domestic, leg, whole (shank and sirloin), separable lean only, trimmed to 1\/4\" fat, choice, cooked, roasted",	LOW	0
Lamb, domestic, leg, whole (shank and sirloin), separable lean only, trimmed to 1\/4\" fat, choice, raw",	LOW	0
Lamb, domestic, loin, separable lean and fat, trimmed to 1\/4\" fat, choice, cooked, broiled",	LOW	0
Lamb, domestic, loin, separable lean and fat, trimmed to 1\/4\" fat, choice, cooked, roasted",	LOW	0
Lamb, domestic, loin, separable lean and fat, trimmed to 1\/4\" fat, choice, raw",	LOW	0
Lamb, domestic, loin, separable lean and fat, trimmed to 1\/8\" fat, choice, cooked, broiled",	LOW	0
Lamb, domestic, loin, separable lean and fat, trimmed to 1\/8\" fat, choice, cooked, roasted",	LOW	0
Lamb, domestic, loin, separable lean and fat, trimmed to 1\/8\" fat, choice, raw",	LOW	0
Lamb, domestic, loin, separable lean only, trimmed to 1\/4\" fat, choice, cooked, broiled",	LOW	0
Lamb, domestic, loin, separable lean only, trimmed to 1\/4\" fat, choice, cooked, roasted",	LOW	0
Lamb, domestic, loin, separable lean only, trimmed to 1\/4\" fat, choice, raw",	LOW	0
Lamb, domestic, rib, separable lean and fat, trimmed to 1\/4\" fat, choice, cooked, broiled",	LOW	0
Lamb, domestic, rib, separable lean and fat, trimmed to 1\/4\" fat, choice, cooked, roasted",	LOW	0
Lamb, domestic, rib, separable lean and fat, trimmed to 1\/4\" fat, choice, raw",	LOW	0
Lamb, domestic, rib, separable lean and fat, trimmed to 1\/8\" fat, choice, cooked, broiled",	LOW	0
Lamb, domestic, rib, separable lean and fat, trimmed to 1\/8\" fat, choice, cooked, roasted",	LOW	0
Lamb, domestic, rib, separable lean and fat, trimmed to 1\/8\" fat, choice, raw",	LOW	0
Lamb, domestic, rib, separable lean only, trimmed to 1\/4\" fat, choice, cooked, broiled",	LOW	0
Lamb, domestic, rib, separable lean only, trimmed to 1\/4\" fat, choice, cooked, roasted",	LOW	0
Lamb, domestic, rib, separable lean only, trimmed to 1\/4\" fat, choice, raw",	LOW	0
Lamb, domestic, shoulder, arm, separable lean and fat, trimmed to 1\/4\" fat, choice, cooked, braised",	LOW	0
Lamb, domestic, shoulder, arm, separable lean and fat, trimmed to 1\/4\" fat, choice, cooked, broiled",	LOW	0
Lamb, domestic, shoulder, arm, separable lean and fat, trimmed to 1\/4\" fat, choice, cooked, roasted",	LOW	0
Lamb, domestic, shoulder, arm, separable lean and fat, trimmed to 1\/4\" fat, choice, raw",	LOW	0
Lamb, domestic, shoulder, arm, separable lean and fat, trimmed to 1\/8\" fat, choice, cooked, braised",	LOW	0
Lamb, domestic, shoulder, arm, separable lean and fat, trimmed to 1\/8\" fat, choice, raw",	LOW	0
Lamb, domestic, shoulder, arm, separable lean and fat, trimmed to 1\/8\" fat, choice, roasted",	LOW	0
Lamb, domestic, shoulder, arm, separable lean and fat, trimmed to 1\/8\" fat, cooked, broiled",	LOW	0

Food name/ Category (100 g)	Status	Carbs content in g
Lamb, domestic, shoulder, arm, separable lean only, trimmed to 1\/4\" fat, choice, cooked, braised",	LOW	0
Lamb, domestic, shoulder, arm, separable lean only, trimmed to 1\/4\" fat, choice, cooked, broiled",	LOW	0
Lamb, domestic, shoulder, arm, separable lean only, trimmed to 1\/4\" fat, choice, cooked, roasted",	LOW	0
Lamb, domestic, shoulder, arm, separable lean only, trimmed to 1\/4\" fat, choice, raw",	LOW	0
Lamb, domestic, shoulder, blade, separable lean and fat, trimmed to 1\/4\" fat, choice, cooked, braised",	LOW	0
Lamb, domestic, shoulder, blade, separable lean and fat, trimmed to 1\/4\" fat, choice, cooked, broiled",	LOW	0
Lamb, domestic, shoulder, blade, separable lean and fat, trimmed to 1\/4\" fat, choice, cooked, roasted",	LOW	0
Lamb, domestic, shoulder, blade, separable lean and fat, trimmed to 1\/4\" fat, choice, raw",	LOW	0
Lamb, domestic, shoulder, blade, separable lean and fat, trimmed to 1\/8\" fat, choice, cooked, braised",	LOW	0
Lamb, domestic, shoulder, blade, separable lean and fat, trimmed to 1\/8\" fat, choice, cooked, broiled",	LOW	0
Lamb, domestic, shoulder, blade, separable lean and fat, trimmed to 1\/8\" fat, choice, cooked, roasted",	LOW	0
Lamb, domestic, shoulder, blade, separable lean and fat, trimmed to 1\/8\" fat, choice, raw",	LOW	0
Lamb, domestic, shoulder, blade, separable lean only, trimmed to 1\/4\" fat, choice, cooked, braised",	LOW	0
Lamb, domestic, shoulder, blade, separable lean only, trimmed to 1\/4\" fat, choice, cooked, broiled",	LOW	0
Lamb, domestic, shoulder, blade, separable lean only, trimmed to 1\/4\" fat, choice, cooked, roasted",	LOW	0
Lamb, domestic, shoulder, blade, separable lean only, trimmed to 1\/4\" fat, choice, raw",	LOW	0
Lamb, domestic, shoulder, whole (arm and blade), separable lean and fat, trimmed to 1\/4\" fat, choice, cooked, braised",	LOW	0
Lamb, domestic, shoulder, whole (arm and blade), separable lean and fat, trimmed to 1\/4\" fat, choice, cooked, broiled",	LOW	0
Lamb, domestic, shoulder, whole (arm and blade), separable lean and fat, trimmed to 1\/4\" fat, choice, cooked, roasted",	LOW	0
Lamb, domestic, shoulder, whole (arm and blade), separable lean and fat, trimmed to 1\/4\" fat, choice, raw",	LOW	0
Lamb, domestic, shoulder, whole (arm and blade), separable lean and fat, trimmed to 1\/8\" fat, choice, cooked, braised",	LOW	0
Lamb, domestic, shoulder, whole (arm and blade), separable lean and fat, trimmed to 1\/8\" fat, choice, cooked, broiled",	LOW	0
Lamb, domestic, shoulder, whole (arm and blade), separable lean and fat, trimmed to 1\/8\" fat, choice, cooked, roasted",	LOW	0
Lamb, domestic, shoulder, whole (arm and blade), separable lean and fat, trimmed to 1\/8\" fat, choice, raw",	LOW	0
Lamb, domestic, shoulder, whole (arm and blade), separable lean only, trimmed to 1\/4\" fat, choice, cooked, braised",	LOW	0
Lamb, domestic, shoulder, whole (arm and blade), separable lean only, trimmed to 1\/4\" fat, choice, cooked, broiled",	LOW	0
Lamb, domestic, shoulder, whole (arm and blade), separable lean only, trimmed to 1\/4\" fat, choice, cooked, roasted",	LOW	0
Lamb, domestic, shoulder, whole (arm and blade), separable lean only, trimmed to 1\/4\" fat, choice, raw",	LOW	0

Food name/ Category (100 g)	Status	Carbs content in g
Lamb, ground, cooked, broiled",	LOW	0
Lamb, ground, raw",	LOW	0
Lamb, New Zealand, imported, brains, cooked, soaked and fried",	LOW	0
Lamb, New Zealand, imported, brains, raw",	LOW	0
Lamb, New Zealand, imported, breast, separable lean only, cooked, braised",	LOW	0
Lamb, New Zealand, imported, breast, separable lean only, raw",	LOW	1.02
Lamb, New Zealand, imported, chump, boneless, separable lean only, cooked, fast roasted",	LOW	0
Lamb, New Zealand, imported, chump, boneless, separable lean only, raw",	LOW	0
Lamb, New Zealand, imported, flap, boneless, separable lean and fat, cooked, braised",	LOW	0.14
Lamb, New Zealand, imported, flap, boneless, separable lean and fat, raw",	LOW	0.27
Lamb, New Zealand, imported, flap, boneless, separable lean only, cooked, braised",	LOW	0
Lamb, New Zealand, imported, flap, boneless, separable lean only, raw",	LOW	0
Lamb, New Zealand, imported, fore-shank, separable lean and fat, cooked, braised",	LOW	0.03
Lamb, New Zealand, imported, fore-shank, separable lean and fat, raw",	LOW	0.09
Lamb, New Zealand, imported, fore-shank, separable lean only, cooked, braised",	LOW	0
Lamb, New Zealand, imported, fore-shank, separable lean only, raw",	LOW	0
Lamb, New Zealand, imported, frozen, composite of trimmed retail cuts, separable lean and fat, cooked",	LOW	0
Lamb, New Zealand, imported, frozen, composite of trimmed retail cuts, separable lean and fat, raw",	LOW	0
Lamb, New Zealand, imported, frozen, composite of trimmed retail cuts, separable lean and fat, trimmed to 1\/8\" fat, cooked",	LOW	0
Lamb, New Zealand, imported, frozen, composite of trimmed retail cuts, separable lean and fat, trimmed to 1\/8\" fat, raw",	LOW	0
Lamb, New Zealand, imported, frozen, composite of trimmed retail cuts, separable lean only, cooked",	LOW	0
Lamb, New Zealand, imported, frozen, composite of trimmed retail cuts, separable lean only, raw",	LOW	0
Lamb, New Zealand, imported, frozen, foreshank, separable lean and fat, trimmed to 1\/8\" fat, cooked, braised",	LOW	0
Lamb, New Zealand, imported, frozen, foreshank, separable lean and fat, trimmed to 1\/8\" fat, raw",	LOW	0
Lamb, New Zealand, imported, frozen, leg, whole (shank and sirloin), separable lean and fat, cooked, roasted",	LOW	0
Lamb, New Zealand, imported, frozen, leg, whole (shank and sirloin), separable lean and fat, trimmed to 1\/8\" fat, cooked, roasted",	LOW	0
Lamb, New Zealand, imported, frozen, leg, whole (shank and sirloin), separable lean and fat, trimmed to 1\/8\" fat, raw",	LOW	0
Lamb, New Zealand, imported, frozen, leg, whole (shank and sirloin), separable lean only, cooked, roasted",	LOW	0

Food name/ Category (100 g)	Status	Carbs content in g
Lamb, New Zealand, imported, frozen, loin, separable lean and fat, cooked, broiled",	LOW	0
Lamb, New Zealand, imported, frozen, loin, separable lean and fat, trimmed to 1\/8\" fat, cooked, broiled",	LOW	0
Lamb, New Zealand, imported, frozen, loin, separable lean and fat, trimmed to 1\/8\" fat, raw",	LOW	0
Lamb, New Zealand, imported, frozen, loin, separable lean only, cooked, broiled",	LOW	0
Lamb, New Zealand, imported, frozen, rib, separable lean and fat, trimmed to 1\/8\" fat, cooked, roasted",	LOW	0
Lamb, new zealand, imported, frozen, rib, separable lean and fat, trimmed to 1\/8\" fat, raw",	LOW	0
Lamb, New Zealand, imported, frozen, shoulder, whole (arm and blade), separable lean and fat, cooked, braised",	LOW	0
Lamb, New Zealand, imported, frozen, shoulder, whole (arm and blade), separable lean and fat, trimmed to 1\/8\" fat, cooked, braised",	LOW	0
Lamb, New Zealand, imported, frozen, shoulder, whole (arm and blade), separable lean and fat, trimmed to 1\/8\" fat, raw",	LOW	0
Lamb, New Zealand, imported, frozen, shoulder, whole (arm and blade), separable lean only, cooked, braised",	LOW	0
Lamb, New Zealand, imported, ground lamb, raw",	LOW	0
Lamb, New Zealand, imported, heart, cooked, soaked and simmered",	LOW	0
Lamb, New Zealand, imported, heart, raw",	LOW	0
Lamb, New Zealand, imported, hind-shank, separable lean and fat, cooked, braised",	LOW	0.04
Lamb, New Zealand, imported, hind-shank, separable lean and fat, raw",	LOW	0.73
Lamb, New Zealand, imported, hind-shank, separable lean only, cooked, braised",	LOW	0
Lamb, New Zealand, imported, hind-shank, separable lean only, raw",	LOW	0.73
Lamb, New Zealand, imported, kidney, cooked, soaked and fried",	LOW	0.18
Lamb, New Zealand, imported, kidney, raw",	LOW	0.03
Lamb, New Zealand, imported, leg chop\/steak, bone-in, separable lean and fat, cooked, fast fried",	LOW	0.04
Lamb, New Zealand, imported, leg chop\/steak, bone-in, separable lean and fat, raw",	LOW	0.13
Lamb, New Zealand, imported, leg chop\/steak, bone-in, separable lean only, cooked, fast fried",	LOW	0
Lamb, New Zealand, imported, leg chop\/steak, bone-in, separable lean only, raw",	LOW	0
Lamb, New Zealand, imported, liver, cooked, soaked and fried",	LOW	1.48
Lamb, New Zealand, imported, liver, raw",	LOW	2.22
Lamb, New Zealand, imported, loin chop, separable lean and fat, cooked, fast fried",	LOW	0.41
Lamb, New Zealand, imported, loin chop, separable lean and fat, raw",	LOW	0.22
Lamb, New Zealand, imported, loin chop, separable lean only, cooked, fast fried",	LOW	0.41

Food name/ Category (100 g)	Status	Carbs content in g
Lamb, New Zealand, imported, loin chop, separable lean only, raw",	LOW	0
Lamb, New Zealand, imported, loin saddle, separable lean and fat, cooked, fast roasted",	LOW	0.1
Lamb, New Zealand, imported, loin saddle, separable lean and fat, raw",	LOW	0.2
Lamb, New Zealand, imported, loin saddle, separable lean only, cooked, fast roasted",	LOW	0
Lamb, New Zealand, imported, loin saddle, separable lean only, raw",	LOW	0
Lamb, New Zealand, imported, loin, boneless, separable lean and fat, cooked, fast roasted",	LOW	0
Lamb, New Zealand, imported, loin, boneless, separable lean and fat, raw",	LOW	0
Lamb, New Zealand, imported, loin, boneless, separable lean only, cooked, fast roasted",	LOW	0
Lamb, New Zealand, imported, loin, boneless, separable lean only, raw",	LOW	0
Lamb, New Zealand, imported, neck chops, separable lean and fat, cooked, braised",	LOW	0.03
Lamb, New Zealand, imported, neck chops, separable lean and fat, raw",	LOW	0.14
Lamb, New Zealand, imported, neck chops, separable lean only, cooked, braised",	LOW	0
Lamb, New Zealand, imported, neck chops, separable lean only, raw",	LOW	0
Lamb, New Zealand, imported, netted shoulder, rolled, boneless, separable lean and fat, cooked, slow roasted",	LOW	0.05
Lamb, New Zealand, imported, netted shoulder, rolled, boneless, separable lean and fat, raw",	LOW	0.2
Lamb, New Zealand, imported, netted shoulder, rolled, boneless, separable lean only, cooked, slow roasted",	LOW	0
Lamb, New Zealand, imported, netted shoulder, rolled, boneless, separable lean only, raw",	LOW	0
Lamb, New Zealand, imported, rack - fully frenched, separable lean and fat, cooked, fast roasted",	LOW	0.01
Lamb, New Zealand, imported, rack - fully frenched, separable lean and fat, raw",	LOW	0.05
Lamb, New Zealand, imported, rack - fully frenched, separable lean only, cooked, fast roasted",	LOW	0
Lamb, New Zealand, imported, rack - fully frenched, separable lean only, raw",	LOW	0
Lamb, New Zealand, imported, rack - partly frenched, separable lean and fat, cooked, fast roasted",	LOW	0.04
Lamb, New Zealand, imported, rack - partly frenched, separable lean and fat, raw",	LOW	0.13
Lamb, New Zealand, imported, rack - partly frenched, separable lean only, cooked, fast roasted",	LOW	0
Lamb, New Zealand, imported, rack - partly frenched, separable lean only, raw",	LOW	0
Lamb, New Zealand, imported, square-cut shoulder chops, separable lean and fat, cooked, braised",	LOW	0.05
Lamb, New Zealand, imported, square-cut shoulder chops, separable lean and fat, raw",	LOW	0.23
Lamb, New Zealand, imported, square-cut shoulder chops, separable lean only, cooked, braised",	LOW	0

Food name/ Category (100 g)	Status	Carbs content in g
Lamb, New Zealand, imported, square-cut shoulder chops, separable lean only, raw",	LOW	0
Lamb, New Zealand, imported, square-cut shoulder, separable lean and fat, cooked, slow roasted",	LOW	0.03
Lamb, New Zealand, imported, square-cut shoulder, separable lean and fat, raw",	LOW	0.24
Lamb, New Zealand, imported, square-cut shoulder, separable lean only, cooked, slow roasted",	LOW	0
Lamb, New Zealand, imported, square-cut shoulder, separable lean only, raw",	LOW	0
Lamb, New Zealand, imported, sweetbread, cooked, soaked and simmered",	LOW	0
Lamb, New Zealand, imported, sweetbread, raw",	LOW	0
Lamb, New Zealand, imported, tenderloin, separable lean and fat, cooked, fast fried",	LOW	0
Lamb, New Zealand, imported, tenderloin, separable lean and fat, raw",	LOW	0.01
Lamb, New Zealand, imported, tenderloin, separable lean only, cooked, fast fried",	LOW	0
Lamb, New Zealand, imported, tenderloin, separable lean only, raw",	LOW	0
Lamb, New Zealand, imported, testes, cooked, soaked and fried",	LOW	0
Lamb, New Zealand, imported, testes, raw",	LOW	0.14
Lamb, New Zealand, imported, tongue - swiss cut, cooked, soaked and simmered",	LOW	0.86
Lamb, New Zealand, imported, tongue - swiss cut, raw",	LOW	0
Lamb, New Zealand, imported, tunnel-boned leg, chump off, shank off, separable lean and fat, cooked, slow roasted",	LOW	0.03
Lamb, New Zealand, imported, tunnel-boned leg, chump off, shank off, separable lean and fat, raw",	LOW	0
Lamb, New Zealand, imported, tunnel-boned leg, chump off, shank off, separable lean only, cooked, slow roasted",	LOW	0
Lamb, New Zealand, imported, tunnel-boned leg, chump off, shank off, separable lean only, raw",	LOW	0
Lamb, variety meats and by-products, brain, cooked, braised",	LOW	0
Lamb, variety meats and by-products, brain, cooked, pan-fried",	LOW	0
Lamb, variety meats and by-products, brain, raw",	LOW	0
Lamb, variety meats and by-products, heart, cooked, braised",	LOW	1.93
Lamb, variety meats and by-products, heart, raw",	LOW	0.21
Lamb, variety meats and by-products, kidneys, cooked, braised",	LOW	0.99
Lamb, variety meats and by-products, kidneys, raw",	LOW	0.82
Lamb, variety meats and by-products, liver, cooked, braised",	LOW	2.53
Lamb, variety meats and by-products, liver, cooked, pan-fried",	LOW	3.78

Food name/ Category (100 g)	Status	Carbs content in g
Lamb, variety meats and by-products, liver, raw",	LOW	1.78
Lamb, variety meats and by-products, lungs, cooked, braised",	LOW	0
Lamb, variety meats and by-products, lungs, raw",	LOW	0
Lamb, variety meats and by-products, mechanically separated, raw",	LOW	0
Lamb, variety meats and by-products, pancreas, cooked, braised",	LOW	0
Lamb, variety meats and by-products, pancreas, raw",	LOW	0
Lamb, variety meats and by-products, spleen, cooked, braised",	LOW	0
Lamb, variety meats and by-products, spleen, raw",	LOW	0
Lamb, variety meats and by-products, tongue, cooked, braised",	LOW	0
Lamb, variety meats and by-products, tongue, raw",	LOW	0
Lambsquarters, cooked, boiled, drained, with salt",	LOW	5
Lambsquarters, steamed (Northern Plains Indians)",	LOW	7.47
Lard",	LOW	0
Lasagna with meat & sauce, frozen entree",	LOW	14.39
Lasagna with meat & sauce, low-fat, frozen entree",	LOW	13.5
Lasagna with meat sauce, frozen, prepared",	LOW	15.36
Lasagna, cheese, frozen, prepared",	LOW	13.84
Lasagna, cheese, frozen, unprepared",	LOW	21.61
Lasagna, Vegetable, frozen, baked",	LOW	14.18
Lean Pockets, Meatballs & Mozzarella",	LOW	32.28
Leavening agents, baking powder, double-acting, sodium aluminum sulfate",	LOW	27.7
Leavening agents, baking powder, double-acting, straight phosphate",	LOW	24.1
Leavening agents, baking powder, low-sodium",	MEDIUM	46.9
Leavening agents, baking soda",	LOW	0
Leavening agents, cream of tartar",	HIGH	61.5
Leavening agents, yeast, baker's, active dry",	MEDIUM	41.22
Lebanon bologna, beef",	LOW	0.44
Leeks, (bulb and lower leaf-portion), cooked, boiled, drained, with salt",	LOW	7.62
Lemon juice, frozen, unsweetened, single strength",	LOW	6.5

Food name/ Category (100 g)	Status	Carbs content in g
Lemon juice, raw",	LOW	6.9
Lemonade, frozen concentrate, pink",	MEDIUM	48.86
Lemonade, frozen concentrate, white, prepared with water",	LOW	10.42
Lemons, raw, without peel",	LOW	9.32
Lentils, mature seeds, cooked, boiled, with salt",	LOW	19.54
Lentils, mature seeds, cooked, boiled, without salt",	LOW	20.13
Lettuce, butterhead (includes boston and bibb types), raw",	LOW	2.23
Light Ice Cream, soft serve, blended with cookie pieces",	LOW	25.55
Light Ice Cream, soft serve, blended with milk chocolate candies",	LOW	26.82
Lima beans, immature seeds, canned, no salt added, solids and liquids",	LOW	13.33
Lima beans, immature seeds, canned, regular pack, solids and liquids",	LOW	13.33
Lima beans, immature seeds, cooked, boiled, drained, with salt",	LOW	23.64
Lima beans, immature seeds, frozen, baby, cooked, boiled, drained, with salt",	LOW	19.45
Lima beans, immature seeds, frozen, baby, unprepared",	LOW	25.14
Lima beans, immature seeds, frozen, fordhook, cooked, boiled, drained, with salt",	LOW	19.32
Lima beans, immature seeds, frozen, fordhook, cooked, boiled, drained, without salt",	LOW	19.32
Lima beans, immature seeds, frozen, fordhook, unprepared",	LOW	19.83
Lima beans, large, mature seeds, canned",	LOW	14.91
Lima beans, large, mature seeds, cooked, boiled, with salt",	LOW	20.88
Lima beans, large, mature seeds, cooked, boiled, without salt",	LOW	20.88
Lima beans, thin seeded (baby), mature seeds, cooked, boiled, with salt",	LOW	23.31
Lima beans, thin seeded (baby), mature seeds, cooked, boiled, without salt",	LOW	23.31
Lime juice, raw",	LOW	8.42
Limeade, frozen concentrate, prepared with water",	LOW	13.79
Limes, raw",	LOW	10.54
Litchis, dried",	HIGH	70.7
Litchis, raw",	LOW	16.53
LITTLE CAESARS 14\" Cheese Pizza, Large Deep Dish Crust",	LOW	30.1
LITTLE CAESARS 14\" Cheese Pizza, Thin Crust",	LOW	22.85

Food name/ Category (100 g)	Status	Carbs content in g
LITTLE CAESARS 14\" Original Round Cheese Pizza, Regular Crust",	LOW	31.5
LITTLE CAESARS 14\" Original Round Meat and Vegetable Pizza, Regular Crust",	LOW	23.1
LITTLE CAESARS 14\" Original Round Pepperoni Pizza, Regular Crust",	LOW	31.01
LITTLE CAESARS 14\" Pepperoni Pizza, Large Deep Dish Crust",	LOW	29.03
Liverwurst spread",	LOW	5.89
Loganberries, frozen",	LOW	13.02
LOMA LINDA Big Franks, canned, unprepared",	LOW	5.8
LOMA LINDA Linketts, canned, unprepared",	LOW	4.4
LOMA LINDA Little Links, canned, unprepared",	LOW	5.5
LOMA LINDA Low Fat Big Franks, canned, unprepared",	LOW	4.9
LOMA LINDA Redi-Burger, canned, unprepared",	LOW	8.2
LOMA LINDA Swiss Stake with Gravy, canned, unprepared",	LOW	10.4
LOMA LINDA Tender Bits, canned, unprepared",	LOW	8.3
LOMA LINDA Tender Rounds with Gravy, canned, unprepared",	LOW	7.4
LOMA LINDA Vege-Burger, canned, unprepared",	LOW	3.7
Longans, dried",	HIGH	74
Longans, raw",	LOW	15.14
Loquats, raw",	LOW	12.14
Lotus root, cooked, boiled, drained, with salt",	LOW	16.02
Lotus root, cooked, boiled, drained, without salt",	LOW	16.02
Lotus root, raw",	LOW	17.23
Luncheon slices, meatless",	LOW	4.44
Lupins, mature seeds, cooked, boiled, with salt",	LOW	9.29
Lupins, mature seeds, cooked, boiled, without salt",	LOW	9.88
Macaroni and cheese dinner with dry sauce mix, boxed, uncooked",	HIGH	70.12
Macaroni and cheese, box mix with cheese sauce, prepared",	LOW	23.1
Macaroni and cheese, box mix with cheese sauce, unprepared",	MEDIUM	46.66
Macaroni and Cheese, canned entree",	LOW	11.52
Macaroni and Cheese, canned, microwavable",	LOW	13.96

Food name/ Category (100 g)	Status	Carbs content in g
Macaroni and cheese, dry mix, prepared with 2% milk and 80% stick margarine from dry mix",	LOW	23.93
Macaroni and cheese, frozen entree",	LOW	17.28
Macaroni or noodles with cheese, made from reduced fat packaged mix, unprepared	MEDIUM	52.06
Macaroni or noodles with cheese, microwaveable, unprepared",	HIGH	70.75
Macaroni, vegetable, enriched, dry",	HIGH	74.88
Malabar spinach, cooked",	LOW	2.71
Mango nectar, canned",	LOW	13.12
Mangos, raw",	LOW	14.98
Maraschino cherries, canned, drained",	MEDIUM	41.97
Margarine Spread, approximately 48% fat, tub",	LOW	0.86
Margarine-like shortening, industrial, soy (partially hydrogenated), cottonseed, and soy, principal use flaky pastries",	LOW	0
Margarine-like spread with yogurt, 70% fat, stick, with salt",	LOW	0.5
Margarine-like spread with yogurt, approximately 40% fat, tub, with salt",	LOW	2
Margarine-like spread, BENECOL Light Spread",	LOW	5.71
Margarine-like spread, SMART BALANCE Light Buttery Spread",	LOW	1.98
Margarine-like spread, SMART BALANCE Omega Plus Spread (with plant sterols & fish oil)",	LOW	0.16
Margarine-like spread, SMART BALANCE Regular Buttery Spread with flax oil",	LOW	0.14
Margarine-like spread, SMART BEAT Smart Squeeze",	LOW	7.1
Margarine-like spread, SMART BEAT Super Light without saturated fat",	LOW	0
Margarine-like vegetable-oil spread, stick\/tub\/bottle, 60% fat, with added vitamin D",	LOW	0
Margarine-like, margarine-butter blend, soybean oil and butter",	LOW	0.77
Margarine-like, vegetable oil spread, 20% fat, with salt",	LOW	0.4
Margarine-like, vegetable oil spread, 20% fat, without salt",	LOW	0.4
Margarine-like, vegetable oil spread, 60% fat, stick, with salt, with added vitamin D",	LOW	0.69
Margarine-like, vegetable oil spread, 60% fat, stick, with salt",	LOW	0.69
Margarine-like, vegetable oil spread, 60% fat, stick\/tub\/bottle, with salt",	LOW	0
Margarine-like, vegetable oil spread, 60% fat, stick\/tub\/bottle, without salt, with added vitamin D",	LOW	0.86
Margarine-like, vegetable oil spread, 60% fat, stick\/tub\/bottle, without salt",	LOW	0.86
Margarine-like, vegetable oil spread, 60% fat, tub, with salt, with added vitamin D",	LOW	0.86
Margarine-like, vegetable oil spread, 60% fat, tub, with salt",	LOW	0.86

Food name/ Category (100 g)	Status	Carbs content in g
Margarine-like, vegetable oil spread, approximately 37% fat, unspecified oils, with salt, with added vitamin D",	LOW	0.66
Margarine-like, vegetable oil spread, fat free, liquid, with salt",	LOW	2.5
Margarine-like, vegetable oil spread, fat-free, tub",	LOW	4.34
Margarine-like, vegetable oil spread, stick or tub, sweetened",	LOW	16.7
Margarine-like, vegetable oil spread, unspecified oils, approximately 37% fat, with salt",	LOW	0.66
Margarine-like, vegetable oil-butter spread, reduced calorie, tub, with salt",	LOW	1
Margarine-like, vegetable oil-butter spread, tub, with salt",	LOW	1
Margarine, 80% fat, stick, includes regular and hydrogenated corn and soybean oils",	LOW	0.7
Margarine, 80% fat, tub, CANOLA HARVEST Soft Spread (canola, palm and palm kernel oils)",	LOW	1.39
Margarine, industrial, non-dairy, cottonseed, soy oil (partially hydrogenated), for flaky pastries",	LOW	0
Margarine, industrial, soy and partially hydrogenated soy oil, use for baking, sauces and candy",	LOW	0.71
Margarine, margarine-like vegetable oil spread, 67-70% fat, tub",	LOW	0.59
Margarine, margarine-type vegetable oil spread, 70% fat, soybean and partially hydrogenated soybean, stick",	LOW	1.53
Margarine, regular, 80% fat, composite, stick, with salt, with added vitamin D",	LOW	0.7
Margarine, regular, 80% fat, composite, stick, with salt",	LOW	0.7
Margarine, regular, 80% fat, composite, stick, without salt, with added vitamin D",	LOW	0.7
Margarine, regular, 80% fat, composite, stick, without salt",	LOW	0.7
Margarine, regular, 80% fat, composite, tub, with salt, with added vitamin D",	LOW	0.75
Margarine, regular, 80% fat, composite, tub, with salt",	LOW	0.75
Margarine, regular, hard, soybean (hydrogenated)",	LOW	0.9
Marmalade, orange",	HIGH	66.3
MARTHA WHITE FOODS, Martha White's Buttermilk Biscuit Mix, dry",	HIGH	59.41
MARTHA WHITE FOODS, Martha White's Chewy Fudge Brownie Mix, dry",	HIGH	83.58
MARY'S GONE CRACKERS, Original Crackers, Organic Gluten Free",	HIGH	64.29
Mayonnaise dressing, no cholesterol",	LOW	0.3
Mayonnaise, low sodium, low calorie or diet",	LOW	16
Mayonnaise, made with tofu",	LOW	3.06
Mayonnaise, reduced fat, with olive oil",	LOW	0
Mayonnaise, reduced-calorie or diet, cholesterol-free",	LOW	6.7
McDONALD'S, Baked Apple Pie",	MEDIUM	43.62

Food name/ Category (100 g)	Status	Carbs content in g
McDONALD'S, Barbeque Sauce",	LOW	36.93
McDONALD'S, BIG BREAKFAST",	LOW	17.5
McDONALD'S, BIG MAC (without Big Mac Sauce)",	LOW	21.01
McDONALD'S, BIG MAC",	LOW	20.08
McDONALD'S, Cheeseburger",	LOW	27.81
McDONALD'S, Chicken McNUGGETS",	LOW	15.09
McDONALD'S, Creamy Ranch Sauce",	LOW	3.49
McDONALD'S, Deluxe Breakfast, with syrup and margarine",	LOW	29.48
McDONALD'S, Double Cheeseburger",	LOW	18.79
McDONALD'S, DOUBLE QUARTER POUNDER with Cheese",	LOW	14.43
McDONALD'S, Egg McMUFFIN",	LOW	21.67
McDONALD'S, FILET-O-FISH (without tartar sauce)",	LOW	31.08
McDONALD'S, FILET-O-FISH",	LOW	26.39
McDONALD'S, french fries",	MEDIUM	42.58
McDONALD'S, Fruit 'n Yogurt Parfait (without granola)",	LOW	17.67
McDONALD'S, Fruit 'n Yogurt Parfait",	LOW	20.72
McDONALD'S, Hash Brown",	LOW	28.56
McDONALD'S, Hot Caramel Sundae",	LOW	33.36
McDONALD'S, Hot Fudge Sundae",	LOW	30.05
McDONALD'S, Hot Mustard Sauce",	LOW	29.08
McDONALD'S, Hotcakes (plain)",	LOW	38.27
McDONALD'S, Hotcakes (with 2 pats margarine & syrup)",	MEDIUM	46.08
McDONALD'S, Hotcakes and Sausage",	LOW	37.55
McDONALD'S, Low Fat Caramel Sauce",	HIGH	71.53
McDONALD'S, McCHICKEN Sandwich (without mayonnaise)",	LOW	30.95
McDONALD'S, McCHICKEN Sandwich",	LOW	27.97
McDONALD'S, McFLURRY with M&M'S CANDIES",	LOW	26.82
McDONALD'S, McFLURRY with OREO cookies",	LOW	25.55
McDONALD'S, NEWMAN'S OWN Cobb Dressing",	LOW	15.49

Food name/ Category (100 g)	Status	Carbs content in g
McDONALD'S, NEWMAN'S OWN Creamy Caesar Dressing",	LOW	6.85
McDONALD'S, NEWMAN'S OWN Low Fat Balsamic Vinaigrette",	LOW	24.65
McDONALD'S, NEWMAN'S OWN Ranch Dressing",	LOW	16.75
McDONALD'S, Peanuts (for Sundaes)",	LOW	16.23
McDONALD'S, Premium Crispy Chicken Classic Sandwich",	LOW	25.46
McDONALD'S, Premium Crispy Chicken Club Sandwich",	LOW	22.61
McDONALD'S, Premium Crispy Chicken Ranch BLT Sandwich",	LOW	24.93
McDONALD'S, Premium Grilled Chicken Classic Sandwich",	LOW	22.28
McDONALD'S, Premium Grilled Chicken Club Sandwich",	LOW	19.87
McDONALD'S, Premium Grilled Chicken Ranch BLT Sandwich",	LOW	21.91
McDONALD'S, QUARTER POUNDER with Cheese",	LOW	19.95
McDONALD'S, QUARTER POUNDER",	LOW	22.17
McDONALD'S, RANCH SNACK WRAP, Crispy",	LOW	23.22
McDONALD'S, RANCH SNACK WRAP, Grilled",	LOW	18.43
McDONALD'S, Sausage Biscuit with Egg",	LOW	19.28
McDONALD'S, Sausage Biscuit",	LOW	27.2
McDONALD'S, Sausage Burrito",	LOW	22.97
McDONALD'S, Sausage McGRIDDLES",	LOW	31.25
McDONALD'S, Sausage McMUFFIN with Egg",	LOW	17.28
McDONALD'S, Sausage McMUFFIN",	LOW	24.52
McDONALD'S, Sausage, Egg & Cheese McGRIDDLES",	LOW	22.04
McDONALD'S, Southern Style Chicken Biscuit",	LOW	30.56
McDONALD'S, Spicy Buffalo Sauce",	LOW	1.81
McDONALD'S, Strawberry Sundae",	LOW	28.09
McDONALD'S, Sweet 'N Sour Sauce",	LOW	39.38
McDONALD'S, Tangy Honey Mustard Sauce",	LOW	28.81
McDONALD'S, Vanilla Reduced Fat Ice Cream Cone",	LOW	26.36
MCKEE BAKING, LITTLE DEBBIE NUTTY BARS, Wafers with Peanut Butter, Chc	MEDIUM	55.2

Food name/ Category (100 g)	Status	Carbs content in g
Meat drippings (lard, beef tallow, mutton tallow)",	LOW	0
Meatballs, frozen, Italian style",	LOW	8.06
Meatballs, meatless",	LOW	8
Milk and cereal bar",	HIGH	72.05
Milk dessert bar, frozen, made from lowfat milk",	LOW	33.09
Milk dessert, frozen, milk-fat free, chocolate",	LOW	37.7
Milk shakes, thick chocolate",	LOW	21.15
Milk shakes, thick vanilla",	LOW	17.75
Milk substitutes, fluid, with lauric acid oil",	LOW	6.16
Milk, buttermilk, dried",	MEDIUM	49
Milk, buttermilk, fluid, cultured, lowfat",	LOW	4.79
Milk, buttermilk, fluid, cultured, reduced fat",	LOW	5.3
Milk, buttermilk, fluid, whole",	LOW	4.88
Milk, canned, condensed, sweetened",	MEDIUM	54.4
Milk, canned, evaporated, nonfat, with added vitamin A and vitamin D",	LOW	11.35
Milk, canned, evaporated, with added vitamin A",	LOW	10.04
Milk, canned, evaporated, with added vitamin D and without added vitamin A",	LOW	10.04
Milk, canned, evaporated, without added vitamin A and vitamin D",	LOW	10.04
Milk, chocolate beverage, hot cocoa, homemade",	LOW	10.74
Milk, chocolate, fluid, commercial, reduced fat, with added calcium",	LOW	12.13
Milk, chocolate, fluid, commercial, reduced fat, with added vitamin A and vitamin D",	LOW	12.13
Milk, chocolate, fluid, commercial, whole, with added vitamin A and vitamin D",	LOW	10.34
Milk, chocolate, lowfat, with added vitamin A and vitamin D",	LOW	9.86
Milk, dry, nonfat, calcium reduced",	MEDIUM	51.8
Milk, dry, nonfat, instant, with added vitamin A and vitamin D",	MEDIUM	52.19
Milk, dry, nonfat, instant, without added vitamin A and vitamin D",	MEDIUM	52.19
Milk, dry, nonfat, regular, with added vitamin A and vitamin D",	MEDIUM	51.98
Milk, dry, nonfat, regular, without added vitamin A and vitamin D",	MEDIUM	51.98
Milk, dry, whole, with added vitamin D",	LOW	38.42
Milk, dry, whole, without added vitamin D",	LOW	38.42
Milk, evaporated, 2% fat, with added vitamin A and vitamin D",	LOW	15.74
Milk, filled, fluid, with blend of hydrogenated vegetable oils",	LOW	4.74

Food name/ Category (100 g)	Status	Carbs content in g
Milk, filled, fluid, with lauric acid oil",	LOW	4.74
Milk, fluid, 1% fat, without added vitamin A and vitamin D",	LOW	4.99
Milk, fluid, nonfat, calcium fortified (fat free or skim)",	LOW	4.85
Milk, goat, fluid, with added vitamin D",	LOW	4.45
Milk, imitation, non-soy",	LOW	5.3
Milk, indian buffalo, fluid",	LOW	5.18
Milk, low sodium, fluid",	LOW	4.46
Milk, lowfat, fluid, 1% milkfat, protein fortified, with added vitamin A and vitamin D",	LOW	5.52
Milk, lowfat, fluid, 1% milkfat, with added nonfat milk solids, vitamin A and vitamin D",	LOW	4.97
Milk, lowfat, fluid, 1% milkfat, with added vitamin A and vitamin D",	LOW	4.99
Milk, nonfat, fluid, protein fortified, with added vitamin A and vitamin D (fat free and skim)",	LOW	5.56
Milk, nonfat, fluid, with added nonfat milk solids, vitamin A and vitamin D (fat free or skim)",	LOW	5.02
Milk, nonfat, fluid, with added vitamin A and vitamin D (fat free or skim)",	LOW	4.96
Milk, nonfat, fluid, without added vitamin A and vitamin D (fat free or skim)",	LOW	4.96
Milk, producer, fluid, 3.7% milkfat",	LOW	4.65
Milk, reduced fat, fluid, 2% milkfat, protein fortified, with added vitamin A and vitamin D",	LOW	5.49
Milk, reduced fat, fluid, 2% milkfat, with added nonfat milk solids and vitamin A and vitamin D",	LOW	4.97
Milk, reduced fat, fluid, 2% milkfat, with added nonfat milk solids, without added vitamin A",	LOW	5.49
Milk, reduced fat, fluid, 2% milkfat, with added vitamin A and vitamin D",	LOW	4.8
Milk, reduced fat, fluid, 2% milkfat, without added vitamin A and vitamin D",	LOW	4.8
Milk, sheep, fluid",	LOW	5.36
Milk, whole, 3.25% milkfat, with added vitamin D",	LOW	4.8
Milk, whole, 3.25% milkfat, without added vitamin A and vitamin D",	LOW	4.78
Millet flour",	HIGH	75.12
Millet, cooked",	LOW	23.67
Millet, puffed",	HIGH	80
Millet, raw",	HIGH	72.85
Miso",	LOW	25.37
MISSION FOODS, MISSION Flour Tortillas, Soft Taco, 8 inch",	MEDIUM	49.6
Molasses",	HIGH	74.73

Food name/ Category (100 g)	Status	Carbs content in g
Mollusks, abalone, mixed species, cooked, fried",	LOW	11.05
Mollusks, abalone, mixed species, raw",	LOW	6.01
Mollusks, clam, mixed species, canned, drained solids",	LOW	5.9
Mollusks, clam, mixed species, canned, liquid",	LOW	0.1
Mollusks, clam, mixed species, cooked, breaded and fried",	LOW	10.33
Mollusks, clam, mixed species, cooked, moist heat",	LOW	5.13
Mollusks, clam, mixed species, raw",	LOW	3.57
Mollusks, conch, baked or broiled",	LOW	1.7
Mollusks, cuttlefish, mixed species, cooked, moist heat",	LOW	1.64
Mollusks, cuttlefish, mixed species, raw",	LOW	0.82
Mollusks, mussel, blue, cooked, moist heat",	LOW	7.39
Mollusks, mussel, blue, raw",	LOW	3.69
Mollusks, octopus, common, cooked, moist heat",	LOW	4.4
Mollusks, octopus, common, raw",	LOW	2.2
Mollusks, oyster, eastern, canned",	LOW	3.91
Mollusks, oyster, eastern, cooked, breaded and fried",	LOW	11.62
Mollusks, oyster, eastern, farmed, cooked, dry heat",	LOW	7.28
Mollusks, oyster, eastern, farmed, raw",	LOW	5.53
Mollusks, oyster, eastern, wild, cooked, dry heat",	LOW	4.23
Mollusks, oyster, eastern, wild, cooked, moist heat",	LOW	5.45
Mollusks, oyster, eastern, wild, raw",	LOW	2.72
Mollusks, oyster, Pacific, cooked, moist heat",	LOW	9.9
Mollusks, oyster, Pacific, raw",	LOW	4.95
Mollusks, scallop, (bay and sea), cooked, steamed",	LOW	5.41
Mollusks, scallop, mixed species, cooked, breaded and fried",	LOW	10.13
Mollusks, scallop, mixed species, imitation, made from surimi",	LOW	10.62
Mollusks, scallop, mixed species, raw",	LOW	3.18
Mollusks, snail, raw",	LOW	2

Food name/ Category (100 g)	Status	Carbs content in g
Mollusks, squid, mixed species, cooked, fried",	LOW	7.79
Mollusks, squid, mixed species, raw",	LOW	3.08
Mollusks, whelk, unspecified, cooked, moist heat",	LOW	15.52
Mollusks, whelk, unspecified, raw",	LOW	7.76
MORI-NU, Tofu, silken, extra firm",	LOW	2
MORI-NU, Tofu, silken, firm",	LOW	2.4
MORI-NU, Tofu, silken, lite extra firm",	LOW	1
MORI-NU, Tofu, silken, lite firm",	LOW	1.1
MORI-NU, Tofu, silken, soft",	LOW	2.9
MORNINGSTAR FARMS Asian Veggie Patties, frozen, unprepared",	LOW	18.2
MORNINGSTAR FARMS BBQ Riblets, frozen, unprepared",	LOW	24.6
MORNINGSTAR FARMS Breakfast Biscuit Sausage, Egg & Cheese, frozen, unprepared",	LOW	37.5
MORNINGSTAR FARMS Breakfast Pattie with Organic Soy, frozen, unprepared",	LOW	12.6
MORNINGSTAR FARMS Breakfast Pattie, frozen, unprepared",	LOW	12.6
MORNINGSTAR FARMS Breakfast Sausage Links, frozen, unprepared",	LOW	6.8
MORNINGSTAR FARMS Breakfast Sausage Patties, frozen, unprepared",	LOW	8.8
MORNINGSTAR FARMS Buffalo Chik Patties, frozen, unprepared",	LOW	25.2
MORNINGSTAR FARMS Buffalo Wings, frozen, unprepared",	LOW	22.6
MORNINGSTAR FARMS California Turk'y Burger, frozen, unprepared",	LOW	12.6
MORNINGSTAR FARMS Chik Patties Original, frozen, unprepared",	LOW	20.5
MORNINGSTAR FARMS Chik Patties, frozen, unprepared",	LOW	22.9
MORNINGSTAR FARMS Chik'n Grill Veggie Patties, frozen, unprepared",	LOW	10.2
MORNINGSTAR FARMS Chik'n Nuggets, frozen, unprepared",	LOW	21.8
MORNINGSTAR FARMS Chipotle Black Bean Crumbles, frozen, unprepared",	LOW	10.2
MORNINGSTAR FARMS Corn Dog Mini, frozen, unprepared",	LOW	32.6
MORNINGSTAR FARMS Corn Dog, frozen, unprepared",	LOW	36
MORNINGSTAR FARMS Garden Veggie Nuggets, frozen, unprepared",	LOW	16.9
MORNINGSTAR FARMS Garden Veggie Patties, frozen, unprepared",	LOW	13.7

Food name/ Category (100 g)	Status	Carbs content in g
MORNINGSTAR FARMS Grillers Burger Style Recipe Crumbles, frozen, unprepared",	LOW	8.3
MORNINGSTAR FARMS Grillers Chik'n Veggie Patties, frozen, unprepared",	LOW	10.2
MORNINGSTAR FARMS Grillers Original, frozen, unprepared",	LOW	8.5
MORNINGSTAR FARMS Grillers Prime, frozen, unprepared",	LOW	5.9
MORNINGSTAR FARMS Grillers Quarter Pound Veggie Burger, frozen, unprepared",	LOW	8.9
MORNINGSTAR FARMS Grillers Vegan, frozen, unprepared",	LOW	9.1
MORNINGSTAR FARMS Hot and Spicy Veggie Sausage Patties, frozen, unprepared",	LOW	8.5
MORNINGSTAR FARMS Lasagna with Veggie Sausage, frozen, unprepared",	LOW	14.4
MORNINGSTAR FARMS Meal Starters Veggie Meatballs, frozen, unprepared",	LOW	9.9
MORNINGSTAR FARMS Mediterranean Chickpea, frozen, unprepared",	LOW	19.8
MORNINGSTAR FARMS Mushroom Lover's Burger, frozen, unprepared",	LOW	9.2
MORNINGSTAR FARMS Parmesan Garlic Wings, frozen, unprepared",	LOW	24.1
MORNINGSTAR FARMS Pizza, Baja Black Bean, single serve, frozen, unprepared",	LOW	36.9
MORNINGSTAR FARMS Roasted Garlic & Quinoa Burger, frozen, unprepared",	LOW	17.8
MORNINGSTAR FARMS Sausage Style Recipe Crumbles, frozen, unprepared",	LOW	9.9
MORNINGSTAR FARMS Sesame Chik'n Entree, frozen, unprepared",	LOW	17.3
MORNINGSTAR FARMS Spicy Black Bean Burger, frozen, unprepared",	LOW	19.1
MORNINGSTAR FARMS Spicy Black Bean Enchilada Entree, frozen, unprepared",	LOW	15.9
MORNINGSTAR FARMS Spicy Indian Veggie Burger, frozen, unprepared",	LOW	17
MORNINGSTAR FARMS Tomato & Basil Pizza Burger, frozen, unprepared",	LOW	14
MORNINGSTAR FARMS Tuscan Greens & Beans, frozen, unprepared",	LOW	11.7
MORNINGSTAR FARMS Veggie Dog, frozen, unprepared",	LOW	11.2
Mothbeans, mature seeds, cooked, boiled, with salt",	LOW	20.96
MOTHER'S, 4th of July Circus Animal Cookies",	HIGH	68.3
MOTHER'S, Chocolate Chip Cookies",	HIGH	67.6
MOTHER'S, Circus Animal Cookies",	HIGH	68.3
MOTHER'S, Coconut Cocadas Cookies",	HIGH	65.1
MOTHER'S, Double Fudge Creme Sandwich Cookies",	HIGH	70
MOTHER'S, English Tea Sandwich Cookies",	HIGH	71
MOTHER'S, Halloween Circus Animals Cookies",	HIGH	68.1
MOTHER'S, Holiday Circus Animal Cookies",	HIGH	68.3
MOTHER'S, Iced Lemonade Cookies",	HIGH	66.3
MOTHER'S, Iced Oatmeal Cookies",	HIGH	71

Food name/ Category (100 g)	Status	Carbs content in g
MOTHER'S, Jungle Animal Cookies",	HIGH	68.3
MOTHER'S, Macaroon Cookies",	MEDIUM	55.7
MOTHER'S, Old Fashioned Chocolate Chip Cookies",	HIGH	66
MOTHER'S, Old Fashioned Iced Oatmeal Cookies",	HIGH	72.8
MOTHER'S, Old Fashioned Oatmeal Cookies",	HIGH	71.2
MOTHER'S, Peanut Butter Gauchos Cookies",	HIGH	65.7
MOTHER'S, Taffy Sandwich Cookies",	HIGH	69.9
MOTHER'S, Vanilla Sandwich Cookies",	HIGH	68.9
Mountain yam, hawaii, cooked, steamed, with salt",	LOW	19.99
Muffin, blueberry, commercially prepared, low-fat",	MEDIUM	50.05
Muffins, blueberry, commercially prepared (Includes mini-muffins)",	MEDIUM	53
Muffins, blueberry, dry mix",	HIGH	61
Muffins, blueberry, prepared from recipe, made with low fat (2%) milk",	MEDIUM	40.7
Muffins, blueberry, toaster-type, toasted",	MEDIUM	56.7
Muffins, blueberry, toaster-type",	MEDIUM	53.3
Muffins, corn, commercially prepared",	MEDIUM	51
Muffins, corn, dry mix, prepared",	MEDIUM	49.1
Muffins, corn, prepared from recipe, made with low fat (2%) milk",	MEDIUM	44.2
Muffins, corn, toaster-type",	HIGH	57.9
Muffins, oat bran",	MEDIUM	48.3
Muffins, plain, prepared from recipe, made with low fat (2%) milk",	MEDIUM	41.4
Muffins, wheat bran, dry mix",	HIGH	73
Muffins, wheat bran, toaster-type with raisins, toasted",	MEDIUM	55.5
Mung beans, mature seeds, cooked, boiled, with salt",	LOW	19.15
Mung beans, mature seeds, cooked, boiled, without salt",	LOW	19.15
Mung beans, mature seeds, sprouted, cooked, boiled, drained, with salt",	LOW	3.6
Mungo beans, mature seeds, cooked, boiled, with salt",	LOW	18.34
Mungo beans, mature seeds, raw",	HIGH	58.99
MURRAY, Chocolate Creme Sandwich Cookies",	HIGH	71.3
MURRAY, Chocolatey Chip Thins Cookies",	HIGH	73.6
MURRAY, COOKIE JAR CLASSICS, Butter Cookies",	HIGH	74.3
MURRAY, COOKIE JAR CLASSICS, Coconut Bars Cookies",	HIGH	73.9
MURRAY, Duplex Creme Sandwich Cookies",	HIGH	72.6
MURRAY, JACKS Vanilla Wafers",	HIGH	78.1
MURRAY, Lemon Creme Sandwich Cookies",	HIGH	73.7
MURRAY, Old Fashioned Gingersnaps Cookies",	HIGH	73.9
MURRAY, Old Fashioned Iced Oatmeal Cookies",	HIGH	71
MURRAY, SOUTHERN KITCHEN, Chocolate Chip Cookies",	HIGH	66.5
MURRAY, SOUTHERN KITCHEN, Coconut Cookies",	HIGH	65.5
MURRAY, SOUTHERN KITCHEN, Iced Oatmeal Cookies",	HIGH	69.5
MURRAY, SOUTHERN KITCHEN, Oatmeal Cookies",	HIGH	67.7
MURRAY, SUGAR FREE, Chocolate Chip & Pecan Cookies",	HIGH	58.6
MURRAY, SUGAR FREE, Chocolate Chip Cookies",	HIGH	63.6
MURRAY, SUGAR FREE, Chocolate Creme Sandwich Cookies",	HIGH	65.9
MURRAY, SUGAR FREE, Fudge Dipped Mint Cookies",	HIGH	63.5
MURRAY, SUGAR FREE, Fudge Dipped Wafers",	HIGH	61.2
MURRAY, SUGAR FREE, Lemon Creme Sandwich Cookies",	HIGH	68.3
MURRAY, SUGAR FREE, Oatmeal Cookies",	HIGH	66.6
MURRAY, SUGAR FREE, Peanut Butter Cookies",	MEDIUM	55.8
MURRAY, SUGAR FREE, Pecan Shortbread Cookies",	HIGH	57.3
MURRAY, SUGAR FREE, Shortbread Bites",	HIGH	75.3
MURRAY, SUGAR FREE, Shortbread Cookies",	HIGH	71.6

Food name/ Category (100 g)	Status	Carbs content in g
MURRAY, SUGAR FREE, Vanilla Creme Sandwich Cookies",	HIGH	70
MURRAY, SUGAR FREE, Vanilla Sugar Wafer",	HIGH	68.5
MURRAY, SUGAR FREE, Vanilla Wafer",	HIGH	74
MURRAY, Vanilla Creme Sandwich Cookies",	HIGH	73.9
MURRAY, Vanilla Sugar Wafer",	HIGH	70
MURRAY, Vanilla Wafer",	HIGH	72.9
Mushroom, white, exposed to ultraviolet light, raw",	LOW	3.26
Mushrooms, canned, drained solids",	LOW	5.09
Mushrooms, enoki, raw",	LOW	7.81
Mushrooms, maitake, raw",	LOW	6.97
Mushrooms, shiitake, cooked, with salt",	LOW	14.39
Mushrooms, shiitake, cooked, without salt",	LOW	14.39
Mushrooms, shiitake, stir-fried",	LOW	7.68
Mushrooms, straw, canned, drained solids",	LOW	4.64
Mushrooms, white, cooked, boiled, drained, with salt",	LOW	5.29
Mushrooms, white, cooked, boiled, drained, without salt",	LOW	5.29
Mushrooms, white, raw",	LOW	3.26
Mustard greens, cooked, boiled, drained, with salt",	LOW	4.51
Mustard greens, frozen, cooked, boiled, drained, with salt",	LOW	3.11
Mustard spinach, (tendergreen), cooked, boiled, drained, with salt",	LOW	2.8
Mustard, prepared, yellow",	LOW	5.83
Mutton, cooked, roasted (Navajo)",	LOW	0.08
NABISCO, NABISCO OREO CRUNCHIES, Cookie Crumb Topping",	HIGH	70.23
NABISCO, NABISCO RITZ Crackers",	HIGH	63.51
NABISCO, NABISCO SNACKWELL'S Fat Free Devil's Food Cookie Cakes",	HIGH	74.25
Nance, frozen, unsweetened",	LOW	16.97
Naranjilla (lulo) pulp, frozen, unsweetened",	LOW	5.9
Nectarines, raw",	LOW	10.55
New zealand spinach, cooked, boiled, drained, with salt",	LOW	2.13
New Zealand spinach, cooked, boiled, drained, without salt",	LOW	2.13
New Zealand spinach, raw",	LOW	2.5
Noodles, chinese, chow mein",	HIGH	72.8
Noodles, egg, cooked, enriched, with added salt",	LOW	25.16

Food name/ Category (100 g)	Status	Carbs content in g
Noodles, egg, cooked, unenriched, with added salt",	LOW	25.16
Noodles, egg, enriched, cooked",	LOW	25.16
Noodles, egg, spinach, enriched, dry",	HIGH	70.32
Noodles, egg, unenriched, cooked, without added salt",	LOW	25.16
Noodles, flat, crunchy, Chinese restaurant",	MEDIUM	51.9
Noodles, japanese, soba, cooked",	LOW	21.44
Noodles, japanese, soba, dry",	HIGH	74.62
Noodles, japanese, somen, cooked",	LOW	27.54
Noodles, japanese, somen, dry",	HIGH	74.1
Nutritional supplement for people with diabetes, liquid",	LOW	11.88
Nuts, acorn flour, full fat",	MEDIUM	54.65
Nuts, acorns, dried",	MEDIUM	53.66
Nuts, acorns, raw",	MEDIUM	40.75
Nuts, almond butter, plain, with salt added",	LOW	18.82
Nuts, almonds, dry roasted, with salt added",	LOW	21.01
Nuts, almonds, dry roasted, without salt added",	LOW	21.01
Nuts, almonds, honey roasted, unblanched",	LOW	27.9
Nuts, almonds, oil roasted, lightly salted",	LOW	17.68
Nuts, almonds, oil roasted, with salt added, smoke flavor",	LOW	17.86
Nuts, almonds, oil roasted, with salt added",	LOW	17.68
Nuts, almonds, oil roasted, without salt added",	LOW	17.68
Nuts, almonds",	LOW	21.55
Nuts, beechnuts, dried",	LOW	33.5
Nuts, brazilnuts, dried, unblanched",	LOW	11.74
Nuts, butternuts, dried",	LOW	12.05
Nuts, cashew butter, plain, with salt added",	LOW	30.3
Nuts, cashew nuts, dry roasted, with salt added",	LOW	32.69
Nuts, cashew nuts, oil roasted, with salt added",	LOW	30.16
Nuts, chestnuts, chinese, boiled and steamed",	LOW	33.64
Nuts, chestnuts, chinese, dried",	HIGH	79.76
Nuts, chestnuts, chinese, raw",	MEDIUM	49.07
Nuts, chestnuts, chinese, roasted",	MEDIUM	52.36
Nuts, chestnuts, european, dried, peeled",	HIGH	78.43
Nuts, chestnuts, european, dried, unpeeled",	HIGH	77.31

Food name/ Category (100 g)	Status	Carbs content in g
Nuts, chestnuts, european, raw, peeled",	MEDIUM	44.17
Nuts, chestnuts, european, raw, unpeeled",	MEDIUM	45.54
Nuts, chestnuts, european, roasted",	MEDIUM	52.96
Nuts, chestnuts, japanese, boiled and steamed",	LOW	12.64
Nuts, coconut cream, canned, sweetened",	MEDIUM	53.21
Nuts, coconut cream, raw (liquid expressed from grated meat)",	LOW	6.65
Nuts, coconut meat, dried (desiccated), creamed",	LOW	21.52
Nuts, coconut meat, dried (desiccated), not sweetened",	LOW	23.65
Nuts, coconut meat, dried (desiccated), sweetened, flaked, packaged",	MEDIUM	51.85
Nuts, coconut meat, dried (desiccated), sweetened, shredded",	MEDIUM	47.67
Nuts, coconut meat, dried (desiccated), toasted",	MEDIUM	44.4
Nuts, coconut water (liquid from coconuts)",	LOW	3.71
Nuts, formulated, wheat-based, all flavors except macadamia, without salt",	LOW	20.79
Nuts, formulated, wheat-based, unflavored, with salt added",	LOW	23.68
Nuts, ginkgo nuts, canned",	LOW	22.1
Nuts, hazelnuts or filberts, blanched",	LOW	17
Nuts, hazelnuts or filberts, dry roasted, without salt added",	LOW	17.6
Nuts, hazelnuts or filberts",	LOW	16.7
Nuts, hickorynuts, dried",	LOW	18.25
Nuts, macadamia nuts, dry roasted, with salt added",	LOW	12.83
Nuts, macadamia nuts, dry roasted, without salt added",	LOW	13.38
Nuts, macadamia nuts, raw",	LOW	13.82
Nuts, mixed nuts, dry roasted, with peanuts, salt added, CHOSEN ROASTER",	LOW	19.02
Nuts, mixed nuts, dry roasted, with peanuts, salt added, PLANTERS pistachio blend",	LOW	22.51
Nuts, mixed nuts, dry roasted, with peanuts, with salt added",	LOW	25.35
Nuts, mixed nuts, dry roasted, with peanuts, without salt added",	LOW	22.42
Nuts, mixed nuts, oil roasted, with peanuts, lightly salted",	LOW	21.05
Nuts, mixed nuts, oil roasted, with peanuts, with salt added",	LOW	21.05
Nuts, mixed nuts, oil roasted, with peanuts, without salt added",	LOW	21.05
Nuts, mixed nuts, oil roasted, without peanuts, lightly salted",	LOW	25
Nuts, mixed nuts, oil roasted, without peanuts, with salt added",	LOW	22.27

Food name/ Category (100 g)	Status	Carbs content in g
Nuts, pecans, dry roasted, with salt added",	LOW	13.55
Nuts, pecans, dry roasted, without salt added",	LOW	13.55
Nuts, pecans, oil roasted, with salt added",	LOW	13.01
Nuts, pecans, oil roasted, without salt added",	LOW	13.01
Nuts, pecans",	LOW	13.86
Nuts, pilinuts, dried",	LOW	3.98
Nuts, pine nuts, dried",	LOW	13.08
Nuts, pine nuts, pinyon, dried",	LOW	19.3
Nuts, pistachio nuts, dry roasted, with salt added",	LOW	27.55
Nuts, pistachio nuts, raw",	LOW	27.17
Nuts, walnuts, black, dried",	LOW	9.58
Nuts, walnuts, dry roasted, with salt added",	LOW	17.86
Nuts, walnuts, english",	LOW	13.71
Nuts, walnuts, glazed",	MEDIUM	47.59
Oat bran, cooked",	LOW	11.44
Oat bran, raw",	HIGH	66.22
Oats",	HIGH	66.27
Oheloberries, raw",	LOW	6.84
Oil, almond",	LOW	0
Oil, apricot kernel",	LOW	0
Oil, avocado",	LOW	0
Oil, babassu",	LOW	0
Oil, canola",	LOW	0
Oil, cocoa butter",	LOW	0
Oil, coconut",	LOW	0
Oil, cooking and salad, ENOVA, 80% diglycerides",	LOW	0
Oil, corn and canola",	LOW	0
Oil, corn, industrial and retail, all purpose salad or cooking",	LOW	0
Oil, corn, peanut, and olive",	LOW	0

Food name/ Category (100 g)	Status	Carbs content in g
Oil, cottonseed, salad or cooking",	LOW	0
Oil, cupu assu",	LOW	0
Oil, flaxseed, cold pressed",	LOW	0
Oil, grapeseed",	LOW	0
Oil, hazelnut",	LOW	0
Oil, industrial, canola (partially hydrogenated) oil for deep fat frying",	LOW	0
Oil, industrial, canola for salads, woks and light frying",	LOW	0
Oil, industrial, canola with antifoaming agent, principal uses salads, woks and light frying",	LOW	0
Oil, industrial, canola, high oleic",	LOW	0
Oil, industrial, coconut, confection fat, typical basis for ice cream coatings",	LOW	0
Oil, industrial, coconut, principal uses candy coatings, oil sprays, roasting nuts",	LOW	0
Oil, industrial, cottonseed, fully hydrogenated",	LOW	0
Oil, industrial, mid-oleic, sunflower",	LOW	0
Oil, industrial, soy (partially hydrogenated), all purpose",	LOW	0
Oil, industrial, soy (partially hydrogenated) and soy (winterized), pourable clear fry",	LOW	0
Oil, industrial, soy (partially hydrogenated), palm, principal uses icings and fillings",	LOW	0
Oil, industrial, soy (partially hydrogenated) and cottonseed, principal use as a tortilla shortening",	LOW	0
Oil, industrial, soy (partially hydrogenated), multiuse for non-dairy butter flavor",	LOW	0
Oil, industrial, soy (partially hydrogenated), principal uses popcorn and flavoring vegetables",	LOW	0
Oil, industrial, soy, fully hydrogenated",	LOW	0
Oil, industrial, soy, low linolenic",	LOW	0
Oil, industrial, soy, refined, for woks and light frying",	LOW	0
Oil, industrial, soy, ultra low linolenic",	LOW	0
Oil, mustard",	LOW	0
Oil, nutmeg butter",	LOW	0
Oil, oat",	LOW	0
Oil, olive, salad or cooking",	LOW	0
Oil, palm",	LOW	0

Food name/ Category (100 g)	Status	Carbs content in g
Oil, PAM cooking spray, original",	LOW	20.69
Oil, peanut, salad or cooking",	LOW	0
Oil, poppyseed",	LOW	0
Oil, rice bran",	LOW	0
Oil, safflower, salad or cooking, high oleic (primary safflower oil of commerce)",	LOW	0
Oil, safflower, salad or cooking, linoleic, (over 70%)",	LOW	0
Oil, sesame, salad or cooking",	LOW	0
Oil, sheanut",	LOW	0
Oil, soybean lecithin",	LOW	0
Oil, soybean, salad or cooking, (partially hydrogenated) and cottonseed",	LOW	0
Oil, soybean, salad or cooking, (partially hydrogenated)",	LOW	0
Oil, soybean, salad or cooking",	LOW	0
Oil, sunflower, high oleic (70% and over)",	LOW	0
Oil, sunflower, linoleic (less than 60%)",	LOW	0
Oil, sunflower, linoleic, (approx. 65%)",	LOW	0
Oil, sunflower, linoleic, (partially hydrogenated)",	LOW	0
Oil, teaseed",	LOW	0
Oil, tomatoseed",	LOW	0
Oil, ucuhuba butter",	LOW	0
Oil, vegetable, Natreon canola, high stability, non trans, high oleic (70%)",	LOW	0
Oil, walnut",	LOW	0
Oil, wheat germ",	LOW	0
Okra, cooked, boiled, drained, with salt",	LOW	4.51
Okra, frozen, cooked, boiled, drained, with salt",	LOW	6.41
Okra, frozen, cooked, boiled, drained, without salt",	LOW	6.41
Okra, frozen, unprepared",	LOW	6.63
OLIVE GARDEN, cheese ravioli with marinara sauce",	LOW	19.64
OLIVE GARDEN, chicken parmigiana without pasta",	LOW	12.28

Food name/ Category (100 g)	Status	Carbs content in g
OLIVE GARDEN, lasagna classico",	LOW	10.33
OLIVE GARDEN, spaghetti with meat sauce",	LOW	17.19
OLIVE GARDEN, spaghetti with pomodoro sauce",	LOW	17.14
Olives, pickled, canned or bottled, green",	LOW	3.84
Olives, ripe, canned (jumbo-super colossal)",	LOW	5.61
Olives, ripe, canned (small-extra large)",	LOW	6.26
ON THE BORDER, cheese enchilada",	LOW	16.2
ON THE BORDER, cheese quesadilla",	LOW	24.25
ON THE BORDER, Mexican rice",	LOW	34.15
ON THE BORDER, refried beans",	LOW	17.52
ON THE BORDER, soft taco with ground beef, cheese and lettuce",	LOW	19.28
Onion rings, breaded, par fried, frozen, prepared, heated in oven",	LOW	33.79
Onion rings, breaded, par fried, frozen, unprepared",	LOW	30.53
Onions, canned, solids and liquids",	LOW	4.02
Onions, cooked, boiled, drained, with salt",	LOW	9.56
Onions, cooked, boiled, drained, without salt",	LOW	10.15
Onions, frozen, chopped, cooked, boiled, drained, with salt",	LOW	6
Onions, frozen, whole, cooked, boiled, drained, with salt",	LOW	6.11
Onions, raw",	LOW	9.34
Orange juice, canned, unsweetened",	LOW	11.01
Orange juice, chilled, includes from concentrate, with added calcium and vitamin D",	LOW	11.27
Orange juice, chilled, includes from concentrate, with added calcium and vitamins A, D, E",	LOW	11.54
Orange juice, chilled, includes from concentrate, with added calcium",	LOW	11.27
Orange juice, chilled, includes from concentrate",	LOW	11.54
Orange juice, frozen concentrate, unsweetened, diluted with 3 volume water, with added calcium",	LOW	8.47
Orange juice, frozen concentrate, unsweetened, diluted with 3 volume water",	LOW	8.8
Orange juice, raw",	LOW	10.4
Orange peel, raw",	LOW	25

Food name/ Category (100 g)	Status	Carbs content in g
Orange Pineapple Juice Blend",	LOW	12.2
Orange-grapefruit juice, canned or bottled, unsweetened",	LOW	10.28
Oranges, raw, all commercial varieties",	LOW	11.75
Oranges, raw, California, valencias",	LOW	11.89
Oranges, raw, Florida",	LOW	11.54
Oranges, raw, navels",	LOW	12.54
Oranges, raw, with peel",	LOW	15.5
OSCAR MAYER, Bologna (beef)",	LOW	2.45
OSCAR MAYER, Braunschweiger Liver Sausage (sliced)",	LOW	2.6
OSCAR MAYER, Chicken Breast (honey glazed)",	LOW	4.3
OSCAR MAYER, Salami (hard)",	LOW	1.6
OSCAR MAYER, Wieners (beef franks)",	LOW	2.78
Ostrich, fan, raw",	LOW	0
Ostrich, ground, cooked, pan-broiled",	LOW	0
Ostrich, ground, raw",	LOW	0
Ostrich, inside leg, cooked",	LOW	0
Ostrich, inside leg, raw",	LOW	0
Ostrich, inside strip, cooked",	LOW	0
Ostrich, inside strip, raw",	LOW	0
Ostrich, outside leg, raw",	LOW	0
Ostrich, outside strip, cooked",	LOW	0
Ostrich, outside strip, raw",	LOW	0
Ostrich, oyster, cooked",	LOW	0
Ostrich, oyster, raw",	LOW	0
Ostrich, round, raw",	LOW	0
Ostrich, tenderloin, raw",	LOW	0
Ostrich, tip trimmed, cooked",	LOW	0
Ostrich, tip trimmed, raw",	LOW	0

Food name/ Category (100 g)	Status	Carbs content in g
Ostrich, top loin, cooked",	LOW	0
Ostrich, top loin, raw",	LOW	0
Oven-roasted chicken breast roll",	LOW	1.79
P REGO Pasta, Roasted Garlic and Herb Italian Sauce, ready-to-serve",	LOW	10
PACE, Chipotle Chunky Salsa",	LOW	6.25
PACE, Cilantro Chunky Salsa",	LOW	6.25
PACE, Diced Green Chilies",	LOW	6.67
PACE, Dry Taco Seasoning Mix",	MEDIUM	56.29
PACE, Enchilada Sauce",	LOW	8.33
PACE, Green Taco Sauce",	LOW	6.25
PACE, Jalapenos Nacho Sliced Peppers",	LOW	3.33
PACE, Lime & Garlic Chunky Salsa",	LOW	9.38
PACE, Organic Picante Sauce",	LOW	6.25
PACE, Picante Sauce",	LOW	6.25
PACE, Pico De Gallo",	LOW	9.38
PACE, Red Taco Sauce",	LOW	12.5
PACE, Salsa Refried Beans",	LOW	11.67
PACE, Salsa Verde",	LOW	6.25
PACE, Spicy Jalapeno Refried Beans",	LOW	11.67
PACE, Tequila Lime Salsa",	LOW	9.38
PACE, Thick & Chunky Salsa",	LOW	6.25
PACE, Traditional Refried Beans",	LOW	10.83
PACE, Triple Pepper Salsa",	LOW	9.38
Pan Dulce, LA RICURA, Salpora de Arroz con Azucar, cookie-like, contains wheat	HIGH	66.28
Pancakes plain, frozen, ready-to-heat (includes buttermilk)",	LOW	37.75
Pancakes, blueberry, prepared from recipe",	LOW	29
Pancakes, buckwheat, dry mix, incomplete",	HIGH	71.3
Pancakes, buttermilk, prepared from recipe",	LOW	28.7
Pancakes, gluten-free, frozen, ready-to-heat",	MEDIUM	40.32
Pancakes, plain, dry mix, complete (includes buttermilk)",	HIGH	73.65

Food name/ Category (100 g)	Status	Carbs content in g
Pancakes, plain, dry mix, complete, prepared",	LOW	36.7
Pancakes, plain, dry mix, incomplete (includes buttermilk)",	HIGH	73.6
Pancakes, plain, dry mix, incomplete, prepared",	LOW	28.9
Pancakes, plain, frozen, ready-to-heat, microwave (includes buttermilk)",	MEDIUM	43.33
Pancakes, plain, low fat, dry mix, incomplete (includes buttermilk)",	HIGH	74.69
Pancakes, plain, prepared from recipe",	LOW	28.3
Pancakes, plain, reduced fat",	HIGH	57.32
Pancakes, special dietary, dry mix",	HIGH	73.9
Pancakes, whole wheat, dry mix, incomplete",	HIGH	74.11
Pancakes, whole-wheat, dry mix, incomplete, prepared",	LOW	29.4
Pancakes, whole-wheat, dry mix, incomplete",	HIGH	71
PAPA JOHN'S 14\" Cheese Pizza, Original Crust",	LOW	32.74
PAPA JOHN'S 14\" Cheese Pizza, Thin Crust",	LOW	26.26
PAPA JOHN'S 14\" Pepperoni Pizza, Original Crust",	LOW	30.04
PAPA JOHN'S 14\" The Works Pizza, Original Crust",	LOW	26.69
Papaya nectar, canned",	LOW	14.51
Parmesan cheese topping, fat free",	MEDIUM	40
Parsley, freeze-dried",	MEDIUM	42.38
Parsley, fresh",	LOW	6.33
Parsnips, cooked, boiled, drained, with salt",	LOW	17.01
Pasta mix, classic beef, unprepared",	HIGH	72.2
Pasta mix, classic cheeseburger macaroni, unprepared",	HIGH	71.51
Pasta mix, Italian four cheese lasagna, unprepared",	HIGH	70.26
Pasta mix, Italian lasagna, unprepared",	HIGH	73.77
Pasta with Sliced Franks in Tomato Sauce, canned entree",	LOW	12.7
Pasta with tomato sauce, no meat, canned",	LOW	14.22
Pasta, cooked, enriched, with added salt",	LOW	30.59
Pasta, cooked, enriched, without added salt",	LOW	30.86
Pasta, cooked, unenriched, with added salt",	LOW	30.59
Pasta, cooked, unenriched, without added salt",	LOW	30.86
Pasta, gluten-free, brown rice flour, cooked, TINKYADA",	LOW	32.2
Pasta, gluten-free, corn and rice flour, cooked",	LOW	38.05
Pasta, gluten-free, corn flour and quinoa flour, cooked, ANCIENT HARVEST",	LOW	31.11
Pasta, gluten-free, corn, cooked",	LOW	27.91
Pasta, gluten-free, corn, dry",	HIGH	79.26

Food name/ Category (100 g)	Status	Carbs content in g
Pasta, gluten-free, rice flour and rice bran extract, cooked, DE BOLES",	MEDIUM	40.75
Pasta, homemade, made with egg, cooked",	LOW	23.54
Pasta, homemade, made without egg, cooked",	LOW	25.12
Pasta, whole grain, 51% whole wheat, remaining enriched semolina, cooked",	LOW	30.87
Pasta, whole-wheat, cooked",	LOW	30.07
Pastrami, beef, 98% fat-free",	LOW	1.54
Pastrami, turkey",	LOW	3.34
Pastry, Pastelitos de Guava (guava pastries)",	MEDIUM	47.76
Pate de foie gras, canned (goose liver pate), smoked",	LOW	4.67
Pate, chicken liver, canned",	LOW	6.55
Pate, goose liver, smoked, canned",	LOW	4.67
Pate, liver, not specified, canned",	LOW	1.5
Pate, truffle flavor",	LOW	6.3
Peaches, canned, extra light syrup, solids and liquids",	LOW	11.1
Peaches, canned, juice pack, solids and liquids",	LOW	11.57
Peaches, canned, light syrup pack, solids and liquids",	LOW	14.55
Peaches, canned, water pack, solids and liquids",	LOW	6.11
Peaches, dehydrated (low-moisture), sulfured, stewed",	LOW	34.14
Peaches, dried, sulfured, stewed, with added sugar",	LOW	26.6
Peaches, dried, sulfured, stewed, without added sugar",	LOW	19.69
Peaches, spiced, canned, heavy syrup pack, solids and liquids",	LOW	20.08
Peaches, yellow, raw",	LOW	9.54
Peanut butter with omega-3, creamy",	LOW	17
Peanut butter, chunk style, with salt",	LOW	21.57
Peanut butter, chunky, vitamin and mineral fortified",	LOW	17.69
Peanut butter, reduced sodium",	LOW	21.83
Peanut butter, smooth style, with salt",	LOW	22.31
Peanut butter, smooth, reduced fat",	LOW	35.65
Peanut butter, smooth, vitamin and mineral fortified",	LOW	18.75

Food name/ Category (100 g)	Status	Carbs content in g
Peanut flour, defatted",	LOW	34.7
Peanut flour, low fat",	LOW	31.27
Peanut spread, reduced sugar",	LOW	14.23
Peanuts, all types, cooked, boiled, with salt",	LOW	21.26
Peanuts, all types, dry-roasted, with salt",	LOW	21.26
Peanuts, all types, oil-roasted, with salt",	LOW	15.26
Peanuts, spanish, oil-roasted, with salt",	LOW	17.45
Peanuts, valencia, oil-roasted, with salt",	LOW	16.3
Peanuts, valencia, raw",	LOW	20.91
Peanuts, virginia, oil-roasted, with salt",	LOW	19.86
Pear nectar, canned, with added ascorbic acid",	LOW	15.76
Pear nectar, canned, without added ascorbic acid",	LOW	15.76
Pears, asian, raw",	LOW	10.65
Pears, canned, extra heavy syrup pack, solids and liquids",	LOW	25.25
Pears, canned, extra light syrup pack, solids and liquids",	LOW	12.2
Pears, canned, heavy syrup pack, solids and liquids",	LOW	19.17
Pears, canned, heavy syrup, drained",	LOW	19.08
Pears, canned, juice pack, solids and liquids",	LOW	12.94
Pears, canned, light syrup pack, solids and liquids",	LOW	15.17
Pears, canned, water pack, solids and liquids",	LOW	7.81
Pears, dried, sulfured, stewed, with added sugar",	LOW	37.14
Pears, dried, sulfured, stewed, without added sugar",	LOW	33.81
Pears, raw, bartlett",	LOW	15.01
Pears, raw, bosc",	LOW	16.1
Pears, raw, green anjou",	LOW	15.79
Pears, raw, red anjou",	LOW	14.94
Pears, raw",	LOW	15.23
Peas and carrots, canned, no salt added, solids and liquids",	LOW	8.48

Food name/ Category (100 g)	Status	Carbs content in g
Peas and carrots, canned, regular pack, solids and liquids",	LOW	8.48
Peas and carrots, frozen, cooked, boiled, drained, with salt",	LOW	10.12
Peas and carrots, frozen, cooked, boiled, drained, without salt",	LOW	10.12
Peas and carrots, frozen, unprepared",	LOW	11.15
Peas and onions, canned, solids and liquids",	LOW	8.57
Peas and onions, frozen, cooked, boiled, drained, with salt",	LOW	8.63
Peas and onions, frozen, cooked, boiled, drained, without salt",	LOW	8.63
Peas and onions, frozen, unprepared",	LOW	13.51
Peas, edible-podded, boiled, drained, without salt",	LOW	7.05
Peas, edible-podded, cooked, boiled, drained, with salt",	LOW	6.46
Peas, edible-podded, frozen, cooked, boiled, drained, with salt",	LOW	8.43
Peas, edible-podded, frozen, cooked, boiled, drained, without salt",	LOW	9.02
Peas, edible-podded, frozen, unprepared",	LOW	7.2
Peas, edible-podded, raw",	LOW	7.55
Peas, green (includes baby and lesuer types), canned, drained solids, unprepared",	LOW	11.36
Peas, green, canned, drained solids, rinsed in tap water",	LOW	11.82
Peas, green, canned, no salt added, drained solids",	LOW	12.58
Peas, green, canned, regular pack, solids and liquids",	LOW	10.6
Peas, green, canned, seasoned, solids and liquids",	LOW	9.25
Peas, green, cooked, boiled, drained, with salt",	LOW	15.63
Peas, green, cooked, boiled, drained, without salt",	LOW	15.63
Peas, green, frozen, cooked, boiled, drained, with salt",	LOW	14.26
Peas, green, frozen, cooked, boiled, drained, without salt",	LOW	14.26
Peas, green, frozen, unprepared",	LOW	13.62
Peas, green, raw",	LOW	14.45
Peas, split, mature seeds, cooked, boiled, with salt",	LOW	20.51
Peas, split, mature seeds, cooked, boiled, without salt",	LOW	21.1
Pectin, unsweetened, dry mix",	HIGH	90.4
Pepeao, dried",	HIGH	81.03

Food name/ Category (100 g)	Status	Carbs content in g
PEPPERIDGE FARM, Cinnamon Swirl Bread",	MEDIUM	52.9
PEPPERIDGE FARM, Deli Swirl Bread",	MEDIUM	44.7
PEPPERIDGE FARM, Farmhouse 100% Whole Wheat Bread",	MEDIUM	46.1
PEPPERIDGE FARM, Farmhouse Hearty White Bread",	HIGH	60.16
PEPPERIDGE FARM, Farmhouse Oatmeal Bread",	MEDIUM	50.7
PEPPERIDGE FARM, Farmhouse Sourdough Bread",	MEDIUM	50.3
PEPPERIDGE FARM, Goldfish, Baked Snack Crackers, Cheddar",	HIGH	66.2
PEPPERIDGE FARM, Goldfish, Baked Snack Crackers, Explosive Pizza",	HIGH	67.2
PEPPERIDGE FARM, Goldfish, Baked Snack Crackers, Original",	HIGH	65.81
PEPPERIDGE FARM, Goldfish, Baked Snack Crackers, Parmesan",	HIGH	64.7
PEPPERIDGE FARM, Goldfish, Baked Snack Crackers, Pizza",	HIGH	65.11
PEPPERIDGE FARM, Jewish Rye Bread (Seedless)",	MEDIUM	45
PEPPERIDGE FARM, Light Style Wheat Bread",	MEDIUM	45.6
PEPPERIDGE FARM, Pumpernickel Bread",	MEDIUM	46.9
PEPPERIDGE FARM, Raisin Cinnamon Swirl Bread",	MEDIUM	52.1
PEPPERIDGE FARM, Seeded Jewish Rye Bread",	MEDIUM	48.4
PEPPERIDGE FARM, White Bread",	MEDIUM	50.2
PEPPERIDGE FARM, White Hoagie Roll",	MEDIUM	50.7
PEPPERIDGE FARM, Whole Grain 15 Grain Bread",	MEDIUM	45.8
PEPPERIDGE FARM, Whole Grain Honey Whole Wheat Bread",	MEDIUM	47.7
PEPPERIDGE FARM, Whole Grain Oatmeal Bread",	MEDIUM	46.5
Peppers, ancho, dried",	MEDIUM	51.42
Peppers, chili, green, canned",	LOW	4.6
Peppers, hot chile, sun-dried",	HIGH	69.86
Peppers, hot chili, green, canned, pods, excluding seeds, solids and liquids",	LOW	5.1
Peppers, hot chili, red, canned, excluding seeds, solids and liquids",	LOW	5.1
Peppers, hot pickled, canned",	LOW	4.56
Peppers, hungarian, raw",	LOW	6.7
Peppers, jalapeno, canned, solids and liquids",	LOW	4.74
Peppers, jalapeno, raw",	LOW	6.5
Peppers, pasilla, dried",	MEDIUM	51.13
Peppers, sweet, green, canned, solids and liquids",	LOW	3.9
Peppers, sweet, green, cooked, boiled, drained, with salt",	LOW	6.11
Peppers, sweet, green, cooked, boiled, drained, without salt",	LOW	6.7
Peppers, sweet, green, freeze-dried",	HIGH	68.7
Peppers, sweet, green, frozen, chopped, cooked, boiled, drained, with salt",	LOW	3.31
Peppers, sweet, green, frozen, chopped, unprepared",	LOW	4.45
Peppers, sweet, green, raw",	LOW	4.64
Peppers, sweet, red, canned, solids and liquids",	LOW	3.9
Peppers, sweet, red, cooked, boiled, drained, with salt",	LOW	6.11
Peppers, sweet, red, cooked, boiled, drained, without salt",	LOW	6.7

Food name/ Category (100 g)	Status	Carbs content in g
Peppers, sweet, red, freeze-dried",	HIGH	68.7
Peppers, sweet, red, frozen, chopped, boiled, drained, with salt",	LOW	3.31
Peppers, sweet, red, frozen, chopped, boiled, drained, without salt",	LOW	3.31
Peppers, sweet, red, frozen, chopped, unprepared",	LOW	4.45
Peppers, sweet, red, raw",	LOW	6.03
Peppers, sweet, yellow, raw",	LOW	6.32
Persimmons, japanese, dried",	HIGH	73.43
Persimmons, japanese, raw",	LOW	18.59
Persimmons, native, raw",	LOW	33.5
Pheasant, cooked, total edible",	LOW	0
Pheasant, leg, meat only, raw",	LOW	0
Pheasant, raw, meat and skin",	LOW	0
Pheasant, raw, meat only",	LOW	0
Phyllo dough",	MEDIUM	52.6
Pickle relish, hot dog",	LOW	23.35
Pickle relish, sweet",	LOW	35.06
Pickles, chowchow, with cauliflower onion mustard, sweet",	LOW	26.64
Pickles, cucumber, dill or kosher dill",	LOW	2.41
Pickles, cucumber, sour",	LOW	2.26
Pickles, cucumber, sweet (includes bread and butter pickles)",	LOW	21.15
Pie Crust, Cookie-type, Chocolate, Ready Crust",	HIGH	64.48
Pie crust, cookie-type, prepared from recipe, vanilla wafer, chilled",	MEDIUM	50.2
Pie crust, deep dish, frozen, baked, made with enriched flour",	MEDIUM	52.47
Pie crust, deep dish, frozen, unbaked, made with enriched flour",	MEDIUM	46.79
Pie crust, refrigerated, regular, baked",	HIGH	58.52
Pie crust, refrigerated, regular, unbaked",	MEDIUM	51.11
Pie crust, standard-type, dry mix, prepared, baked",	MEDIUM	50.4
Pie crust, standard-type, dry mix",	MEDIUM	52.1
Pie crust, standard-type, frozen, ready-to-bake, enriched, baked",	MEDIUM	56.24
Pie crust, standard-type, frozen, ready-to-bake, enriched",	MEDIUM	48.62
Pie crust, standard-type, frozen, ready-to-bake, unenriched",	MEDIUM	44.1
Pie crust, standard-type, prepared from recipe, baked",	MEDIUM	47.5
Pie crust, standard-type, prepared from recipe, unbaked",	MEDIUM	42.3
Pie fillings, apple, canned",	LOW	26.1
Pie, apple, commercially prepared, enriched flour",	LOW	34
Pie, apple, commercially prepared, unenriched flour",	LOW	34

Food name/ Category (100 g)	Status	Carbs content in g
Pie, apple, prepared from recipe",	LOW	37.1
Pie, banana cream, prepared from mix, no-bake type",	LOW	31.6
Pie, banana cream, prepared from recipe",	LOW	32.9
Pie, blueberry, commercially prepared",	LOW	34.9
Pie, blueberry, prepared from recipe",	LOW	33.5
Pie, cherry, commercially prepared",	LOW	39.8
Pie, cherry, prepared from recipe",	LOW	38.5
Pie, chocolate creme, commercially prepared",	LOW	38.44
Pie, chocolate mousse, prepared from mix, no-bake type",	LOW	29.6
Pie, coconut cream, prepared from mix, no-bake type",	LOW	28.5
Pie, coconut creme, commercially prepared",	LOW	37.3
Pie, coconut custard, commercially prepared",	LOW	30.2
Pie, Dutch Apple, Commercially Prepared",	MEDIUM	44.54
Pie, egg custard, commercially prepared",	LOW	20.8
Pie, fried pies, cherry",	MEDIUM	42.6
Pie, fried pies, fruit",	MEDIUM	42.6
Pie, fried pies, lemon",	MEDIUM	42.6
Pie, lemon meringue, commercially prepared",	MEDIUM	47.2
Pie, lemon meringue, prepared from recipe",	LOW	39.1
Pie, mince, prepared from recipe",	MEDIUM	48
Pie, peach",	LOW	32.9
Pie, pecan, commercially prepared",	HIGH	59.61
Pie, pecan, prepared from recipe",	MEDIUM	52.2
Pie, pumpkin, commercially prepared",	LOW	34.83
Pie, pumpkin, prepared from recipe",	LOW	26.4
Pie, vanilla cream, prepared from recipe",	LOW	32.6
Pigeon peas (red gram), mature seeds, cooked, boiled, with salt",	LOW	23.25
Pigeon peas (red gram), mature seeds, cooked, boiled, without salt",	LOW	23.25
Pigeonpeas, immature seeds, cooked, boiled, drained, with salt",	LOW	19.49
Pigeonpeas, immature seeds, cooked, boiled, drained, without salt",	LOW	19.49
Pigeonpeas, immature seeds, raw",	LOW	23.88
Piki bread, made from blue cornmeal (Hopi)",	HIGH	72.22
PILLSBURY Golden Layer Buttermilk Biscuits, Artificial Flavor, refrigerated dough",	MEDIUM	41.18

Food name/ Category (100 g)	Status	Carbs content in g
PILLSBURY GRANDS, Buttermilk Biscuits, refrigerated dough",	MEDIUM	42.41
PILLSBURY, Buttermilk Biscuits, Artificial Flavor, refrigerated dough",	MEDIUM	47.07
PILLSBURY, Chocolate Chip Cookies, refrigerated dough",	HIGH	60.75
PILLSBURY, Cinnamon Rolls with Icing, refrigerated dough",	MEDIUM	53.42
PILLSBURY, Crusty French Loaf, refrigerated dough",	MEDIUM	46.35
PILLSBURY, Traditional Fudge Brownie Mix, dry",	HIGH	78.3
Pineapple juice, canned or bottled, unsweetened, with added ascorbic acid",	LOW	12.87
Pineapple juice, canned or bottled, unsweetened, without added ascorbic acid",	LOW	12.87
Pineapple juice, canned, not from concentrate, unsweetened, with added vitamins A, C and E",	LOW	12.18
Pineapple juice, frozen concentrate, unsweetened, diluted with 3 volume water",	LOW	12.67
Pineapple juice, frozen concentrate, unsweetened, undiluted",	MEDIUM	44.3
Pineapple, canned, extra heavy syrup pack, solids and liquids",	LOW	21.5
Pineapple, canned, heavy syrup pack, solids and liquids",	LOW	20.2
Pineapple, canned, juice pack, drained",	LOW	15.56
Pineapple, canned, juice pack, solids and liquids",	LOW	15.7
Pineapple, canned, light syrup pack, solids and liquids",	LOW	13.45
Pineapple, canned, water pack, solids and liquids",	LOW	8.3
Pineapple, frozen, chunks, sweetened",	LOW	22.2
Pineapple, raw, all varieties",	LOW	13.12
Pineapple, raw, extra sweet variety",	LOW	13.5
Pineapple, raw, traditional varieties",	LOW	11.82
Pitanga, (surinam-cherry), raw",	LOW	7.49
PIZZA HUT 12\" Cheese Pizza, Hand-Tossed Crust",	LOW	31.22
PIZZA HUT 12\" Cheese Pizza, Pan Crust",	LOW	29.93
PIZZA HUT 12\" Cheese Pizza, THIN 'N CRISPY Crust",	LOW	28.64
PIZZA HUT 12\" Pepperoni Pizza, Hand-Tossed Crust",	LOW	31.55
PIZZA HUT 12\" Pepperoni Pizza, Pan Crust",	LOW	30.49
PIZZA HUT 12\" Super Supreme Pizza, Hand-Tossed Crust",	LOW	25.62
PIZZA HUT 14\" Cheese Pizza, Hand-Tossed Crust",	LOW	33.42
PIZZA HUT 14\" Cheese Pizza, Pan Crust",	LOW	32.85
PIZZA HUT 14\" Cheese Pizza, Stuffed Crust",	LOW	30

Food name/ Category (100 g)	Status	Carbs content in g
PIZZA HUT 14\" Cheese Pizza, THIN 'N CRISPY Crust",	LOW	34.22
PIZZA HUT 14\" Pepperoni Pizza, Hand-Tossed Crust",	LOW	32.11
PIZZA HUT 14\" Pepperoni Pizza, Pan Crust",	LOW	31.79
PIZZA HUT 14\" Pepperoni Pizza, THIN 'N CRISPY Crust",	LOW	32.66
PIZZA HUT 14\" Sausage Pizza, Hand-Tossed Crust",	LOW	29.39
PIZZA HUT 14\" Sausage Pizza, Pan Crust",	LOW	29.56
PIZZA HUT 14\" Sausage Pizza, THIN 'N CRISPY Crust",	LOW	28.7
PIZZA HUT 14\" Super Supreme Pizza, Hand-Tossed Crust",	LOW	26.01
PIZZA HUT, breadstick, parmesan garlic",	MEDIUM	44.48
Pizza rolls, frozen, unprepared",	MEDIUM	50.72
Pizza, cheese topping, regular crust, frozen, cooked",	LOW	29.02
Pizza, cheese topping, rising crust, frozen, cooked",	LOW	32.91
Pizza, cheese topping, thin crust, frozen, cooked",	LOW	28.8
Pizza, meat and vegetable topping, regular crust, frozen, cooked",	LOW	25.14
Pizza, meat and vegetable topping, rising crust, frozen, cooked",	LOW	28.78
Pizza, meat topping, thick crust, frozen, cooked",	LOW	30.76
Pizza, pepperoni topping, regular crust, frozen, cooked",	LOW	24.69
Plantains, cooked",	LOW	31.15
Plantains, green, fried",	MEDIUM	49.17
Plantains, raw",	LOW	31.89
Plums, canned, purple, juice pack, solids and liquids",	LOW	15.15
Plums, canned, purple, water pack, solids and liquids",	LOW	11.03
Plums, dried (prunes), stewed, with added sugar",	LOW	32.88
Plums, dried (prunes), stewed, without added sugar",	LOW	28.08
Plums, dried (prunes), uncooked",	HIGH	63.88
Plums, raw",	LOW	11.42
Plums, wild (Northern Plains Indians)",	LOW	21.95
Pokeberry shoots, (poke), cooked, boiled, drained, with salt",	LOW	3.1
Pomegranates, raw",	LOW	18.7
Popcorn, microwave, low fat and sodium",	HIGH	73.39
Popcorn, microwave, regular (butter) flavor, made with palm oil",	HIGH	57.26

Food name/ Category (100 g)	Status	Carbs content in g
Popcorn, sugar syrup\/caramel, fat-free",	HIGH	90.06
POPEYES, biscuit",	MEDIUM	40.95
POPEYES, Coleslaw",	LOW	14.12
POPEYES, Fried Chicken, Mild, Breast, meat and skin with breading",	LOW	9.83
POPEYES, Fried Chicken, Mild, Breast, meat only, skin and breading removed",	LOW	0
POPEYES, Fried Chicken, Mild, Drumstick, meat and skin with breading",	LOW	9.84
POPEYES, Fried Chicken, Mild, Drumstick, meat only, skin and breading removed",	LOW	0.04
POPEYES, Fried Chicken, Mild, Thigh, meat and skin with breading",	LOW	11.2
POPEYES, Fried Chicken, Mild, Thigh, meat only, skin and breading removed",	LOW	0.85
POPEYES, Fried Chicken, Mild, Wing, meat and skin with breading",	LOW	13.52
POPEYES, Fried Chicken, Mild, Wing, meat only, skin and breading removed",	LOW	2.9
POPEYES, Mild Chicken Strips, analyzed 2006",	LOW	19.31
POPEYES, Spicy Chicken Strips, analyzed 2006",	LOW	18.52
Popovers, dry mix, enriched",	HIGH	71
Popovers, dry mix, unenriched",	HIGH	71
Potato flour",	HIGH	83.1
Potato pancakes",	LOW	27.81
Potato puffs, frozen, oven-heated",	LOW	27.29
Potato puffs, frozen, unprepared",	LOW	24.8
Potato salad with egg",	LOW	16.18
Potato salad, home-prepared",	LOW	11.17
Potato soup, instant, dry mix",	HIGH	76.14
Potatoes, au gratin, dry mix, prepared with water, whole milk and butter",	LOW	12.84
Potatoes, au gratin, dry mix, unprepared",	HIGH	74.31
Potatoes, au gratin, home-prepared from recipe using butter",	LOW	11.27
Potatoes, au gratin, home-prepared from recipe using margarine",	LOW	11.27
Potatoes, baked, flesh, with salt",	LOW	21.55
Potatoes, baked, flesh, without salt",	LOW	21.55
Potatoes, baked, skin only, with salt",	MEDIUM	46.06
Potatoes, boiled, cooked in skin, flesh, with salt",	LOW	20.13
Potatoes, boiled, cooked in skin, flesh, without salt",	LOW	20.13
Potatoes, boiled, cooked in skin, skin, with salt",	LOW	17.2

Food name/ Category (100 g)	Status	Carbs content in g
Potatoes, boiled, cooked without skin, flesh, with salt",	LOW	20.01
Potatoes, boiled, cooked without skin, flesh, without salt",	LOW	20.01
Potatoes, canned, drained solids, no salt added",	LOW	13.6
Potatoes, canned, drained solids",	LOW	13.61
Potatoes, canned, solids and liquids",	LOW	9.89
Potatoes, french fried, all types, salt added in processing, frozen, home-prepared, oven heated",	LOW	25.55
Potatoes, french fried, all types, salt added in processing, frozen, unprepared",	LOW	24.81
Potatoes, french fried, cottage-cut, salt not added in processing, frozen, oven-heated",	LOW	34.03
Potatoes, french fried, crinkle or regular cut, salt added in processing, frozen, as purchased",	LOW	23.96
Potatoes, french fried, crinkle or regular cut, salt added in processing, frozen, oven-heated",	LOW	27.5
Potatoes, french fried, cross cut, frozen, unprepared",	LOW	22.95
Potatoes, french fried, shoestring, salt added in processing, frozen, as purchased",	LOW	25.59
Potatoes, french fried, shoestring, salt added in processing, frozen, oven-heated",	LOW	31.66
Potatoes, french fried, steak fries, salt added in processing, frozen, as purchased",	LOW	23.51
Potatoes, french fried, steak fries, salt added in processing, frozen, oven-heated",	LOW	26.98
Potatoes, french fried, wedge cut, frozen, unprepared",	LOW	22.22
Potatoes, frozen, french fried, par fried, cottage-cut, prepared, heated in oven, with salt",	LOW	34.03
Potatoes, frozen, french fried, par fried, extruded, prepared, heated in oven, without salt",	LOW	39.68
Potatoes, frozen, french fried, par fried, extruded, unprepared",	LOW	30.15
Potatoes, hash brown, frozen, with butter sauce, unprepared",	LOW	18.28
Potatoes, hash brown, home-prepared",	LOW	35.11
Potatoes, hash brown, refrigerated, prepared, pan-fried in canola oil",	LOW	33.99
Potatoes, hash brown, refrigerated, unprepared",	LOW	19.16
Potatoes, mashed, dehydrated, flakes without milk, dry form",	HIGH	81.17
Potatoes, mashed, dehydrated, granules with milk, dry form",	HIGH	77.7
Potatoes, mashed, dehydrated, granules without milk, dry form",	HIGH	85.51
Potatoes, mashed, dehydrated, prepared from flakes without milk, whole milk and butter added",	LOW	10.87
Potatoes, mashed, dehydrated, prepared from flakes without milk, whole milk and margarine added",	LOW	15.02
Potatoes, mashed, dehydrated, prepared from granules with milk, water and margarine added",	LOW	16.13

Food name/ Category (100 g)	Status	Carbs content in g
Potatoes, mashed, dehydrated, prepared from granules without milk, whole milk and butter added",	LOW	14.36
Potatoes, mashed, home-prepared, whole milk added",	LOW	17.57
Potatoes, mashed, home-prepared, whole milk and butter added",	LOW	16.81
Potatoes, mashed, home-prepared, whole milk and margarine added",	LOW	16.94
Potatoes, mashed, prepared from granules, without milk, whole milk and margarine",	LOW	14.4
Potatoes, mashed, ready-to-eat",	LOW	13.29
Potatoes, microwaved, cooked in skin, flesh, with salt",	LOW	23.28
Potatoes, microwaved, cooked, in skin, flesh and skin, with salt",	LOW	24.24
Potatoes, microwaved, cooked, in skin, skin with salt",	LOW	29.63
Potatoes, o'brien, home-prepared",	LOW	15.47
Potatoes, roasted, salt added in processing, frozen, unprepared",	LOW	26.15
Potatoes, russet, flesh and skin, raw",	LOW	18.07
Potatoes, scalloped, dry mix, prepared with water, whole milk and butter",	LOW	12.77
Potatoes, scalloped, dry mix, unprepared",	HIGH	73.93
Potatoes, scalloped, home-prepared with butter",	LOW	10.78
Potatoes, scalloped, home-prepared with margarine",	LOW	10.78
Potatoes, yellow fleshed, french fried, frozen, unprepared",	LOW	25.01
Potatoes, yellow fleshed, hash brown, shredded, salt added in processing, frozen, unprepared",	LOW	17.98
Potatoes, yellow fleshed, roasted, salt added in processing, frozen, unprepared",	LOW	23.44
Poultry salad sandwich spread",	LOW	7.41
Poultry, mechanically deboned, from backs and necks with skin, raw",	LOW	0
Poultry, mechanically deboned, from backs and necks without skin, raw",	LOW	0
Poultry, mechanically deboned, from mature hens, raw",	LOW	0
Prairie Turnips, boiled (Northern Plains Indians)",	LOW	29.99
Prairie Turnips, raw (Northern Plains Indians)",	LOW	35.67
PREGO Pasta, Chunky Garden Combination Italian Sauce, ready-to-serve",	LOW	10
PREGO Pasta, Chunky Garden Mushroom and Green Pepper Italian Sauce, ready-to-serve",	LOW	10
PREGO Pasta, Chunky Garden Mushroom Supreme Italian Sauce, ready-to-serve",	LOW	10

Food name/ Category (100 g)	Status	Carbs content in g
PREGO Pasta, Chunky Garden Tomato, Onion and Garlic Italian Sauce, ready-to-serve",	LOW	10.4
PREGO Pasta, Diced Onion and Garlic Italian Sauce, ready-to-serve",	LOW	13.85
PREGO Pasta, Flavored with Meat Italian Sauce, ready-to-serve",	LOW	10
PREGO Pasta, Fresh Mushroom Italian Sauce, ready-to-serve",	LOW	10
PREGO Pasta, Garlic Supreme Italian Sauce, ready-to-serve",	LOW	13.08
PREGO Pasta, Heart Smart- Ricotta Parmesan Italian Sauce, ready-to-serve",	LOW	10.4
PREGO Pasta, Heart Smart- Roasted Red Pepper and Garlic Italian Sauce, ready-to-serve",	LOW	10.4
PREGO Pasta, Heart Smart- Traditional Sauce, ready-to-serve",	LOW	10
PREGO Pasta, Italian Sausage and Garlic Italian Sauce, ready-to-serve",	LOW	10.4
PREGO Pasta, Mini Meatball Italian Sauce, ready-to-serve",	LOW	10
PREGO Pasta, Mushroom and Garlic Italian Sauce, ready-to-serve",	LOW	10
PREGO Pasta, Mushroom and Parmesan Italian Sauce, ready-to-serve",	LOW	17.6
PREGO Pasta, Organic Mushroom Italian Sauce, ready-to-serve",	LOW	10.4
PREGO Pasta, Organic Tomato and Basil Italian Sauce, ready-to-serve",	LOW	10.4
PREGO Pasta, Roasted Garlic Parmesan Italian Sauce, ready-to-serve",	LOW	10
PREGO Pasta, Tomato, Basil and Garlic Italian Sauce, ready-to-serve",	LOW	9.6
PREGO Pasta, Traditional Italian Sauce, ready-to-serve",	LOW	10
PREGO Pasta, Zesty Mushroom Italian Sauce, ready-to-serve",	LOW	13.85
Pretzels, soft, unsalted",	HIGH	71.04
Pretzels, soft",	HIGH	69.39
Prickly pears, raw (Northern Plains Indians)",	LOW	10.17
Prickly pears, raw",	LOW	9.57
Protein supplement, milk based, Muscle Milk Light, powder",	LOW	22
Protein supplement, milk based, Muscle Milk, powder",	LOW	18.5
Prune juice, canned",	LOW	17.45
Prunes, canned, heavy syrup pack, solids and liquids",	LOW	27.8
Prunes, dehydrated (low-moisture), stewed",	LOW	29.7
Prunes, dehydrated (low-moisture), uncooked",	HIGH	89.07
Pudding, lemon, dry mix, regular, prepared with sugar, egg yolk and water",	LOW	24.2
Puddings, all flavors except chocolate, low calorie, instant, dry mix",	HIGH	84.66

Food name/ Category (100 g)	Status	Carbs content in g
Puddings, all flavors except chocolate, low calorie, regular, dry mix",	HIGH	86.04
Puddings, banana, dry mix, instant, prepared with 2% milk",	LOW	19.74
Puddings, banana, dry mix, instant, prepared with whole milk",	LOW	19.76
Puddings, banana, dry mix, instant, with added oil",	HIGH	89
Puddings, banana, dry mix, instant",	HIGH	92.7
Puddings, banana, dry mix, regular, prepared with 2% milk",	LOW	18.43
Puddings, banana, dry mix, regular, prepared with whole milk",	LOW	18.44
Puddings, banana, dry mix, regular, with added oil",	HIGH	88.4
Puddings, banana, dry mix, regular",	HIGH	93
Puddings, chocolate flavor, low calorie, instant, dry mix",	HIGH	78.2
Puddings, chocolate flavor, low calorie, regular, dry mix",	HIGH	74.42
Puddings, chocolate, dry mix, instant, prepared with 2% milk",	LOW	18.89
Puddings, chocolate, dry mix, instant, prepared with whole milk",	LOW	18.8
Puddings, chocolate, dry mix, instant",	HIGH	87.9
Puddings, chocolate, dry mix, regular, prepared with 2% milk",	LOW	19.76
Puddings, chocolate, dry mix, regular, prepared with whole milk",	LOW	19.64
Puddings, chocolate, dry mix, regular",	HIGH	89.3
Puddings, chocolate, ready-to-eat, fat free",	LOW	20.87
Puddings, chocolate, ready-to-eat",	LOW	23.01
Puddings, coconut cream, dry mix, instant, prepared with 2% milk",	LOW	19.2
Puddings, coconut cream, dry mix, instant, prepared with whole milk",	LOW	19.1
Puddings, coconut cream, dry mix, instant",	HIGH	83.5
Puddings, coconut cream, dry mix, regular, prepared with 2% milk",	LOW	17.8
Puddings, coconut cream, dry mix, regular, prepared with whole milk",	LOW	17.7
Puddings, coconut cream, dry mix, regular",	HIGH	81.84
Puddings, lemon, dry mix, instant, prepared with 2% milk",	LOW	20.2
Puddings, lemon, dry mix, instant, prepared with whole milk",	LOW	20.1
Puddings, lemon, dry mix, instant",	HIGH	95.4
Puddings, lemon, dry mix, regular, with added oil, potassium, sodium",	HIGH	90.3
Puddings, lemon, dry mix, regular",	HIGH	91.8
Puddings, rice, dry mix, prepared with 2% milk",	LOW	20.81
Puddings, rice, dry mix, prepared with whole milk",	LOW	20.68
Puddings, rice, dry mix",	HIGH	91.2
Puddings, rice, ready-to-eat",	LOW	18.39
Puddings, tapioca, dry mix, prepared with 2% milk",	LOW	19.56

Food name/ Category (100 g)	Status	Carbs content in g
Puddings, tapioca, dry mix, prepared with whole milk",	LOW	19.43
Puddings, tapioca, dry mix",	HIGH	94.3
Puddings, tapioca, ready-to-eat, fat free",	LOW	21.31
Puddings, tapioca, ready-to-eat",	LOW	21.69
Puddings, vanilla, dry mix, instant, prepared with whole milk",	LOW	19.7
Puddings, vanilla, dry mix, instant",	HIGH	92.9
Puddings, vanilla, dry mix, regular, prepared with 2% milk",	LOW	18.53
Puddings, vanilla, dry mix, regular, prepared with whole milk",	LOW	18.92
Puddings, vanilla, dry mix, regular, with added oil",	HIGH	92.4
Puddings, vanilla, dry mix, regular",	HIGH	93.5
Puddings, vanilla, ready-to-eat, fat free",	LOW	20.16
Puddings, vanilla, ready-to-eat",	LOW	22.6
Puff pastry, frozen, ready-to-bake, baked",	MEDIUM	45.7
Puff pastry, frozen, ready-to-bake",	MEDIUM	45.1
Pummelo, raw",	LOW	9.62
Pumpkin flowers, raw",	LOW	3.28
Pumpkin leaves, cooked, boiled, drained, with salt",	LOW	3.39
Pumpkin pie mix, canned",	LOW	26.39
Pumpkin, canned, with salt",	LOW	8.09
Pumpkin, canned, without salt",	LOW	8.09
Pumpkin, cooked, boiled, drained, with salt",	LOW	4.31
Pumpkin, cooked, boiled, drained, without salt",	LOW	4.9
Pumpkin, flowers, cooked, boiled, drained, with salt",	LOW	3.18
Pumpkin, raw",	LOW	6.5
Purslane, cooked, boiled, drained, with salt",	LOW	3.55
Purslane, cooked, boiled, drained, without salt",	LOW	3.55
Purslane, raw",	LOW	3.39
Quail, breast, meat only, raw",	LOW	0
Quail, cooked, total edible",	LOW	0
Quail, meat and skin, raw",	LOW	0
Quail, meat only, raw",	LOW	0

Food name/ Category (100 g)	Status	Carbs content in g
Quinces, raw",	LOW	15.3
Quinoa, uncooked",	HIGH	64.16
Radishes, hawaiian style, pickled",	LOW	5.2
Radishes, oriental, cooked, boiled, drained, with salt",	LOW	3.43
Radishes, oriental, dried",	HIGH	63.37
Radishes, raw",	LOW	3.4
Raspberries, canned, red, heavy syrup pack, solids and liquids",	LOW	23.36
Raspberries, frozen, red, sweetened",	LOW	26.16
Raspberries, frozen, unsweetened",	LOW	11.94
Raspberries, raw",	LOW	11.94
Raspberries, wild (Northern Plains Indians)",	LOW	13.85
Ravioli, cheese with tomato sauce, frozen, not prepared, includes regular and light entrees",	LOW	17.31
Ravioli, cheese-filled, canned",	LOW	13.64
Ravioli, meat-filled, with tomato sauce or meat sauce, canned",	LOW	13.26
Reddi Wip Fat Free Whipped Topping",	LOW	25
Refried beans, canned, fat-free",	LOW	13.5
Refried beans, canned, traditional style (includes USDA commodity)",	LOW	13.55
Refried beans, canned, traditional, reduced sodium",	LOW	13.55
Refried beans, canned, vegetarian",	LOW	13.5
Restaurant, Chinese, beef and vegetables",	LOW	7.29
Restaurant, Chinese, chicken and vegetables",	LOW	5.38
Restaurant, Chinese, chicken chow mein",	LOW	8.29
Restaurant, Chinese, egg rolls, assorted",	LOW	27.29
Restaurant, Chinese, fried rice, without meat",	LOW	32.79
Restaurant, Chinese, general tso's chicken",	LOW	23.99
Restaurant, Chinese, kung pao chicken",	LOW	6.87
Restaurant, Chinese, lemon chicken",	LOW	20.61
Restaurant, Chinese, orange chicken",	LOW	22.46
Restaurant, Chinese, sesame chicken",	LOW	26.88

Food name/ Category (100 g)	Status	Carbs content in g
Restaurant, Chinese, shrimp and vegetables",	LOW	4.52
Restaurant, Chinese, sweet and sour chicken",	LOW	23.86
Restaurant, Chinese, vegetable chow mein, without meat or noodles",	LOW	5.74
Restaurant, Chinese, vegetable lo mein, without meat",	LOW	20.16
Restaurant, family style, chicken fingers, from kid's menu",	LOW	18.77
Restaurant, family style, chicken tenders",	LOW	19.29
Restaurant, family style, chili with meat and beans",	LOW	4.57
Restaurant, family style, coleslaw",	LOW	12.35
Restaurant, family style, fish fillet, battered or breaded, fried",	LOW	16.89
Restaurant, family style, french fries",	LOW	37.2
Restaurant, family style, fried mozzarella sticks",	LOW	25.14
Restaurant, family style, hash browns",	LOW	26.59
Restaurant, family style, macaroni & cheese, from kids' menu",	LOW	18.8
Restaurant, family style, onion rings",	MEDIUM	40.72
Restaurant, family style, shrimp, breaded and fried",	LOW	22.29
Restaurant, family style, sirloin steak",	LOW	0
Restaurant, family style, spaghetti and meatballs",	LOW	15.51
Restaurant, Italian, cheese ravioli with marinara sauce",	LOW	18.5
Restaurant, Italian, chicken parmesan without pasta",	LOW	10.92
Restaurant, Italian, lasagna with meat",	LOW	11.36
Restaurant, Italian, spaghetti with meat sauce",	LOW	16.4
Restaurant, Italian, spaghetti with pomodoro sauce (no meat)",	LOW	17.77
Restaurant, Latino, arepa (unleavened cornmeal bread)",	LOW	37.14
Restaurant, Latino, Arroz con frijoles negros (rice and black beans)",	LOW	24.4
Restaurant, Latino, Arroz con grandules (rice and pigeonpeas)",	LOW	30.75
Restaurant, Latino, Arroz con habichuelas colorados (Rice And Red Beans)",	LOW	23.74
Restaurant, Latino, arroz con leche (rice pudding)",	LOW	24.92
Restaurant, Latino, black bean soup",	LOW	14.79
Restaurant, Latino, bunuelos (fried yeast bread)",	MEDIUM	48.57

Food name/ Category (100 g)	Status	Carbs content in g
Restaurant, Latino, chicken and rice, entree, prepared",	LOW	20.03
Restaurant, Latino, empanadas, beef, prepared",	LOW	31.19
Restaurant, Latino, pupusas con frijoles (pupusas, bean)",	LOW	31.49
Restaurant, Latino, pupusas con queso (pupusas, cheese)",	LOW	22.39
Restaurant, Latino, tamale, corn",	LOW	26.68
Restaurant, Latino, tripe soup",	LOW	4.07
Restaurant, Mexican, cheese enchilada",	LOW	15.45
Restaurant, Mexican, cheese quesadilla",	LOW	24.11
Restaurant, Mexican, cheese tamales",	LOW	17.97
Restaurant, Mexican, refried beans",	LOW	16.79
Restaurant, Mexican, soft taco with ground beef, cheese and lettuce",	LOW	17.92
Restaurant, Mexican, spanish rice",	LOW	31.16
Rhubarb, frozen, cooked, with sugar",	LOW	31.2
Rhubarb, frozen, uncooked",	LOW	5.1
Rhubarb, raw",	LOW	4.54
Rice and vermicelli mix, beef flavor, prepared with 80% margarine",	LOW	22.03
Rice and vermicelli mix, beef flavor, unprepared",	HIGH	76.02
Rice and vermicelli mix, chicken flavor, prepared with 80% margarine",	LOW	23.54
Rice and vermicelli mix, chicken flavor, unprepared",	HIGH	75.8
Rice and vermicelli mix, rice pilaf flavor, prepared with 80% margarine",	LOW	25.67
Rice and vermicelli mix, rice pilaf flavor, unprepared",	HIGH	76.31
Rice and Wheat cereal bar",	HIGH	72.73
Rice bowl with chicken, frozen entree, prepared (includes fried, teriyaki, and sweet and sour varieties)",	LOW	22.46
Rice bran, crude",	MEDIUM	49.69
Rice cake, cracker (include hain mini rice cakes)",	HIGH	81.1
Rice flour, white, unenriched",	HIGH	80.13
Rice mix, cheese flavor, dry mix, unprepared",	HIGH	73.88
Rice mix, white and wild, flavored, unprepared",	HIGH	76.14
Rice noodles, dry",	HIGH	80.18
Rice, brown, long-grain, cooked",	LOW	25.58
Rice, brown, long-grain, raw",	HIGH	76.25
Rice, brown, medium-grain, cooked",	LOW	23.51
Rice, brown, medium-grain, raw",	HIGH	76.17
Rice, brown, parboiled, cooked, UNCLE BENS",	LOW	31.33

Food name/ Category (100 g)	Status	Carbs content in g
Rice, white, glutinous, unenriched, cooked",	LOW	21.09
Rice, white, long-grain, parboiled, enriched, cooked",	LOW	26.05
Rice, white, long-grain, parboiled, enriched, dry",	HIGH	80.89
Rice, white, long-grain, parboiled, unenriched, cooked",	LOW	26.05
Rice, white, long-grain, parboiled, unenriched, dry",	HIGH	80.89
Rice, white, long-grain, precooked or instant, enriched, prepared",	LOW	26.76
Rice, white, long-grain, regular, cooked, enriched, with salt",	LOW	28.17
Rice, white, long-grain, regular, cooked, unenriched, with salt",	LOW	28.17
Rice, white, long-grain, regular, enriched, cooked",	LOW	28.17
Rice, white, long-grain, regular, raw, enriched",	HIGH	79.95
Rice, white, long-grain, regular, raw, unenriched",	HIGH	79.95
Rice, white, long-grain, regular, unenriched, cooked without salt",	LOW	28.17
Rice, white, medium-grain, cooked, unenriched",	LOW	28.59
Rice, white, medium-grain, enriched, cooked",	LOW	28.59
Rice, white, medium-grain, raw, enriched",	HIGH	79.34
Rice, white, medium-grain, raw, unenriched",	HIGH	79.34
Rice, white, short-grain, cooked, unenriched",	LOW	28.73
Rice, white, short-grain, enriched, cooked",	LOW	28.73
Rice, white, short-grain, enriched, uncooked",	HIGH	79.15
Rice, white, short-grain, raw, unenriched",	HIGH	79.15
Rice, white, steamed, Chinese restaurant",	LOW	33.88
Roast beef spread",	LOW	3.73
Roast beef, deli style, prepackaged, sliced",	LOW	0.64
Rolls, dinner, egg",	MEDIUM	52
Rolls, dinner, oat bran",	MEDIUM	40.2
Rolls, dinner, plain, commercially prepared (includes brown-and-serve)",	MEDIUM	52.04
Rolls, dinner, plain, prepared from recipe, made with low fat (2%) milk",	MEDIUM	53.4
Rolls, dinner, rye",	MEDIUM	53.1
Rolls, dinner, sweet",	MEDIUM	53.58
Rolls, dinner, wheat",	MEDIUM	46
Rolls, dinner, whole-wheat",	MEDIUM	51.1
Rolls, french",	MEDIUM	50.2
Rolls, gluten-free, white, made with brown rice flour, tapioca starch, and potato star	MEDIUM	55.1
Rolls, gluten-free, white, made with brown rice flour, tapioca starch, and sorghum fl	MEDIUM	40.24
Rolls, gluten-free, white, made with rice flour, rice starch, and corn starch",	MEDIUM	50.47
Rolls, gluten-free, whole grain, made with tapioca starch and brown rice flour",	MEDIUM	44.29
Rolls, hard (includes kaiser)",	MEDIUM	52.7
Rolls, pumpernickel",	MEDIUM	51.87
Rose Hips, wild (Northern Plains Indians)",	LOW	38.22

Food name/ Category (100 g)	Status	Carbs content in g
Rowal, raw",	LOW	23.9
RUDI'S, Gluten-Free Bakery, Original Sandwich Bread",	MEDIUM	52.83
Ruffed Grouse, breast meat, skinless, raw",	LOW	0
Rutabagas, cooked, boiled, drained, with salt",	LOW	6.84
Rutabagas, cooked, boiled, drained, without salt",	LOW	6.84
Rye flour, dark",	HIGH	68.63
Rye flour, light",	HIGH	76.68
Rye flour, medium",	HIGH	75.43
Rye grain",	HIGH	75.86
SAGE VALLEY, Gluten Free Vanilla Sandwich Cookies",	HIGH	71.88
Salad dressing, blue or roquefort cheese dressing, commercial, regular",	LOW	4.77
Salad dressing, blue or roquefort cheese dressing, fat-free",	LOW	25.6
Salad dressing, blue or roquefort cheese dressing, light",	LOW	13.2
Salad dressing, blue or roquefort cheese, low calorie",	LOW	2.9
Salad dressing, buttermilk, lite",	LOW	21.33
Salad dressing, caesar dressing, regular",	LOW	3.3
Salad dressing, caesar, fat-free",	LOW	30.73
Salad dressing, caesar, low calorie",	LOW	18.6
Salad Dressing, coleslaw dressing, reduced fat",	MEDIUM	40
Salad dressing, coleslaw",	LOW	23.8
Salad dressing, french dressing, commercial, regular, without salt",	LOW	15.58
Salad dressing, french dressing, commercial, regular",	LOW	15.58
Salad dressing, french dressing, fat-free",	LOW	32.14
Salad dressing, french dressing, reduced calorie",	LOW	27
Salad dressing, french dressing, reduced fat",	LOW	31.22
Salad dressing, french, cottonseed, oil, home recipe",	LOW	3.4
Salad dressing, french, home recipe",	LOW	3.4
Salad dressing, green goddess, regular",	LOW	7.36
Salad dressing, home recipe, vinegar and oil",	LOW	2.5
Salad dressing, honey mustard dressing, reduced calorie",	LOW	28.26
Salad dressing, honey mustard, regular",	LOW	23.33

Food name/ Category (100 g)	Status	Carbs content in g
Salad dressing, italian dressing, commercial, reduced fat",	LOW	9.99
Salad dressing, italian dressing, commercial, regular",	LOW	12.12
Salad dressing, italian dressing, fat-free",	LOW	8.75
Salad dressing, italian dressing, reduced calorie",	LOW	6.7
Salad dressing, KRAFT Mayo Fat Free Mayonnaise Dressing",	LOW	15.8
Salad dressing, KRAFT Mayo Light Mayonnaise",	LOW	8.5
Salad dressing, KRAFT MIRACLE WHIP FREE Nonfat Dressing",	LOW	15.5
Salad dressing, mayonnaise and mayonnaise-type, low calorie",	LOW	23.9
Salad dressing, mayonnaise type, regular, with salt",	LOW	14.78
Salad Dressing, mayonnaise-like, fat-free",	LOW	15.5
Salad dressing, mayonnaise, imitation, milk cream",	LOW	11.1
Salad dressing, mayonnaise, imitation, soybean without cholesterol",	LOW	15.8
Salad dressing, mayonnaise, imitation, soybean",	LOW	16
Salad Dressing, mayonnaise, light, SMART BALANCE, Omega Plus light",	LOW	9.39
Salad dressing, mayonnaise, light",	LOW	9.23
Salad dressing, mayonnaise, regular",	LOW	0.57
Salad dressing, mayonnaise, soybean and safflower oil, with salt",	LOW	2.7
Salad dressing, peppercorn dressing, commercial, regular",	LOW	3.5
Salad dressing, poppyseed, creamy",	LOW	23.73
Salad dressing, ranch dressing, fat-free",	LOW	26.51
Salad dressing, ranch dressing, reduced fat",	LOW	21.33
Salad dressing, ranch dressing, regular",	LOW	5.9
Salad dressing, russian dressing, low calorie",	LOW	27.6
Salad dressing, russian dressing",	LOW	31.9
Salad dressing, sesame seed dressing, regular",	LOW	8.6
Salad dressing, spray-style dressing, assorted flavors",	LOW	16.6
Salad dressing, sweet and sour",	LOW	3.7
Salad dressing, thousand island dressing, fat-free",	LOW	29.27

Food name/ Category (100 g)	Status	Carbs content in g
Salad dressing, thousand island dressing, reduced fat",	LOW	24.06
Salad dressing, thousand island, commercial, regular",	LOW	14.64
Salami, cooked, beef",	LOW	1.9
Salami, cooked, turkey",	LOW	1.55
Salisbury steak with gravy, frozen",	LOW	6.78
Salmon, red (sockeye), filets with skin, smoked (Alaska Native)",	LOW	0
Salmon, sockeye, canned, drained solids, without skin and bones",	LOW	0
Salmon, sockeye, canned, total can contents",	LOW	0
Salsify, cooked, boiled, drained, with salt",	LOW	15.36
Salt, table",	LOW	0
Sandwich spread, meatless",	LOW	9
Sandwich spread, with chopped pickle, regular, unspecified oils",	LOW	22.4
Sauce, barbecue, BULL'S-EYE, original",	LOW	39.95
Sauce, barbecue, KC MASTERPIECE, original",	LOW	37.92
Sauce, barbecue, KRAFT, original",	MEDIUM	40.77
Sauce, barbecue, OPEN PIT, original",	LOW	29.45
Sauce, barbecue, SWEET BABY RAY'S, original",	MEDIUM	46.08
Sauce, barbecue",	MEDIUM	40.77
Sauce, cheese, ready-to-serve",	LOW	6.83
Sauce, cocktail, ready-to-serve",	LOW	28.22
Sauce, duck, ready-to-serve",	HIGH	60.61
Sauce, enchilada, red, mild, ready to serve",	LOW	4.87
Sauce, fish, ready-to-serve",	LOW	3.64
Sauce, hoisin, ready-to-serve",	MEDIUM	44.08
Sauce, homemade, white, medium",	LOW	9.17
Sauce, homemade, white, thick",	LOW	11.61
Sauce, homemade, white, thin",	LOW	7.4
Sauce, horseradish",	LOW	10.05
Sauce, hot chile, sriracha, CHA! BY TEXAS PETE",	LOW	22.73
Sauce, hot chile, sriracha, TUONG OT SRIRACHA",	LOW	15.87

Food name/ Category (100 g)	Status	Carbs content in g
Sauce, hot chile, sriracha",	LOW	19.16
Sauce, OLD EL PASO, enchilada, red, mild, ready to serve",	LOW	5.04
Sauce, oyster, ready-to-serve",	LOW	10.92
Sauce, pasta, spaghetti/marinara, ready-to-serve",	LOW	7.43
Sauce, peanut, made from coconut, water, sugar, peanuts",	LOW	28.46
Sauce, peanut, made from peanut butter, water, soy sauce",	LOW	22.02
Sauce, pesto, BUITONI, pesto with basil, ready-to-serve, refrigerated",	LOW	10.09
Sauce, pesto, CLASSICO, basil pesto, ready-to-serve",	LOW	6.93
Sauce, pesto, MEZZETTA, NAPA VALLEY BISTRO, basil pesto, ready-to-serve",	LOW	5.12
Sauce, pesto, ready-to-serve, refrigerated",	LOW	10.09
Sauce, pesto, ready-to-serve, shelf stable",	LOW	6.14
Sauce, pizza, canned, ready-to-serve",	LOW	8.66
Sauce, plum, ready-to-serve",	MEDIUM	42.81
Sauce, ready-to-serve, pepper or hot",	LOW	1.75
Sauce, ready-to-serve, pepper, TABASCO",	LOW	0.8
Sauce, salsa, ready-to-serve",	LOW	6.64
Sauce, salsa, verde, ready-to-serve",	LOW	6.36
Sauce, sofrito, prepared from recipe",	LOW	5.46
Sauce, steak, tomato based",	LOW	22.04
Sauce, sweet and sour, ready-to-serve",	LOW	38.22
Sauce, tartar, ready-to-serve",	LOW	13.3
Sauce, teriyaki, ready-to-serve, reduced sodium",	LOW	15.58
Sauce, teriyaki, ready-to-serve",	LOW	15.56
Sauce, tomato chili sauce, bottled, with salt",	LOW	19.79
Sauce, worcestershire",	LOW	19.46
Sauerkraut, canned, solids and liquids",	LOW	4.28
Sausage, egg and cheese breakfast biscuit",	LOW	21.57
Sausage, Italian, sweet, links",	LOW	2.1

Food name/ Category (100 g)	Status	Carbs content in g
Sausage, Italian, turkey, smoked",	LOW	4.65
Sausage, meatless",	LOW	8.09
Sausage, Polish, beef with chicken, hot",	LOW	3.6
Sausage, turkey, breakfast links, mild",	LOW	1.56
Sausage, turkey, hot, smoked",	LOW	4.65
SCHAR, Gluten-Free, Classic White Rolls",	MEDIUM	50.47
School Lunch, chicken nuggets, whole grain breaded",	LOW	22.86
School Lunch, chicken patty, whole grain breaded",	LOW	12.5
School Lunch, pizza, BIG DADDY'S LS 16\" 51% Whole Grain Rolled Edge Cheese Pizza, frozen",	LOW	27.1
School Lunch, pizza, BIG DADDY'S LS 16\" 51% Whole Grain Rolled Edge Turkey Pepperoni Pizza, frozen",	LOW	27.35
School Lunch, pizza, cheese topping, thick crust, whole grain, frozen, cooked",	LOW	28.08
School Lunch, pizza, cheese topping, thin crust, whole grain, frozen, cooked",	LOW	31.31
School Lunch, pizza, pepperoni topping, thick crust, whole grain, frozen, cooked",	LOW	28.3
School Lunch, pizza, pepperoni topping, thin crust, whole grain, frozen, cooked",	LOW	31.24
School Lunch, pizza, sausage topping, thick crust, whole grain, frozen, cooked",	LOW	30.58
School Lunch, pizza, sausage topping, thin crust, whole grain, frozen, cooked",	LOW	32.24
School Lunch, pizza, TONY'S Breakfast Pizza Sausage, frozen",	LOW	26.99
School Lunch, pizza, TONY'S SMARTPIZZA Whole Grain 4x6 Cheese Pizza 50\/50 Cheese, frozen",	LOW	29.27
School Lunch, pizza, TONY'S SMARTPIZZA Whole Grain 4x6 Pepperoni Pizza 50\/50 Cheese, frozen",	LOW	28.84
Seasoning mix, dry, chili, original",	MEDIUM	56.56
Seasoning mix, dry, sazon, coriander & annatto",	LOW	0
Seasoning mix, dry, taco, original",	HIGH	58
Seaweed, Canadian Cultivated EMI-TSUNOMATA, dry",	MEDIUM	46.24
Seaweed, Canadian Cultivated EMI-TSUNOMATA, rehydrated",	LOW	5.62
Seaweed, irishmoss, raw",	LOW	12.29
Seaweed, kelp, raw",	LOW	9.57
Seaweed, laver, raw",	LOW	5.11
Seaweed, spirulina, dried",	LOW	23.9
Seaweed, wakame, raw",	LOW	9.14
Seeds, breadnut tree seeds, dried",	HIGH	79.39

Food name/ Category (100 g)	Status	Carbs content in g
Seeds, cottonseed meal, partially defatted (glandless)",	LOW	38.43
Seeds, hemp seed, hulled",	LOW	8.67
Seeds, lotus seeds, dried",	HIGH	64.47
Seeds, lotus seeds, raw",	LOW	17.28
Seeds, pumpkin and squash seed kernels, roasted, with salt added",	LOW	14.71
Seeds, pumpkin and squash seeds, whole, roasted, with salt added",	MEDIUM	53.75
Seeds, safflower seed kernels, dried",	LOW	34.29
Seeds, safflower seed meal, partially defatted",	MEDIUM	48.73
Seeds, sesame butter, tahini, from raw and stone ground kernels",	LOW	26.19
Seeds, sesame butter, tahini, from roasted and toasted kernels (most common type)",	LOW	21.19
Seeds, sesame butter, tahini, from unroasted kernels (non-chemically removed seed coat)",	LOW	17.89
Seeds, sesame flour, high-fat",	LOW	26.62
Seeds, sesame flour, low-fat",	LOW	35.51
Seeds, sesame flour, partially defatted",	LOW	35.14
Seeds, sesame meal, partially defatted",	LOW	26.04
Seeds, sesame seed kernels, dried (decorticated)",	LOW	11.73
Seeds, sesame seed kernels, toasted, with salt added (decorticated)",	LOW	26.04
Seeds, sesame seed kernels, toasted, without salt added (decorticated)",	LOW	26.04
Seeds, sisymbrium sp. seeds, whole, dried",	HIGH	58.26
Seeds, sunflower seed butter, with salt added",	LOW	23.32
Seeds, sunflower seed butter, without salt",	LOW	23.32
Seeds, sunflower seed flour, partially defatted",	LOW	35.83
Seeds, sunflower seed kernels from shell, dry roasted, with salt added",	LOW	15.31
Seeds, sunflower seed kernels, dry roasted, with salt added",	LOW	24.07
Seeds, sunflower seed kernels, dry roasted, without salt",	LOW	24.07
Seeds, sunflower seed kernels, oil roasted, with salt added",	LOW	22.89
Seeds, sunflower seed kernels, oil roasted, without salt",	LOW	22.89
Seeds, sunflower seed kernels, toasted, with salt added",	LOW	20.59
Seeds, sunflower seed kernels, toasted, without salt",	LOW	20.59
Seeds, watermelon seed kernels, dried",	LOW	15.31

Food name/ Category (100 g)	Status	Carbs content in g
Semolina, enriched",	HIGH	72.83
Semolina, unenriched",	HIGH	72.83
Sesbania flower, cooked, steamed, with salt",	LOW	5.1
Shake, fast food, vanilla",	LOW	19.59
Shallots, freeze-dried",	HIGH	80.7
Sherbet, orange",	LOW	30.4
Shortening bread, soybean (hydrogenated) and cottonseed",	LOW	0
Shortening cake mix, soybean (hydrogenated) and cottonseed (hydrogenated)",	LOW	0
Shortening confectionery, coconut (hydrogenated) and or palm kernel (hydrogenated)",	LOW	0
Shortening frying (heavy duty), beef tallow and cottonseed",	LOW	0
Shortening frying (heavy duty), palm (hydrogenated)",	LOW	0
Shortening frying (heavy duty), soybean (hydrogenated), linoleic (less than 1%)",	LOW	0
Shortening household soybean (hydrogenated) and palm",	LOW	0
Shortening industrial, lard and vegetable oil",	LOW	0
Shortening industrial, soybean (hydrogenated) and cottonseed",	LOW	0
Shortening, confectionery, fractionated palm",	LOW	0
Shortening, household, lard and vegetable oil",	LOW	0
Shortening, household, soybean (partially hydrogenated)-cottonseed (partially hydrogenated)",	LOW	0
Shortening, industrial, soy (partially hydrogenated) and corn for frying",	LOW	0
Shortening, industrial, soy (partially hydrogenated) for baking and confections",	LOW	0
Shortening, industrial, soy (partially hydrogenated), pourable liquid fry shortening",	LOW	0
Shortening, multipurpose, soybean (hydrogenated) and palm (hydrogenated)",	LOW	0
Shortening, special purpose for baking, soybean (hydrogenated) palm and cottonseed",	LOW	0
Shortening, special purpose for cakes and frostings, soybean (hydrogenated)",	LOW	0
Shortening, vegetable, household, composite",	LOW	0
Side dishes, potato salad",	LOW	13.53
SILK Chai, soymilk",	LOW	7.82
SILK Chocolate, soymilk",	LOW	9.47
SILK Coffee, soymilk",	LOW	10.29

Food name/ Category (100 g)	Status	Carbs content in g
SILK French Vanilla Creamer",	LOW	20
SILK Hazelnut Creamer",	LOW	20
SILK Light Chocolate, soymilk",	LOW	9.05
SILK Light Plain, soymilk",	LOW	3.29
SILK Light Vanilla, soymilk",	LOW	4.12
SILK Mocha, soymilk",	LOW	9.05
SILK Nog, soymilk",	LOW	12.3
SILK Original Creamer",	LOW	6.67
SILK Plain, soymilk",	LOW	3.29
SILK Plus Fiber, soymilk",	LOW	5.76
SILK Plus for Bone Health, soymilk",	LOW	4.53
SILK Plus Omega-3 DHA, soymilk",	LOW	3.29
SILK Vanilla, soymilk",	LOW	4.12
SILK Very Vanilla, soymilk",	LOW	7.82
SMART SOUP, French Lentil",	LOW	9.5
SMART SOUP, Greek Minestrone",	LOW	8.4
SMART SOUP, Indian Bean Masala",	LOW	10.5
SMART SOUP, Moroccan Chick Pea",	LOW	9.7
SMART SOUP, Santa Fe Corn Chowder",	LOW	11.2
SMART SOUP, Thai Coconut Curry",	LOW	6.5
SMART SOUP, Vietnamese Carrot Lemongrass",	LOW	8.2
Snack, Mixed Berry Bar",	HIGH	58.84
Snack, potato chips, made from dried potatoes, plain",	MEDIUM	55.38
Snack, Pretzel, hard chocolate coated",	HIGH	70.07
Snacks, bagel chips, plain",	HIGH	66.36
Snacks, beef jerky, chopped and formed",	LOW	11
Snacks, beef sticks, smoked",	LOW	5.4
Snacks, brown rice chips",	HIGH	81.5
Snacks, candy bits, yogurt covered with vitamin C",	HIGH	86.9
Snacks, CLIF BAR, mixed flavors",	HIGH	65.44
Snacks, corn cakes",	HIGH	83.4
Snacks, corn-based, extruded, chips, barbecue-flavor, made with enriched masa flc	MEDIUM	56.2
Snacks, corn-based, extruded, chips, barbecue-flavor",	MEDIUM	56.2

Food name/ Category (100 g)	Status	Carbs content in g
Snacks, corn-based, extruded, chips, plain",	MEDIUM	56.9
Snacks, corn-based, extruded, cones, plain",	HIGH	62.9
Snacks, corn-based, extruded, onion-flavor",	HIGH	65.1
Snacks, corn-based, extruded, puffs or twists, cheese-flavor, unenriched",	MEDIUM	54.1
Snacks, corn-based, extruded, puffs or twists, cheese-flavor",	MEDIUM	53.53
Snacks, cornnuts, barbecue-flavor",	HIGH	71.7
Snacks, crisped rice bar, almond",	HIGH	64.6
Snacks, crisped rice bar, chocolate chip",	HIGH	73
Snacks, FARLEY CANDY, FARLEY Fruit Snacks, with vitamins A, C, and E",	HIGH	80.9
Snacks, FRITOLAY, SUNCHIPS, Multigrain Snack, Harvest Cheddar flavor",	HIGH	64.7
Snacks, FRITOLAY, SUNCHIPS, Multigrain Snack, original flavor",	HIGH	67.26
Snacks, FRITOLAY, SUNCHIPS, multigrain, French onion flavor",	HIGH	65.49
Snacks, fruit leather, pieces, with vitamin C",	HIGH	85.2
Snacks, fruit leather, pieces",	HIGH	82.82
Snacks, fruit leather, rolls",	HIGH	85.8
Snacks, GENERAL MILLS, BETTY CROCKER Fruit Roll Ups, berry flavored, with	HIGH	85.2
Snacks, GENERAL MILLS, CHEX MIX, traditional flavor",	HIGH	75.69
Snacks, granola bar, chewy, reduced sugar, all flavors",	HIGH	69.4
Snacks, granola bar, GENERAL MILLS NATURE VALLEY, SWEET&SALTY NUT,	HIGH	61.14
Snacks, granola bar, GENERAL MILLS, NATURE VALLEY, CHEWY TRAIL MIX",	HIGH	72.27
Snacks, granola bar, GENERAL MILLS, NATURE VALLEY, with yogurt coating",	HIGH	74.29
Snacks, granola bar, KASHI GOLEAN, chewy, mixed flavors",	HIGH	63.42
Snacks, granola bar, KASHI GOLEAN, crunchy, mixed flavors",	HIGH	59.58
Snacks, granola bar, KASHI TLC Bar, chewy, mixed flavors",	MEDIUM	53.26
Snacks, granola bar, KASHI TLC Bar, crunchy, mixed flavors",	HIGH	62.78
Snacks, granola bar, QUAKER, chewy, 90 Calorie Bar",	HIGH	79.17
Snacks, granola bar, QUAKER, DIPPS, all flavors",	HIGH	64.96
Snacks, granola bar, with coconut, chocolate coated",	MEDIUM	55.2
Snacks, granola bars, hard, almond",	HIGH	62
Snacks, granola bars, hard, chocolate chip",	HIGH	72.1
Snacks, granola bars, hard, peanut butter",	HIGH	62.3
Snacks, granola bars, hard, plain",	HIGH	64.4
Snacks, granola bars, QUAKER OATMEAL TO GO, all flavors",	HIGH	75.47
Snacks, granola bars, soft, almond, confectioners coating",	HIGH	60.13
Snacks, granola bars, soft, coated, milk chocolate coating, chocolate chip",	HIGH	63.8
Snacks, granola bars, soft, coated, milk chocolate coating, peanut butter",	MEDIUM	53.4
Snacks, granola bars, soft, uncoated, chocolate chip",	HIGH	70.2
Snacks, granola bars, soft, uncoated, nut and raisin",	HIGH	63.6
Snacks, granola bars, soft, uncoated, peanut butter and chocolate chip",	HIGH	62.2
Snacks, granola bars, soft, uncoated, peanut butter",	HIGH	64.4
Snacks, granola bars, soft, uncoated, plain",	HIGH	67.3
Snacks, granola bars, soft, uncoated, raisin",	HIGH	66.4
Snacks, granola bites, mixed flavors",	HIGH	66.27
Snacks, KELLOGG, KELLOGG'S Low Fat Granola Bar, Crunchy Almond\/Brown Su	HIGH	78
Snacks, KELLOGG, KELLOGG'S RICE KRISPIES TREATS Squares",	HIGH	80.5
Snacks, KRAFT, CORNNUTS, plain",	HIGH	71.86
Snacks, M&M MARS, COMBOS Snacks Cheddar Cheese Pretzel",	HIGH	66.5
Snacks, M&M MARS, KUDOS Whole Grain Bar, chocolate chip",	HIGH	72.31
Snacks, M&M MARS, KUDOS Whole Grain Bar, M&M's milk chocolate",	HIGH	73.01
Snacks, M&M MARS, KUDOS Whole Grain Bars, peanut butter",	HIGH	64.69
Snacks, NUTRI-GRAIN FRUIT AND NUT BAR",	HIGH	66.72
Snacks, oriental mix, rice-based",	MEDIUM	51.62
Snacks, pita chips, salted",	HIGH	68.26
Snacks, plantain chips, salted",	HIGH	63.84
Snacks, popcorn, air-popped (Unsalted)",	HIGH	77.9
Snacks, popcorn, cakes",	HIGH	80.1
Snacks, popcorn, caramel-coated, with peanuts",	HIGH	80.7

Food name/ Category (100 g)	Status	Carbs content in g
Snacks, popcorn, caramel-coated, without peanuts",	HIGH	79.1
Snacks, popcorn, cheese-flavor",	MEDIUM	51.6
Snacks, popcorn, home-prepared, oil-popped, unsalted",	HIGH	58.1
Snacks, popcorn, microwave, 94% fat free",	HIGH	76.04
Snacks, popcorn, microwave, low fat",	HIGH	72
Snacks, popcorn, microwave, regular (butter) flavor, made with partially hydrogenat	MEDIUM	55.16
Snacks, popcorn, oil-popped, microwave, regular flavor, no trans fat",	MEDIUM	45.06
Snacks, popcorn, oil-popped, white popcorn, salt added",	HIGH	57.2
Snacks, potato chips, barbecue-flavor",	MEDIUM	55.92
Snacks, potato chips, cheese-flavor",	HIGH	57.7
Snacks, potato chips, fat free, salted",	HIGH	83.76
Snacks, potato chips, fat-free, made with olestra",	HIGH	65
Snacks, potato chips, lightly salted",	MEDIUM	53.54
Snacks, potato chips, made from dried potatoes (preformed), multigrain",	HIGH	65.34
Snacks, potato chips, made from dried potatoes, cheese-flavor",	MEDIUM	50.6
Snacks, potato chips, made from dried potatoes, fat-free, made with olestra",	MEDIUM	56
Snacks, potato chips, made from dried potatoes, reduced fat",	HIGH	64.76
Snacks, potato chips, made from dried potatoes, sour-cream and onion-flavor",	MEDIUM	51.3
Snacks, potato chips, plain, made with partially hydrogenated soybean oil, salted",	MEDIUM	52.9
Snacks, potato chips, plain, salted",	MEDIUM	53.83
Snacks, potato chips, reduced fat",	HIGH	66.9
Snacks, potato chips, sour-cream-and-onion-flavor",	MEDIUM	51.5
Snacks, potato chips, white, restructured, baked",	HIGH	71.4
Snacks, potato sticks",	MEDIUM	53.3
Snacks, pretzels, hard, confectioner's coating, chocolate-flavor",	HIGH	70.9
Snacks, pretzels, hard, plain, made with enriched flour, unsalted",	HIGH	79.2
Snacks, pretzels, hard, plain, made with unenriched flour, salted",	HIGH	79.2
Snacks, pretzels, hard, plain, made with unenriched flour, unsalted",	HIGH	79.2
Snacks, pretzels, hard, plain, salted",	HIGH	80.39
Snacks, pretzels, hard, whole-wheat including both salted and unsalted",	HIGH	81.3
Snacks, rice cakes, brown rice, buckwheat, unsalted",	HIGH	80.1
Snacks, rice cakes, brown rice, buckwheat",	HIGH	80.1
Snacks, rice cakes, brown rice, corn",	HIGH	81.2
Snacks, rice cakes, brown rice, multigrain, unsalted",	HIGH	80.1
Snacks, rice cakes, brown rice, multigrain",	HIGH	80.1
Snacks, rice cakes, brown rice, rye",	HIGH	79.9
Snacks, rice cakes, brown rice, sesame seed, unsalted",	HIGH	81.5
Snacks, rice cakes, brown rice, sesame seed",	HIGH	81.5
Snacks, rice cracker brown rice, plain",	HIGH	81.5
Snacks, sesame sticks, wheat-based, salted",	MEDIUM	46.5
Snacks, soy chips or crisps, salted",	MEDIUM	53.15
Snacks, SUNKIST, SUNKIST Fruit Roll, strawberry, with vitamins A, C, and E",	HIGH	82.7
Snacks, taro chips",	HIGH	68.1
Snacks, tortilla chips, light (baked with less oil)",	HIGH	73.4
Snacks, tortilla chips, low fat, made with olestra, nacho cheese",	HIGH	65.22
Snacks, tortilla chips, nacho cheese",	HIGH	60.81
Snacks, tortilla chips, nacho-flavor, made with enriched masa flour",	HIGH	62.4
Snacks, tortilla chips, nacho-flavor, reduced fat",	HIGH	71.6
Snacks, tortilla chips, plain, white corn, salted",	HIGH	67.78
Snacks, tortilla chips, ranch-flavor",	HIGH	62.74
Snacks, tortilla chips, taco-flavor",	HIGH	63.1
Snacks, trail mix, regular, with chocolate chips, salted nuts and seeds",	MEDIUM	44.9
Snacks, trail mix, regular",	MEDIUM	44.9
Snacks, trail mix, tropical",	HIGH	65.6
Snacks, vegetable chips, HAIN CELESTIAL GROUP, TERRA CHIPS",	HIGH	57.97
Snacks, vegetable chips, made from garden vegetables",	HIGH	60.43
Snacks, yucca (cassava) chips, salted",	HIGH	69.23

Food name/ Category (100 g)	Status	Carbs content in g
Sorghum flour, refined, unenriched",	HIGH	76.85
Sorghum flour, whole-grain",	HIGH	76.64
Sorghum grain",	HIGH	72.09
Soup, bean with frankfurters, canned, condensed",	LOW	16.75
Soup, bean with frankfurters, canned, prepared with equal volume water",	LOW	8.8
Soup, beef and vegetables, canned, ready-to-serve",	LOW	6.16
Soup, beef and vegetables, reduced sodium, canned, ready-to-serve",	LOW	4.99
Soup, beef barley, ready to serve",	LOW	7.94
Soup, beef broth bouillon and consomme, canned, condensed",	LOW	0.32
Soup, beef broth or bouillon canned, ready-to-serve",	LOW	0.04
Soup, beef broth or bouillon, powder, dry",	LOW	17.4
Soup, beef broth or bouillon, powder, prepared with water",	LOW	0.25
Soup, beef broth, bouillon, consomme, prepared with equal volume water",	LOW	0.73
Soup, beef broth, cubed, dry",	LOW	16.1
Soup, beef broth, cubed, prepared with water",	LOW	0.25
Soup, beef broth, less\/reduced sodium, ready to serve",	LOW	0.2
Soup, beef mushroom, canned, condensed",	LOW	5.2
Soup, beef mushroom, canned, prepared with equal volume water",	LOW	2.6
Soup, beef noodle, canned, condensed",	LOW	7.16
Soup, beef noodle, canned, prepared with equal volume water",	LOW	3.58
Soup, beef stroganoff, canned, chunky style, ready-to-serve",	LOW	9
Soup, beef with vegetables and barley, canned, condensed, single brand",	LOW	8.2
Soup, black bean, canned, condensed",	LOW	15.42
Soup, black bean, canned, prepared with equal volume water",	LOW	7.71
Soup, bouillon cubes and granules, low sodium, dry",	HIGH	64.88
Soup, broccoli cheese, canned, condensed, commercial",	LOW	7.7
Soup, cheese, canned, condensed",	LOW	11.3
Soup, cheese, canned, prepared with equal volume milk",	LOW	6.47
Soup, cheese, canned, prepared with equal volume water",	LOW	4.26
Soup, chicken and vegetable, canned, ready-to-serve",	LOW	4.68

Food name/ Category (100 g)	Status	Carbs content in g
Soup, chicken broth cubes, dry, prepared with water",	LOW	0.62
Soup, chicken broth cubes, dry",	LOW	23.5
Soup, chicken broth or bouillon, dry, prepared with water",	LOW	0.3
Soup, chicken broth or bouillon, dry",	LOW	18.01
Soup, chicken broth, canned, condensed",	LOW	0.75
Soup, chicken broth, canned, prepared with equal volume water",	LOW	0.38
Soup, chicken broth, less\/reduced sodium, ready to serve",	LOW	0.38
Soup, chicken broth, ready-to-serve",	LOW	0.44
Soup, chicken corn chowder, chunky, ready-to-serve, single brand",	LOW	7.5
Soup, chicken gumbo, canned, condensed",	LOW	6.67
Soup, chicken gumbo, canned, prepared with equal volume water",	LOW	3.43
Soup, chicken mushroom chowder, chunky, ready-to-serve, single brand",	LOW	7.1
Soup, chicken mushroom, canned, condensed",	LOW	11.95
Soup, chicken mushroom, canned, prepared with equal volume water",	LOW	3.8
Soup, chicken noodle, canned, condensed",	LOW	6.07
Soup, chicken noodle, canned, prepared with equal volume water",	LOW	2.97
Soup, chicken noodle, dry, mix, prepared with water",	LOW	3.67
Soup, chicken noodle, dry, mix",	HIGH	62.32
Soup, chicken noodle, low sodium, canned, prepared with equal volume water",	LOW	2.95
Soup, chicken noodle, reduced sodium, canned, ready-to-serve",	LOW	3.84
Soup, chicken rice, canned, chunky, ready-to-serve",	LOW	5.41
Soup, chicken vegetable with potato and cheese, chunky, ready-to-serve",	LOW	5.2
Soup, chicken vegetable, canned, condensed",	LOW	7.01
Soup, chicken vegetable, chunky, reduced fat, reduced sodium, ready-to-serve, single brand",	LOW	6.3
Soup, chicken with rice, canned, condensed",	LOW	11.57
Soup, chicken with rice, canned, prepared with equal volume water",	LOW	2.92
Soup, chicken with star-shaped pasta, canned, condensed, single brand",	LOW	7.1
Soup, chicken, canned, chunky, ready-to-serve",	LOW	6.88

Food name/ Category (100 g)	Status	Carbs content in g
Soup, chili beef, canned, condensed",	LOW	18.86
Soup, chili beef, canned, prepared with equal volume water",	LOW	9.23
Soup, chunky beef, canned, ready-to-serve",	LOW	10.08
Soup, chunky chicken noodle, canned, ready-to-serve",	LOW	4.46
Soup, chunky vegetable, canned, ready-to-serve",	LOW	7.9
Soup, chunky vegetable, reduced sodium, canned, ready-to-serve",	LOW	10.28
Soup, clam chowder, manhattan style, canned, chunky, ready-to-serve",	LOW	7.84
Soup, clam chowder, manhattan, canned, condensed",	LOW	9.74
Soup, clam chowder, manhattan, canned, prepared with equal volume water",	LOW	4.77
Soup, clam chowder, new england, canned, condensed",	LOW	10.32
Soup, clam chowder, new england, canned, prepared with equal volume low fat (2%) milk",	LOW	7.46
Soup, clam chowder, new england, canned, prepared with equal volume water",	LOW	5.05
Soup, clam chowder, new england, canned, ready-to-serve",	LOW	8.28
Soup, clam chowder, new england, reduced sodium, canned, ready-to-serve",	LOW	5.68
Soup, cream of asparagus, canned, condensed",	LOW	8.52
Soup, cream of asparagus, canned, prepared with equal volume milk",	LOW	6.61
Soup, cream of asparagus, canned, prepared with equal volume water",	LOW	4.38
Soup, cream of celery, canned, condensed",	LOW	7.03
Soup, cream of celery, canned, prepared with equal volume milk",	LOW	5.86
Soup, cream of celery, canned, prepared with equal volume water",	LOW	3.62
Soup, cream of chicken, canned, condensed, reduced sodium",	LOW	9.5
Soup, cream of chicken, canned, condensed, single brand",	LOW	7.7
Soup, cream of chicken, canned, condensed",	LOW	7.16
Soup, cream of chicken, canned, prepared with equal volume milk",	LOW	6.04
Soup, cream of chicken, canned, prepared with equal volume water",	LOW	3.8
Soup, cream of chicken, dry, mix, prepared with water",	LOW	5.11
Soup, cream of mushroom, canned, condensed, reduced sodium",	LOW	8.1
Soup, cream of mushroom, canned, condensed",	LOW	6.8

Food name/ Category (100 g)	Status	Carbs content in g
Soup, cream of mushroom, canned, prepared with equal volume low fat (2%) milk",	LOW	5.76
Soup, cream of mushroom, canned, prepared with equal volume water",	LOW	3.33
Soup, cream of onion, canned, condensed",	LOW	10.4
Soup, cream of onion, canned, prepared with equal volume milk",	LOW	7.4
Soup, cream of onion, canned, prepared with equal volume water",	LOW	5.2
Soup, cream of potato, canned, condensed",	LOW	12.79
Soup, cream of potato, canned, prepared with equal volume milk",	LOW	6.92
Soup, cream of potato, canned, prepared with equal volume water",	LOW	4.7
Soup, cream of shrimp, canned, condensed",	LOW	6.53
Soup, cream of shrimp, canned, prepared with equal volume low fat (2%) milk",	LOW	5.64
Soup, cream of shrimp, canned, prepared with equal volume water",	LOW	3.27
Soup, cream of vegetable, dry, powder",	MEDIUM	52.1
Soup, egg drop, Chinese restaurant",	LOW	4.29
Soup, HEALTHY CHOICE Chicken and Rice Soup, canned",	LOW	5.71
Soup, HEALTHY CHOICE Chicken Noodle Soup, canned",	LOW	5.2
Soup, HEALTHY CHOICE Garden Vegetable Soup, canned",	LOW	10.04
Soup, hot and sour, Chinese restaurant",	LOW	4.35
Soup, minestrone, canned, chunky, ready-to-serve",	LOW	8.64
Soup, minestrone, canned, condensed",	LOW	9.17
Soup, minestrone, canned, prepared with equal volume water",	LOW	4.66
Soup, minestrone, canned, reduced sodium, ready-to-serve",	LOW	9
Soup, mushroom barley, canned, condensed",	LOW	9.6
Soup, mushroom barley, canned, prepared with equal volume water",	LOW	4.8
Soup, mushroom with beef stock, canned, condensed",	LOW	7.41
Soup, mushroom with beef stock, canned, prepared with equal volume water",	LOW	3.81
Soup, onion, canned, condensed",	LOW	6.68
Soup, onion, dry, mix, prepared with water",	LOW	2.77
Soup, onion, dry, mix",	HIGH	65.07
Soup, oyster stew, canned, condensed",	LOW	3.32

Food name/ Category (100 g)	Status	Carbs content in g
Soup, oyster stew, canned, prepared with equal volume milk",	LOW	3.99
Soup, oyster stew, canned, prepared with equal volume water",	LOW	1.69
Soup, pea, green, canned, condensed",	LOW	20.18
Soup, pea, green, canned, prepared with equal volume milk",	LOW	12.69
Soup, pea, green, canned, prepared with equal volume water",	LOW	9.88
Soup, PROGRESSO, beef barley, traditional, ready to serve",	LOW	6.69
Soup, ramen noodle, any flavor, dry",	HIGH	60.26
Soup, ramen noodle, beef flavor, dry",	HIGH	60.34
Soup, ramen noodle, chicken flavor, dry",	HIGH	60.23
Soup, ramen noodle, dry, any flavor, reduced fat, reduced sodium",	HIGH	70.95
Soup, shark fin, restaurant-prepared",	LOW	3.8
Soup, sirloin burger with vegetables, ready-to-serve, single brand",	LOW	6.8
Soup, stock, beef, home-prepared",	LOW	1.2
Soup, stock, chicken, home-prepared",	LOW	3.53
Soup, stock, fish, home-prepared",	LOW	0
Soup, SWANSON Chicken Broth 99% Fat Free",	LOW	0.14
Soup, SWANSON, beef broth, lower sodium",	LOW	0.21
Soup, SWANSON, vegetable broth",	LOW	1.02
Soup, tomato beef with noodle, canned, condensed",	LOW	16.87
Soup, tomato beef with noodle, canned, prepared with equal volume water",	LOW	8.44
Soup, tomato bisque, canned, condensed",	LOW	18.47
Soup, tomato bisque, canned, prepared with equal volume milk",	LOW	11.73
Soup, tomato bisque, canned, prepared with equal volume water",	LOW	9.6
Soup, tomato rice, canned, condensed",	LOW	17.08
Soup, tomato rice, canned, prepared with equal volume water",	LOW	8.54
Soup, tomato, canned, condensed",	LOW	15.22
Soup, tomato, canned, prepared with equal volume low fat (2%) milk",	LOW	9.82
Soup, tomato, canned, prepared with equal volume water, commercial",	LOW	7.45
Soup, tomato, dry, mix, prepared with water",	LOW	7.17
Soup, turkey noodle, canned, prepared with equal volume water",	LOW	3.54

Food name/ Category (100 g)	Status	Carbs content in g
Soup, turkey vegetable, canned, prepared with equal volume water",	LOW	3.58
Soup, turkey, chunky, canned, ready-to-serve",	LOW	5.96
Soup, vegetable beef, canned, condensed, single brand",	LOW	7.7
Soup, vegetable beef, canned, condensed",	LOW	8.11
Soup, vegetable beef, canned, prepared with equal volume water",	LOW	4.06
Soup, vegetable beef, microwavable, ready-to-serve, single brand",	LOW	3.3
Soup, vegetable broth, ready to serve",	LOW	0.93
Soup, vegetable soup, condensed, low sodium, prepared with equal volume water",	LOW	6.06
Soup, vegetable with beef broth, canned, condensed",	LOW	10.7
Soup, vegetable with beef broth, canned, prepared with equal volume water",	LOW	5.35
Soup, vegetable, canned, low sodium, condensed",	LOW	12.11
Soup, vegetarian vegetable, canned, condensed",	LOW	9.78
Soup, vegetarian vegetable, canned, prepared with equal volume water",	LOW	4.89
Soup, wonton, Chinese restaurant",	LOW	5.25
Sour cream, fat free",	LOW	15.6
Sour cream, imitation, cultured",	LOW	6.63
Sour cream, light",	LOW	7.1
Sour cream, reduced fat",	LOW	7
Sour dressing, non-butterfat, cultured, filled cream-type",	LOW	4.68
Soy meal, defatted, raw",	LOW	35.89
Soy protein concentrate, produced by acid wash",	LOW	25.41
Soy protein concentrate, produced by alcohol extraction",	LOW	25.41
Soy protein isolate, potassium type",	LOW	2.59
Soy protein isolate",	LOW	0
Soy sauce made from hydrolyzed vegetable protein",	LOW	7.84
Soy sauce made from soy (tamari)",	LOW	5.57
Soy sauce made from soy and wheat (shoyu), low sodium",	LOW	5.59
Soy sauce made from soy and wheat (shoyu)",	LOW	4.93

Food name/ Category (100 g)	Status	Carbs content in g
Soy sauce, reduced sodium, made from hydrolyzed vegetable protein",	LOW	14.44
Soybeans, green, cooked, boiled, drained, with salt",	LOW	11.05
Soybeans, mature cooked, boiled, without salt",	LOW	8.36
Soybeans, mature seeds, cooked, boiled, with salt",	LOW	8.36
Soybeans, mature seeds, dry roasted",	LOW	28.98
Soybeans, mature seeds, raw",	LOW	30.16
Soybeans, mature seeds, roasted, no salt added",	LOW	30.22
Soybeans, mature seeds, roasted, salted",	LOW	30.22
Soybeans, mature seeds, sprouted, cooked, steamed, with salt",	LOW	6.53
Soymilk (All flavors), enhanced",	LOW	3.45
Soymilk (All flavors), lowfat, with added calcium, vitamins A and D",	LOW	7.2
Soymilk (all flavors), nonfat, with added calcium, vitamins A and D",	LOW	4.14
Soymilk (all flavors), unsweetened, with added calcium, vitamins A and D",	LOW	1.74
Soymilk, chocolate and other flavors, light, with added calcium, vitamins A and D",	LOW	8.24
Soymilk, chocolate, nonfat, with added calcium, vitamins A and D",	LOW	8.51
Soymilk, chocolate, unfortified",	LOW	9.95
Soymilk, chocolate, with added calcium, vitamins A and D",	LOW	9.95
Soymilk, original and vanilla, light, unsweetened, with added calcium, vitamins A and D",	LOW	3.85
Soymilk, original and vanilla, light, with added calcium, vitamins A and D",	LOW	3.51
Soymilk, original and vanilla, unfortified",	LOW	6.28
Soymilk, original and vanilla, with added calcium, vitamins A and D",	LOW	4.92
Spaghetti with meat sauce, frozen entree",	LOW	15.24
Spaghetti, protein-fortified, cooked, enriched (n x 6.25)",	LOW	30.88
Spaghetti, spinach, dry",	HIGH	74.81
Spaghetti, with meatballs in tomato sauce, canned",	LOW	11.45
SPAGHETTIOS, Mini Beef Ravioli in Meat Sauce",	LOW	16.6
SPAGHETTIOS, Spaghetti in Tomato & Cheese Sauce",	LOW	15.87
SPAGHETTIOS, SpaghettiOs A to Z's with Meatballs",	LOW	12.7

Food name/ Category (100 g)	Status	Carbs content in g
SPAGHETTIOS, SpaghettiOs A to Z's",	LOW	13.89
SPAGHETTIOS, SpaghettiOs in Meat Sauce",	LOW	12.3
SPAGHETTIOS, SpaghettiOs Original, easy open",	LOW	14.55
SPAGHETTIOS, SpaghettiOs Original",	LOW	13.89
SPAGHETTIOS, SpaghettiOs plus Calcium",	LOW	13.89
SPAGHETTIOS, SpaghettiOs RavioliOs Beef Ravioli in Meat Sauce",	LOW	15.08
SPAGHETTIOS, SpaghettiOs with Meatballs - Easy Open",	LOW	11.65
SPAGHETTIOS, SpaghettiOs with Meatballs",	LOW	12.7
SPAGHETTIOS, SpaghettiOs with Sliced Franks",	LOW	12.7
Spanish rice mix, dry mix, prepared (with canola\/vegetable oil blend or diced tomatoes and margarine)",	LOW	22.74
Spanish rice mix, dry mix, unprepared",	HIGH	76.45
Spearmint, dried",	MEDIUM	52.04
Spelt, cooked",	LOW	26.44
Spices, allspice, ground",	HIGH	72.12
Spices, basil, dried",	MEDIUM	47.75
Spices, celery seed",	MEDIUM	41.35
Spices, chervil, dried",	MEDIUM	49.1
Spices, chili powder",	MEDIUM	49.7
Spices, cloves, ground",	HIGH	65.53
Spices, coriander leaf, dried",	MEDIUM	52.1
Spices, cumin seed",	MEDIUM	44.24
Spices, curry powder",	MEDIUM	55.83
Spices, dill weed, dried",	MEDIUM	55.82
Spices, fennel seed",	MEDIUM	52.29
Spices, fenugreek seed",	HIGH	58.35
Spices, garlic powder",	HIGH	72.73
Spices, mace, ground",	MEDIUM	50.5
Spices, marjoram, dried",	HIGH	60.56
Spices, onion powder",	HIGH	79.12
Spices, paprika",	MEDIUM	53.99
Spices, parsley, dried",	MEDIUM	50.64
Spices, pepper, white",	HIGH	68.61
Spices, pumpkin pie spice",	HIGH	69.28
Spices, rosemary, dried",	HIGH	64.06
Spices, saffron",	HIGH	65.37
Spices, tarragon, dried",	MEDIUM	50.22
Spices, thyme, dried",	HIGH	63.94
Spinach souffle",	LOW	5.9
Spinach, canned, no salt added, solids and liquids",	LOW	2.92
Spinach, canned, regular pack, drained solids",	LOW	3.4
Spinach, canned, regular pack, solids and liquids",	LOW	2.92

Food name/ Category (100 g)	Status	Carbs content in g
Spinach, cooked, boiled, drained, with salt",	LOW	3.75
Spinach, cooked, boiled, drained, without salt",	LOW	3.75
Spinach, frozen, chopped or leaf, cooked, boiled, drained, with salt",	LOW	4.8
Spinach, frozen, chopped or leaf, cooked, boiled, drained, without salt",	LOW	4.8
Spinach, frozen, chopped or leaf, unprepared",	LOW	4.21
Spinach, raw",	LOW	3.63
Split pea soup, canned, reduced sodium, prepared with water or ready-to serve",	LOW	11.83
Squab, (pigeon), light meat without skin, raw",	LOW	0
Squab, (pigeon), meat and skin, raw",	LOW	0
Squab, (pigeon), meat only, raw",	LOW	0
Squash, summer, all varieties, cooked, boiled, drained, with salt",	LOW	4.31
Squash, summer, all varieties, cooked, boiled, drained, without salt",	LOW	4.31
Squash, summer, all varieties, raw",	LOW	3.35
Squash, summer, crookneck and straightneck, canned, drained, solid, without salt",	LOW	2.96
Squash, summer, crookneck and straightneck, cooked, boiled, drained, with salt",	LOW	3.79
Squash, summer, crookneck and straightneck, cooked, boiled, drained, without salt",	LOW	3.79
Squash, summer, crookneck and straightneck, frozen, cooked, boiled, drained, with salt",	LOW	5.54
Squash, summer, crookneck and straightneck, frozen, unprepared",	LOW	4.8
Squash, summer, crookneck and straightneck, raw",	LOW	3.88
Squash, summer, scallop, cooked, boiled, drained, with salt",	LOW	3.3
Squash, summer, scallop, cooked, boiled, drained, without salt",	LOW	3.3
Squash, summer, scallop, raw",	LOW	3.84
Squash, summer, zucchini, includes skin, cooked, boiled, drained, with salt",	LOW	2.69
Squash, summer, zucchini, includes skin, cooked, boiled, drained, without salt",	LOW	2.69
Squash, summer, zucchini, includes skin, frozen, cooked, boiled, drained, with salt",	LOW	2.97
Squash, summer, zucchini, includes skin, frozen, cooked, boiled, drained, without salt",	LOW	3.56
Squash, summer, zucchini, includes skin, frozen, unprepared",	LOW	3.58
Squash, summer, zucchini, italian style, canned",	LOW	6.85

Food name/ Category (100 g)	Status	Carbs content in g
Squash, winter, acorn, cooked, baked, with salt",	LOW	14.58
Squash, winter, acorn, cooked, baked, without salt",	LOW	14.58
Squash, winter, acorn, cooked, boiled, mashed, with salt",	LOW	8.79
Squash, winter, acorn, cooked, boiled, mashed, without salt",	LOW	8.79
Squash, winter, acorn, raw",	LOW	10.42
Squash, winter, all varieties, cooked, baked, with salt",	LOW	8.85
Squash, winter, all varieties, cooked, baked, without salt",	LOW	8.85
Squash, winter, all varieties, raw",	LOW	8.59
Squash, winter, butternut, cooked, baked, with salt",	LOW	10.49
Squash, winter, butternut, cooked, baked, without salt",	LOW	10.49
Squash, winter, butternut, frozen, cooked, boiled, with salt",	LOW	10.04
Squash, winter, butternut, frozen, cooked, boiled, without salt",	LOW	10.05
Squash, winter, butternut, frozen, unprepared",	LOW	14.41
Squash, winter, butternut, raw",	LOW	11.69
Squash, winter, hubbard, baked, with salt",	LOW	10.81
Squash, winter, hubbard, cooked, boiled, mashed, with salt",	LOW	6.46
Squash, winter, hubbard, cooked, boiled, mashed, without salt",	LOW	6.46
Squash, winter, spaghetti, cooked, boiled, drained, or baked, with salt",	LOW	6.46
Squash, zucchini, baby, raw",	LOW	3.11
Stew, dumpling with mutton (Navajo)",	LOW	8.03
Stew, hominy with mutton (Navajo)",	LOW	9.38
Stew, mutton, corn, squash (Navajo)",	LOW	7.27
Stew, pinto bean and hominy, badufsuki (Hopi)",	LOW	5.38
Stinging Nettles, blanched (Northern Plains Indians)",	LOW	7.49
Strawberries, canned, heavy syrup pack, solids and liquids",	LOW	23.53
Strawberries, frozen, sweetened, sliced",	LOW	25.92
Strawberries, frozen, sweetened, whole",	LOW	21
Strawberries, frozen, unsweetened",	LOW	9.13

Food name/ Category (100 g)	Status	Carbs content in g
Strawberries, raw",	LOW	7.68
Strawberry-flavor beverage mix, powder",	HIGH	99.1
Strudel, apple",	MEDIUM	41.1
SUBWAY, cold cut sub on white bread with lettuce and tomato",	LOW	20.43
SUBWAY, meatball marinara sub on white bread (no toppings)",	LOW	26.01
SUBWAY, oven roasted chicken sub on white bread with lettuce and tomato",	LOW	21.35
SUBWAY, roast beef sub on white bread with lettuce and tomato",	LOW	20.34
SUBWAY, steak & cheese sub on white bread with American cheese, lettuce and tomato",	LOW	21.49
SUBWAY, SUBWAY CLUB sub on white bread with lettuce and tomato",	LOW	20.36
SUBWAY, sweet onion chicken teriyaki sub on white bread with lettuce, tomato and sweet onion sauce",	LOW	22.54
SUBWAY, tuna sub on white bread with lettuce and tomato",	LOW	15.95
SUBWAY, turkey breast sub on white bread with lettuce and tomato",	LOW	22.42
Succotash, (corn and limas), canned, with cream style corn",	LOW	17.61
Succotash, (corn and limas), canned, with whole kernel corn, solids and liquids",	LOW	13.98
Succotash, (corn and limas), cooked, boiled, drained, with salt",	LOW	24.37
Succotash, (corn and limas), frozen, cooked, boiled, drained, with salt",	LOW	19.95
Succotash, (corn and limas), frozen, cooked, boiled, drained, without salt",	LOW	19.95
Succotash, (corn and limas), frozen, unprepared",	LOW	19.94
Sugar, turbinado",	HIGH	99.8
Sugars, granulated",	HIGH	99.98
Sugars, powdered",	HIGH	99.77
SUNSHINE, CHEEZ-IT, 100 Calorie RIGHT BITES, Extra Cheesy Party Mix",	HIGH	65.3
SUNSHINE, CHEEZ-IT, 100 Calorie Right Bites, Reduced Fat",	HIGH	67
SUNSHINE, CHEEZ-IT, Asiago Crackers",	HIGH	62.6
SUNSHINE, CHEEZ-IT, Baby Swiss Crackers",	HIGH	63.1
SUNSHINE, CHEEZ-IT, BIG Crackers",	HIGH	57.4
SUNSHINE, CHEEZ-IT, Cheddar Jack Crackers",	HIGH	57.6
SUNSHINE, CHEEZ-IT, Colby Crackers",	HIGH	59.25
SUNSHINE, CHEEZ-IT, Crackers (made with Whole Grain)",	HIGH	58.2
SUNSHINE, CHEEZ-IT, Duoz Sharp Cheddar Parmesan Crackers",	HIGH	60.5
SUNSHINE, CHEEZ-IT, Duoz Smoked Cheddar Monterey Jack Crackers",	HIGH	60.8
SUNSHINE, CHEEZ-IT, Hot & Spicy Crackers",	HIGH	61.2
SUNSHINE, CHEEZ-IT, Italian Four Cheese Crackers",	HIGH	62.4
SUNSHINE, CHEEZ-IT, Mozzarella Crackers",	HIGH	64.1
SUNSHINE, CHEEZ-IT, Original Crackers",	HIGH	57.4
SUNSHINE, CHEEZ-IT, Parmesan Garlic Crackers",	HIGH	62
SUNSHINE, CHEEZ-IT, Pepper Jack Crackers",	HIGH	61.9
SUNSHINE, CHEEZ-IT, Reduced Fat Crackers",	HIGH	67
SUNSHINE, CHEEZ-IT, Scrabble Jr. Crackers",	HIGH	67.9
SUNSHINE, CHEEZ-IT, Snack Mix, White Cheddar",	HIGH	65.7
SUNSHINE, CHEEZ-IT, Snack Mix",	HIGH	66.7

Food name/ Category (100 g)	Status	Carbs content in g
SUNSHINE, CHEEZ-IT, White Cheddar, Reduced Fat Crackers",	HIGH	72
SUNSHINE, GRIPZ, Cheez-It Crackers",	HIGH	61
SUNSHINE, GRIPZ, Cheez-It Mixx and Cheesy Pizza Crackers",	HIGH	63.7
SUNSHINE, KRISPY, Soup & Oyster Crackers (large)",	HIGH	76.1
SUPPER BAKES MEAL KITS, Cheesy Chicken with pasta (chicken not included)",	LOW	31.76
SUPPER BAKES MEAL KITS, Creamy Stroganoff Sauce with pasta",	LOW	24.8
SUPPER BAKES MEAL KITS, Garlic Chicken with pasta (chicken not included)",	MEDIUM	42.93
SUPPER BAKES MEAL KITS, Herb Chicken with rice (chicken not included)",	MEDIUM	42.55
SUPPER BAKES MEAL KITS, Lemon Chicken with herb rice (chicken not included	MEDIUM	45.74
SUPPER BAKES MEAL KITS, Southwestern-Style Chicken w\rice (chicken not included)",	LOW	39.51
SUPPER BAKES MEAL KITS, Traditional Roast Chicken with stuffing (chicken not included)",	LOW	34.44
Swamp cabbage (skunk cabbage), cooked, boiled, drained, with salt",	LOW	3.7
Swamp cabbage (skunk cabbage), cooked, boiled, drained, without salt",	LOW	3.7
Swamp cabbage, (skunk cabbage), raw",	LOW	3.14
SWANSON BROTH, Certified Organic Vegetable Broth",	LOW	1.28
SWANSON, Chicken A La King",	LOW	4.03
SWANSON, Chicken and Dumplings",	LOW	9.72
Sweet potato leaves, cooked, steamed, with salt",	LOW	7.38
Sweet Potato puffs, frozen, unprepared",	LOW	30.72
Sweet potato, canned, mashed",	LOW	23.19
Sweet potato, canned, syrup pack, drained solids",	LOW	25.36
Sweet potato, canned, vacuum pack",	LOW	21.12
Sweet potato, cooked, baked in skin, flesh, with salt",	LOW	20.71
Sweet potato, cooked, baked in skin, flesh, without salt",	LOW	20.71
Sweet potato, cooked, boiled, without skin, with salt",	LOW	17.72
Sweet potato, cooked, candied, home-prepared",	LOW	32.12
Sweet potato, frozen, cooked, baked, with salt",	LOW	23.4
Sweet potato, raw, unprepared",	LOW	20.12
Sweet Potatoes, french fried, crosscut, frozen, unprepared",	LOW	25.52
Sweet Potatoes, french fried, frozen as packaged, salt added in processing",	LOW	35.58
Sweet rolls, cheese",	MEDIUM	43.7
Sweet rolls, cinnamon, commercially prepared with raisins",	MEDIUM	50.9
Sweet rolls, cinnamon, refrigerated dough with frosting, baked",	MEDIUM	56.1

Food name/ Category (100 g)	Status	Carbs content in g
Sweet rolls, cinnamon, refrigerated dough with frosting",	MEDIUM	51.6
Sweetener, herbal extract powder from Stevia leaf",	HIGH	100
Sweetener, syrup, agave",	HIGH	76.37
Sweeteners, for baking, contains sugar and sucralose",	HIGH	99.53
Sweeteners, sugar substitute, granulated, brown",	HIGH	84.77
Sweeteners, tabletop, aspartame, EQUAL, packets",	HIGH	89.08
Sweeteners, tabletop, fructose, liquid",	HIGH	76.1
Sweeteners, tabletop, saccharin (sodium saccharin)",	HIGH	89.11
Sweeteners, tabletop, sucralose, SPLENDA packets",	HIGH	91.17
Syrup, Cane",	HIGH	73.14
Syrup, fruit flavored",	HIGH	65.1
Syrup, NESTLE, chocolate",	HIGH	67.21
Syrups, chocolate, fudge-type",	HIGH	62.9
Syrups, chocolate, HERSHEY'S Genuine Chocolate Flavored Lite Syrup",	LOW	34.56
Syrups, chocolate, HERSHEY'S Sugar free, Genuine Chocolate Flavored, Lite Syrup",	LOW	14.2
Syrups, corn, dark",	HIGH	77.59
Syrups, corn, high-fructose",	HIGH	76
Syrups, corn, light",	HIGH	76.79
Syrups, sugar free",	LOW	12.13
Syrups, table blends, cane and 15% maple",	HIGH	69.52
Syrups, table blends, corn, refiner, and sugar",	HIGH	83.9
Syrups, table blends, pancake, reduced-calorie",	MEDIUM	44.55
Syrups, table blends, pancake, with 2% maple, with added potassium",	HIGH	69.6
Syrups, table blends, pancake, with 2% maple",	HIGH	69.6
Syrups, table blends, pancake, with butter",	HIGH	72.43
Syrups, table blends, pancake",	HIGH	61.47
T.G.I. FRIDAY'S, chicken fingers, from kids' menu",	LOW	17.72
T.G.I. FRIDAY'S, chicken fingers",	LOW	16.84
T.G.I. FRIDAY'S, classic sirloin steak (10 oz)",	LOW	0.47
T.G.I. FRIDAY'S, french fries",	LOW	36.9
T.G.I. FRIDAY'S, FRIDAY'S Shrimp, breaded",	LOW	20.87
T.G.I. FRIDAY'S, fried mozzarella",	LOW	25.33
T.G.I. FRIDAY'S, macaroni & cheese, from kid's menu",	LOW	17.4
TACO BELL, Bean Burrito",	LOW	31.23
TACO BELL, BURRITO SUPREME with beef",	LOW	23.37
TACO BELL, BURRITO SUPREME with chicken",	LOW	20.51
TACO BELL, BURRITO SUPREME with steak",	LOW	20.32
TACO BELL, Nachos Supreme",	LOW	21.39
TACO BELL, Nachos",	LOW	34.91

Food name/ Category (100 g)	Status	Carbs content in g
TACO BELL, Original Taco with beef, cheese and lettuce",	LOW	19.85
TACO BELL, Soft Taco with beef, cheese and lettuce",	LOW	20.23
TACO BELL, Soft Taco with chicken, cheese and lettuce",	LOW	19.69
TACO BELL, Soft Taco with steak",	LOW	17.22
TACO BELL, Taco Salad",	LOW	15.1
Taco shells, baked",	HIGH	63.49
Tamales (Navajo)",	LOW	18.12
Tangerine juice, canned, sweetened",	LOW	12
Tangerine juice, raw",	LOW	10.1
Tangerines, (mandarin oranges), canned, juice pack, drained",	LOW	9.41
Tangerines, (mandarin oranges), canned, juice pack",	LOW	9.57
Tangerines, (mandarin oranges), raw",	LOW	13.34
Tapioca, pearl, dry",	HIGH	88.69
Taquitos, frozen, beef and cheese, oven-heated",	LOW	33.46
Taquitos, frozen, chicken and cheese, oven-heated",	LOW	33.63
Taro leaves, cooked, steamed, without salt",	LOW	4.02
Taro leaves, raw",	LOW	6.7
Taro shoots, cooked, without salt",	LOW	3.2
Taro shoots, raw",	LOW	2.32
Taro, cooked, with salt",	LOW	34.6
Taro, leaves, cooked, steamed, with salt",	LOW	3.89
Taro, shoots, cooked, with salt",	LOW	3.19
Taro, tahitian, cooked, with salt",	LOW	6.85
Taro, tahitian, cooked, without salt",	LOW	6.85
Taro, tahitian, raw",	LOW	6.91
Toaster pastries, brown-sugar-cinnamon",	HIGH	72.64
Toaster pastries, fruit (includes apple, blueberry, cherry, strawberry)",	HIGH	70.32
Toaster Pastries, fruit, frosted (include apples, blueberry, cherry, strawberry)",	HIGH	71.83
Toaster pastries, fruit, toasted (include apple, blueberry, cherry, strawberry)",	HIGH	72.7
Toaster Pastries, KELLOGG, KELLOGG'S LOW FAT POP TARTS, Frosted brown	HIGH	73.7
Toaster Pastries, KELLOGG, KELLOGG'S LOW FAT POP TARTS, Frosted strawb	HIGH	74.4
Toaster Pastries, KELLOGG, KELLOGG'S POP TARTS, Blueberry",	HIGH	68.41
Toaster Pastries, KELLOGG, KELLOGG'S POP TARTS, Brown sugar cinnamon",	HIGH	64.4

Food name/ Category (100 g)	Status	Carbs content in g
Toaster Pastries, KELLOGG, KELLOGG'S POP TARTS, Frosted blueberry",	HIGH	71.77
Toaster Pastries, KELLOGG, KELLOGG'S POP TARTS, Frosted brown sugar cinn	HIGH	69
Toaster Pastries, KELLOGG, KELLOGG'S POP TARTS, Frosted cherry",	HIGH	72
Toaster Pastries, KELLOGG, KELLOGG'S POP TARTS, Frosted chocolate fudge",	HIGH	70.4
Toaster Pastries, KELLOGG, KELLOGG'S POP TARTS, Frosted raspberry",	HIGH	71.62
Toaster Pastries, KELLOGG, KELLOGG'S POP TARTS, Frosted strawberry",	HIGH	71.7
Toaster Pastries, KELLOGG, KELLOGG'S POP TARTS, Frosted wild berry",	HIGH	72.4
Toaster Pastries, KELLOGG, KELLOGG'S POP TARTS, S'mores",	HIGH	69.6
Toaster Pastries, KELLOGG, KELLOGG'S POP TARTS, Strawberry",	HIGH	71.1
Toddler formula, MEAD JOHNSON, ENFAGROW, PREMIUM (formerly ENFAMIL,	MEDIUM	56
Tofu, extra firm, prepared with nigari",	LOW	1.18
Tofu, hard, prepared with nigari",	LOW	4.39
Tofu, salted and fermented (fuyu), prepared with calcium sulfate",	LOW	5.15
Tofu, salted and fermented (fuyu)",	LOW	4.38
Tomatillos, raw",	LOW	5.84
Tomato and vegetable juice, low sodium",	LOW	4.59
Tomato juice, canned, with salt added",	LOW	3.53
Tomato products, canned, paste, without salt added",	LOW	18.91
Tomato products, canned, puree, with salt added",	LOW	8.98
Tomato products, canned, sauce, spanish style",	LOW	7.24
Tomato products, canned, sauce, with herbs and cheese",	LOW	10.24
Tomato products, canned, sauce, with mushrooms",	LOW	8.43
Tomato products, canned, sauce, with onions, green peppers, and celery",	LOW	8.77
Tomato products, canned, sauce, with onions",	LOW	9.94
Tomato products, canned, sauce",	LOW	5.31
Tomatoes, crushed, canned",	LOW	7.29
Tomatoes, orange, raw",	LOW	3.18
Tomatoes, red, ripe, canned, packed in tomato juice",	LOW	3.47
Tomatoes, red, ripe, canned, stewed",	LOW	6.19
Tomatoes, red, ripe, canned, with green chilies",	LOW	3.62
Tomatoes, red, ripe, cooked, stewed",	LOW	13.05
Tomatoes, red, ripe, cooked, with salt",	LOW	4.01
Tomatoes, red, ripe, raw, year round average",	LOW	3.89

Food name/ Category (100 g)	Status	Carbs content in g
Tomatoes, sun-dried, packed in oil, drained",	LOW	23.33
Tomatoes, sun-dried",	MEDIUM	55.76
Toppings, butterscotch or caramel",	HIGH	57.01
Toppings, marshmallow cream",	HIGH	79
Toppings, nuts in syrup",	HIGH	58.08
Toppings, pineapple",	HIGH	66.4
Tortellini, pasta with cheese filling, fresh-refrigerated, as purchased",	MEDIUM	47
Tortilla chips, low fat, baked without fat",	HIGH	80
Tortilla chips, yellow, plain, salted",	HIGH	67.38
Tortilla, blue corn, Sakwavikaviki (Hopi)",	HIGH	58.12
Tortilla, includes plain and from mutton sandwich (Navajo)",	MEDIUM	49.94
Tortillas, ready-to-bake or -fry, corn",	MEDIUM	44.64
Tortillas, ready-to-bake or -fry, flour, refrigerated",	MEDIUM	49.38
Tortillas, ready-to-bake or -fry, flour, shelf stable",	MEDIUM	49.27
Tortillas, ready-to-bake or -fry, flour, without added calcium",	MEDIUM	55.6
Tortillas, ready-to-bake or -fry, whole wheat",	MEDIUM	45.89
Tostada shells, corn",	HIGH	64.43
Tree fern, cooked, with salt",	LOW	10.78
Tree fern, cooked, without salt",	LOW	10.98
Triticale flour, whole-grain",	HIGH	73.14
Triticale",	HIGH	72.13
Turkey and gravy, frozen",	LOW	4.61
Turkey breast, low salt, prepackaged or deli, luncheon meat",	LOW	3.51
Turkey breast, pre-basted, meat and skin, cooked, roasted",	LOW	0
Turkey breast, sliced, prepackaged",	LOW	2.34
Turkey from whole, dark meat, meat only, raw",	LOW	0.15
Turkey from whole, light meat, meat and skin, cooked, roasted",	LOW	0.05
Turkey from whole, light meat, meat and skin, raw",	LOW	0.15
Turkey from whole, light meat, meat and skin, with added solution, cooked, roasted",	LOW	0
Turkey from whole, light meat, meat and skin, with added solution, raw",	LOW	0.14
Turkey from whole, light meat, meat only, with added solution, cooked, roasted",	LOW	0
Turkey from whole, light meat, meat only, with added solution, raw",	LOW	0
Turkey from whole, light meat, raw",	LOW	0.14
Turkey from whole, neck, meat only, cooked, simmered",	LOW	0
Turkey from whole, neck, meat only, raw",	LOW	0
Turkey Pot Pie, frozen entree",	LOW	17.7
Turkey roast, boneless, frozen, seasoned, light and dark meat, raw",	LOW	6.4

Food name/ Category (100 g)	Status	Carbs content in g
Turkey sausage, fresh, cooked",	LOW	0
Turkey sausage, fresh, raw",	LOW	0.47
Turkey sausage, reduced fat, brown and serve, cooked (include BUTTERBALL breakfast links turkey sausage)",	LOW	10.92
Turkey sticks, breaded, battered, fried",	LOW	17
Turkey thigh, pre-basted, meat and skin, cooked, roasted",	LOW	0
Turkey, all classes, back, meat and skin, cooked, roasted",	LOW	0.16
Turkey, all classes, breast, meat and skin, cooked, roasted",	LOW	0
Turkey, all classes, breast, meat and skin, raw",	LOW	0
Turkey, all classes, leg, meat and skin, cooked, roasted",	LOW	0
Turkey, all classes, leg, meat and skin, raw",	LOW	0
Turkey, all classes, light meat, cooked, roasted",	LOW	0
Turkey, all classes, wing, meat and skin, cooked, roasted",	LOW	0
Turkey, all classes, wing, meat and skin, raw",	LOW	0
Turkey, back from whole bird, meat only, raw",	LOW	0.15
Turkey, back, from whole bird, meat and skin, with added solution, raw",	LOW	0.15
Turkey, back, from whole bird, meat and skin, with added solution, roasted",	LOW	0
Turkey, back, from whole bird, meat only, roasted",	LOW	0
Turkey, back, from whole bird, meat only, with added solution, raw",	LOW	0.15
Turkey, back, from whole bird, meat only, with added solution, roasted",	LOW	0
Turkey, breast, from whole bird, meat only, raw",	LOW	0.14
Turkey, breast, from whole bird, meat only, roasted",	LOW	0
Turkey, breast, from whole bird, meat only, with added solution, raw",	LOW	0.14
Turkey, breast, from whole bird, meat only, with added solution, roasted",	LOW	0
Turkey, breast, smoked, lemon pepper flavor, 97% fat-free",	LOW	1.31
Turkey, canned, meat only, with broth",	LOW	1.47
Turkey, dark meat from whole, meat and skin, cooked, roasted",	LOW	0.07
Turkey, dark meat from whole, meat and skin, with added solution, cooked, roasted",	LOW	0
Turkey, dark meat from whole, meat and skin, with added solution, raw",	LOW	0.15

Food name/ Category (100 g)	Status	Carbs content in g
Turkey, dark meat from whole, meat only, with added solution, raw",	LOW	**0.1**
Turkey, dark meat, meat and skin, raw",	LOW	**0.15**
Turkey, dark meat, meat only, with added solution, cooked, roasted",	LOW	**0**
Turkey, diced, light and dark meat, seasoned",	LOW	**1**
Turkey, drumstick, from whole bird, meat only, raw",	LOW	**0.14**
Turkey, drumstick, from whole bird, meat only, roasted",	LOW	**0**
Turkey, drumstick, from whole bird, meat only, with added solution, raw",	LOW	**0.15**
Turkey, drumstick, from whole bird, meat only, with added solution, roasted",	LOW	**0**
Turkey, drumstick, smoked, cooked, with skin, bone removed",	LOW	**0**
Turkey, from whole, dark meat, cooked, roasted",	LOW	**0**
Turkey, fryer-roasters, meat and skin, cooked, roasted",	LOW	**0**
Turkey, gizzard, all classes, cooked, simmered",	LOW	**0**
Turkey, gizzard, all classes, raw",	LOW	**0**
Turkey, heart, all classes, cooked, simmered",	LOW	**0**
Turkey, heart, all classes, raw",	LOW	**0.4**
Turkey, light or dark meat, smoked, cooked, skin and bone removed",	LOW	**0**
Turkey, light or dark meat, smoked, cooked, with skin, bone removed",	LOW	**0**
Turkey, liver, all classes, cooked, simmered",	LOW	**0**
Turkey, liver, all classes, raw",	LOW	**0**
Turkey, mechanically deboned, from turkey frames, raw",	LOW	**0**
Turkey, retail parts, breast, meat and skin, cooked, roasted",	LOW	**0.05**
Turkey, retail parts, breast, meat and skin, raw",	LOW	**0**
Turkey, retail parts, breast, meat and skin, with added solution, raw",	LOW	**0.03**
Turkey, retail parts, breast, meat only, cooked, roasted",	LOW	**0**
Turkey, retail parts, breast, meat only, raw",	LOW	**0**
Turkey, retail parts, breast, meat only, with added solution, cooked, roasted",	LOW	**0**
Turkey, retail parts, breast, meat only, with added solution, raw",	LOW	**0**
Turkey, retail parts, drumstick, meat and skin, cooked, roasted",	LOW	**0**

Food name/ Category (100 g)	Status	Carbs content in g
Turkey, retail parts, drumstick, meat and skin, raw",	LOW	0
Turkey, retail parts, drumstick, meat only, cooked, roasted",	LOW	0
Turkey, retail parts, drumstick, meat only, raw",	LOW	0
Turkey, retail parts, thigh, meat and skin, cooked, roasted",	LOW	0.41
Turkey, retail parts, thigh, meat and skin, raw",	LOW	0
Turkey, retail parts, thigh, meat only, cooked, roasted",	LOW	0.46
Turkey, retail parts, thigh, meat only, raw",	LOW	0
Turkey, retail parts, wing, meat and skin, cooked, roasted",	LOW	0.13
Turkey, retail parts, wing, meat and skin, raw",	LOW	0.05
Turkey, retail parts, wing, meat only, cooked, roasted",	LOW	0
Turkey, retail parts, wing, meat only, raw",	LOW	0
Turkey, skin from whole (light and dark), roasted",	LOW	0.57
Turkey, skin from whole (light and dark), with added solution, raw",	LOW	0.21
Turkey, skin from whole, (light and dark), raw",	LOW	0.16
Turkey, skin from whole, (light and dark), with added solution, roasted",	LOW	0
Turkey, skin, from retail parts, from dark meat, cooked, roasted",	LOW	0
Turkey, skin, from retail parts, from dark meat, raw",	LOW	0
Turkey, stuffing, mashed potatoes w\/gravy, assorted vegetables, frozen, microwaved",	LOW	16.32
Turkey, thigh, from whole bird, meat only, raw",	LOW	0.15
Turkey, thigh, from whole bird, meat only, roasted",	LOW	0
Turkey, thigh, from whole bird, meat only, with added solution, raw",	LOW	0.15
Turkey, thigh, from whole bird, meat only, with added solution, roasted",	LOW	0
Turkey, white, rotisserie, deli cut",	LOW	7.7
Turkey, whole, giblets, cooked, simmered",	LOW	0
Turkey, whole, giblets, raw",	LOW	0.07
Turkey, whole, meat and skin, cooked, roasted",	LOW	0.06
Turkey, whole, meat and skin, raw",	LOW	0.13
Turkey, whole, meat and skin, with added solution, raw",	LOW	0.15

Food name/ Category (100 g)	Status	Carbs content in g
Turkey, whole, meat and skin, with added solution, roasted",	LOW	0
Turkey, whole, meat only, cooked, roasted",	LOW	0
Turkey, whole, meat only, raw",	LOW	0.14
Turkey, whole, meat only, with added solution, raw",	LOW	0.14
Turkey, whole, meat only, with added solution, roasted",	LOW	0
Turkey, wing, from whole bird, meat only, raw",	LOW	0.14
Turkey, wing, from whole bird, meat only, roasted",	LOW	0
Turkey, wing, from whole bird, meat only, with added solution, raw",	LOW	0.14
Turkey, wing, from whole bird, meat only, with added solution, roasted",	LOW	0
Turkey, wing, smoked, cooked, with skin, bone removed",	LOW	0
Turkey, young hen, skin only, cooked, roasted",	LOW	0
Turnip greens and turnips, frozen, cooked, boiled, drained, with salt",	LOW	4.74
Turnip greens, canned, solids and liquids",	LOW	2.42
Turnip greens, cooked, boiled, drained, with salt",	LOW	4.36
Turnip greens, frozen, cooked, boiled, drained, with salt",	LOW	4.98
Turnip greens, raw",	LOW	7.13
Turnips, cooked, boiled, drained, with salt",	LOW	5.06
Turnips, frozen, cooked, boiled, drained, with salt",	LOW	3.73
Turnips, frozen, cooked, boiled, drained, without salt",	LOW	4.35
Turnips, raw",	LOW	6.43
Turnover, cheese-filled, tomato-based sauce, frozen, unprepared",	LOW	27.29
Turnover, chicken- or turkey-, and vegetable-filled, reduced fat, frozen",	LOW	21.74
Turnover, filled with egg, meat and cheese, frozen",	LOW	20.67
Turnover, meat- and cheese-filled, tomato-based sauce, reduced fat, frozen",	LOW	31.89
Turtle, green, raw",	LOW	0
UDI'S, Gluten Free, Classic French Dinner Rolls",	MEDIUM	55.1
UDI'S, Gluten Free, Soft & Delicious White Sandwich Bread",	MEDIUM	51.15
UDI'S, Gluten Free, Soft & Hearty Whole Grain Bread",	MEDIUM	49.09
UDI'S, Gluten Free, Whole Grain Dinner Rolls",	MEDIUM	44.29
USDA Commodity Chicken, canned, meat only, drained",	LOW	0

Food name/ Category (100 g)	Status	Carbs content in g
USDA Commodity Food, oil, vegetable, low saturated fat",	LOW	0
USDA Commodity Food, oil, vegetable, soybean, refined",	LOW	0
USDA Commodity, beef patties with VPP, frozen, cooked",	LOW	7.89
USDA Commodity, beef patties with VPP, frozen, raw",	LOW	3.84
USDA Commodity, beef, canned",	LOW	0
USDA Commodity, beef, ground bulk\/coarse ground, frozen, cooked",	LOW	0
USDA Commodity, beef, ground, bulk\/coarse ground, frozen, raw",	LOW	0
USDA Commodity, beef, patties (100%), frozen, cooked",	LOW	0.91
USDA Commodity, beef, patties (100%), frozen, raw",	LOW	0
USDA Commodity, cheese, cheddar, reduced fat",	LOW	2
USDA Commodity, chicken fajita strips, frozen",	LOW	2.23
USDA Commodity, Chicken, canned, meat only, with broth",	LOW	0.23
USDA Commodity, Chicken, canned, meat only, with water",	LOW	0
USDA Commodity, luncheon meat, canned",	LOW	1.04
USDA Commodity, Peanut Butter, smooth",	LOW	23.98
USDA Commodity, salmon nuggets, breaded, frozen, heated",	LOW	13.96
USDA Commodity, salmon nuggets, cooked as purchased, unheated",	LOW	11.85
USDA Commodity, turkey taco meat, frozen, cooked",	LOW	3.03
VAN'S, Gluten Free, Totally Original Pancakes",	MEDIUM	40.32
VAN'S, Gluten Free, Totally Original Waffles",	MEDIUM	40.54
VAN'S, The Perfect 10, Crispy Six Whole Grain + Four Seed Baked Crackers, Glut	HIGH	67.57
Vanilla extract, imitation, alcohol",	LOW	2.41
Vanilla extract, imitation, no alcohol",	LOW	14.4
Veal, Australian, rib, rib roast, separable lean and fat, raw",	LOW	1.15
Veal, Australian, rib, rib roast, separable lean only, raw",	LOW	1.4
Veal, Australian, separable fat, raw",	LOW	0
Veal, Australian, shank, fore, bone-in, separable lean and fat, raw",	LOW	0
Veal, Australian, shank, fore, bone-in, separable lean only, raw",	LOW	0
Veal, Australian, shank, hind, bone-in, separable lean and fat",	LOW	0

Food name/ Category (100 g)	Status	Carbs content in g
Veal, Australian, shank, hind, bone-in, separable lean only, raw",	LOW	0
Veal, breast, plate half, boneless, separable lean and fat, cooked, braised",	LOW	0
Veal, breast, point half, boneless, separable lean and fat, cooked, braised",	LOW	0
Veal, breast, separable fat, cooked",	LOW	0
Veal, breast, whole, boneless, separable lean and fat, cooked, braised",	LOW	0
Veal, breast, whole, boneless, separable lean and fat, raw",	LOW	0
Veal, breast, whole, boneless, separable lean only, cooked, braised",	LOW	0
Veal, composite of trimmed retail cuts, separable fat, cooked",	LOW	0
Veal, composite of trimmed retail cuts, separable lean and fat, cooked",	LOW	0
Veal, composite of trimmed retail cuts, separable lean and fat, raw",	LOW	0
Veal, composite of trimmed retail cuts, separable lean only, cooked",	LOW	0
Veal, composite of trimmed retail cuts, separable lean only, raw",	LOW	0
Veal, cubed for stew (leg and shoulder), separable lean only, cooked, braised",	LOW	0
Veal, cubed for stew (leg and shoulder), separable lean only, raw",	LOW	0
Veal, foreshank, osso buco, separable lean and fat, cooked, braised",	LOW	0.11
Veal, foreshank, osso buco, separable lean only, cooked, braised",	LOW	0
Veal, ground, cooked, broiled",	LOW	0
Veal, ground, cooked, pan-fried",	LOW	1.51
Veal, ground, raw",	LOW	0
Veal, leg (top round), separable lean and fat, cooked, braised",	LOW	0
Veal, leg (top round), separable lean and fat, cooked, pan-fried, breaded",	LOW	9.91
Veal, leg (top round), separable lean and fat, cooked, pan-fried, not breaded",	LOW	0
Veal, leg (top round), separable lean and fat, cooked, roasted",	LOW	0
Veal, leg (top round), separable lean and fat, raw",	LOW	0
Veal, leg (top round), separable lean only, cooked, braised",	LOW	0
Veal, leg (top round), separable lean only, cooked, pan-fried, breaded",	LOW	9.84
Veal, leg (top round), separable lean only, cooked, pan-fried, not breaded",	LOW	0
Veal, leg (top round), separable lean only, cooked, roasted",	LOW	0

Food name/ Category (100 g)	Status	Carbs content in g
Veal, leg (top round), separable lean only, raw",	LOW	0
Veal, leg, top round, cap off, cutlet, boneless, cooked, grilled",	LOW	0
Veal, leg, top round, cap off, cutlet, boneless, raw",	LOW	0
Veal, loin, chop, separable lean and fat, cooked, grilled",	LOW	0.16
Veal, loin, chop, separable lean only, cooked, grilled",	LOW	0.07
Veal, loin, separable lean and fat, cooked, braised",	LOW	0
Veal, loin, separable lean and fat, cooked, roasted",	LOW	0
Veal, loin, separable lean and fat, raw",	LOW	0.07
Veal, loin, separable lean only, cooked, braised",	LOW	0
Veal, loin, separable lean only, cooked, roasted",	LOW	0
Veal, loin, separable lean only, raw",	LOW	0
Veal, rib, separable lean and fat, cooked, braised",	LOW	0
Veal, rib, separable lean and fat, cooked, roasted",	LOW	0
Veal, rib, separable lean and fat, raw",	LOW	0
Veal, rib, separable lean only, cooked, braised",	LOW	0
Veal, rib, separable lean only, cooked, roasted",	LOW	0
Veal, rib, separable lean only, raw",	LOW	0
Veal, shank (fore and hind), separable lean and fat, cooked, braised",	LOW	0
Veal, shank (fore and hind), separable lean and fat, raw",	LOW	0
Veal, shank (fore and hind), separable lean only, cooked, braised",	LOW	0
Veal, shank (fore and hind), separable lean only, raw",	LOW	0
Veal, shank, separable lean and fat, raw",	LOW	0
Veal, shank, separable lean only, raw",	LOW	0
Veal, shoulder, arm, separable lean and fat, cooked, braised",	LOW	0
Veal, shoulder, arm, separable lean and fat, cooked, roasted",	LOW	0
Veal, shoulder, arm, separable lean and fat, raw",	LOW	0
Veal, shoulder, arm, separable lean only, cooked, braised",	LOW	0
Veal, shoulder, arm, separable lean only, cooked, roasted",	LOW	0

Food name/ Category (100 g)	Status	Carbs content in g
Veal, shoulder, arm, separable lean only, raw",	LOW	0
Veal, shoulder, blade chop, separable lean and fat, cooked, grilled",	LOW	0.15
Veal, shoulder, blade chop, separable lean and fat, raw",	LOW	0.03
Veal, shoulder, blade chop, separable lean only, cooked, grilled",	LOW	0
Veal, shoulder, blade chop, separable lean only, raw",	LOW	0
Veal, shoulder, blade, separable lean and fat, cooked, braised",	LOW	0
Veal, shoulder, blade, separable lean and fat, cooked, roasted",	LOW	0
Veal, shoulder, blade, separable lean only, cooked, braised",	LOW	0
Veal, shoulder, blade, separable lean only, cooked, roasted",	LOW	0
Veal, shoulder, whole (arm and blade), separable lean and fat, cooked, braised",	LOW	0
Veal, shoulder, whole (arm and blade), separable lean and fat, cooked, roasted",	LOW	0
Veal, shoulder, whole (arm and blade), separable lean and fat, raw",	LOW	0
Veal, shoulder, whole (arm and blade), separable lean only, cooked, braised",	LOW	0
Veal, shoulder, whole (arm and blade), separable lean only, cooked, roasted",	LOW	0
Veal, shoulder, whole (arm and blade), separable lean only, raw",	LOW	0
Veal, sirloin, separable lean and fat, cooked, braised",	LOW	0
Veal, sirloin, separable lean and fat, cooked, roasted",	LOW	0
Veal, sirloin, separable lean and fat, raw",	LOW	0
Veal, sirloin, separable lean only, cooked, braised",	LOW	0
Veal, sirloin, separable lean only, cooked, roasted",	LOW	0
Veal, sirloin, separable lean only, raw",	LOW	0
Veal, variety meats and by-products, brain, cooked, braised",	LOW	0
Veal, variety meats and by-products, brain, cooked, pan-fried",	LOW	0
Veal, variety meats and by-products, brain, raw",	LOW	0
Veal, variety meats and by-products, heart, cooked, braised",	LOW	0.13
Veal, variety meats and by-products, heart, raw",	LOW	0.08
Veal, variety meats and by-products, kidneys, cooked, braised",	LOW	0
Veal, variety meats and by-products, kidneys, raw",	LOW	0.85

Food name/ Category (100 g)	Status	Carbs content in g
Veal, variety meats and by-products, liver, cooked, braised",	LOW	3.77
Veal, variety meats and by-products, liver, cooked, pan-fried",	LOW	4.47
Veal, variety meats and by-products, liver, raw",	LOW	2.91
Veal, variety meats and by-products, lungs, cooked, braised",	LOW	0
Veal, variety meats and by-products, lungs, raw",	LOW	0
Veal, variety meats and by-products, pancreas, cooked, braised",	LOW	0
Veal, variety meats and by-products, pancreas, raw",	LOW	0
Veal, variety meats and by-products, spleen, cooked, braised",	LOW	0
Veal, variety meats and by-products, spleen, raw",	LOW	0
Veal, variety meats and by-products, thymus, cooked, braised",	LOW	0
Veal, variety meats and by-products, thymus, raw",	LOW	0
Veal, variety meats and by-products, tongue, cooked, braised",	LOW	0
Veal, variety meats and by-products, tongue, raw",	LOW	1.91
Vegetable juice cocktail, canned",	LOW	3.87
Vegetable juice cocktail, low sodium, canned",	LOW	3.83
Vegetable oil-butter spread, reduced calorie",	LOW	0
Vegetable oil, palm kernel",	LOW	0
Vegetables, mixed, canned, drained solids",	LOW	9.26
Vegetables, mixed, canned, solids and liquids",	LOW	7.13
Vegetables, mixed, frozen, cooked, boiled, drained, with salt",	LOW	13.09
Vegetables, mixed, frozen, unprepared",	LOW	13.47
Vegetarian fillets",	LOW	9
Vegetarian meatloaf or patties",	LOW	8
Veggie burgers or soyburgers, unprepared",	LOW	14.27
Vermicelli, made from soy",	HIGH	82.32
Vinegar, cider",	LOW	0.93
Vinegar, distilled",	LOW	0.04
Vitasoy USA Azumaya, Silken Tofu",	LOW	0.58

Food name/ Category (100 g)	Status	Carbs content in g
Vitasoy USA Nasoya, Lite Silken Tofu",	LOW	0
Vitasoy USA Organic Nasoya, Soft Tofu",	LOW	0.74
Vitasoy USA Organic Nasoya, Tofu Plus Firm",	LOW	1.71
Vitasoy USA, Organic Nasoya Extra Firm Tofu",	LOW	2.6
Vitasoy USA, Organic Nasoya Firm Tofu",	LOW	2.3
Vitasoy USA, Organic Nasoya Silken Tofu",	LOW	1.4
Vitasoy USA, Vitasoy Light Vanilla Soymilk",	LOW	4.1
Vitasoy USA, Vitasoy Organic Classic Original Soymilk",	LOW	4.5
Vitasoy USA, Vitasoy Organic Creamy Original Soymilk",	LOW	4.5
Waffle, buttermilk, frozen, ready-to-heat, microwaved",	MEDIUM	44.16
Waffle, buttermilk, frozen, ready-to-heat, toasted",	MEDIUM	48.39
Waffle, plain, frozen, ready-to-heat, microwave",	MEDIUM	45.41
Waffles, buttermilk, frozen, ready-to-heat",	MEDIUM	41.05
Waffles, chocolate chip, frozen, ready-to-heat",	MEDIUM	45.68
Waffles, gluten-free, frozen, ready-to-heat",	MEDIUM	43.05
Waffles, plain, frozen, ready -to-heat, toasted",	MEDIUM	49.29
Waffles, plain, frozen, ready-to-heat",	MEDIUM	42.98
Waffles, plain, prepared from recipe",	LOW	32.9
Waffles, whole wheat, lowfat, frozen, ready-to-heat",	MEDIUM	49.16
Wasabi",	MEDIUM	46.13
Water, bottled, generic",	LOW	0
Water, bottled, non-carbonated, NAYA",	LOW	0
Watercress, raw",	LOW	1.29
Watermelon, raw",	LOW	7.55
Waxgourd, (chinese preserving melon), cooked, boiled, drained, with salt",	LOW	2.45
Waxgourd, (chinese preserving melon), cooked, boiled, drained, without salt",	LOW	3.04
Waxgourd, (chinese preserving melon), raw",	LOW	3
WEND'YS, Crispy Chicken Sandwich",	LOW	26.36
WENDY'S, Chicken Nuggets",	LOW	14.31
WENDY'S, CLASSIC DOUBLE, with cheese",	LOW	11.71
WENDY'S, DAVE'S Hot 'N Juicy 1\/4 LB, single",	LOW	17.73
WENDY'S, Double Stack, with cheese",	LOW	15.35
WENDY'S, Frosty Dairy Dessert",	LOW	23.62

Food name/ Category (100 g)	Status	Carbs content in g
WENDY'S, Homestyle Chicken Fillet Sandwich",	LOW	21.55
WENDY'S, Ultimate Chicken Grill Sandwich",	LOW	18.88
Whale, beluga, meat, dried (Alaska Native)",	LOW	0
Wheat bran, crude",	HIGH	64.51
Wheat flour, white, all-purpose, enriched, bleached",	HIGH	76.31
Wheat flour, white, all-purpose, enriched, calcium-fortified",	HIGH	76.31
Wheat flour, white, all-purpose, enriched, unbleached",	HIGH	76.31
Wheat flour, white, all-purpose, self-rising, enriched",	HIGH	74.22
Wheat flour, white, all-purpose, unenriched",	HIGH	76.31
Wheat flour, white, bread, enriched",	HIGH	72.53
Wheat flour, white, cake, enriched",	HIGH	78.03
Wheat flour, white, tortilla mix, enriched",	HIGH	67.14
Wheat flour, whole-grain",	HIGH	71.97
Wheat flours, bread, unenriched",	HIGH	72.53
Wheat, durum",	HIGH	71.13
Wheat, hard red spring",	HIGH	68.03
Wheat, hard red winter",	HIGH	71.18
Wheat, hard white",	HIGH	75.9
Wheat, KAMUT khorasan, uncooked",	HIGH	70.58
Wheat, soft red winter",	HIGH	74.24
Wheat, soft white",	HIGH	75.36
Whey, acid, dried",	HIGH	73.45
Whey, acid, fluid",	LOW	5.12
Whey, sweet, dried",	HIGH	74.46
Whey, sweet, fluid",	LOW	5.14
Whipped cream substitute, dietetic, made from powdered mix",	LOW	10.6
Whipped topping, frozen, low fat",	LOW	23.6
Wild rice, cooked",	LOW	21.34
Winged bean, immature seeds, cooked, boiled, drained, with salt",	LOW	3.21
Winged beans, immature seeds, cooked, boiled, drained, without salt",	LOW	3.21
Winged beans, immature seeds, raw",	LOW	4.31
Winged beans, mature seeds, cooked, boiled, with salt",	LOW	14.94
Winged beans, mature seeds, raw",	MEDIUM	41.71
Wonton wrappers (includes egg roll wrappers)",	HIGH	57.9
WORTHINGTON Chic-Ketts, frozen, unprepared",	LOW	5.1
WORTHINGTON Chili, canned, unprepared",	LOW	10.9
WORTHINGTON Choplets, canned, unprepared",	LOW	4.1
WORTHINGTON Diced Chik, canned, unprepared",	LOW	3.7
WORTHINGTON Dinner Roast, frozen, unprepared",	LOW	6.9

Food name/ Category (100 g)	Status	Carbs content in g
WORTHINGTON FriChik Original, canned, unprepared",	LOW	3.4
WORTHINGTON FriPats, frozen, unprepared",	LOW	8
WORTHINGTON Leanies, frozen, unprepared",	LOW	6.1
WORTHINGTON Low Fat Fri Chik, canned, unprepared",	LOW	4.9
WORTHINGTON Low Fat Veja-Links, canned, unprepared",	LOW	4.3
WORTHINGTON Meatless Chicken Roll, frozen, unprepared",	LOW	4.3
WORTHINGTON Meatless Corned Beef Roll, frozen, unprepared",	LOW	9.9
WORTHINGTON Multigrain Cutlets, canned, unprepared",	LOW	7.3
WORTHINGTON Prime Stakes, canned, unprepared",	LOW	7.5
WORTHINGTON Prosage Links, frozen, unprepared",	LOW	5
WORTHINGTON Prosage Roll, frozen, unprepared",	LOW	6
WORTHINGTON Saucettes, canned, unprepared",	LOW	5.6
WORTHINGTON Smoked Turkey Roll, frozen, unprepared",	LOW	7.9
WORTHINGTON Stakelets, frozen, unprepared",	LOW	9.6
WORTHINGTON Stripples, frozen, unprepared",	LOW	14.3
WORTHINGTON Super Links, canned, unprepared",	LOW	5.5
WORTHINGTON Vegetable Skallops, canned, unprepared",	LOW	4.6
WORTHINGTON Vegetable Steaks, canned, unprepared",	LOW	5.1
WORTHINGTON Vegetarian Burger, canned, unprepared",	LOW	6.2
WORTHINGTON Veja-Links, canned, unprepared",	LOW	4.1
Yachtwurst, with pistachio nuts, cooked",	LOW	1.4
Yam, cooked, boiled, drained, or baked, with salt",	LOW	26.99
Yambean (jicama), raw",	LOW	8.82
Yardlong bean, cooked, boiled, drained, with salt",	LOW	9.17
Yardlong bean, cooked, boiled, drained, without salt",	LOW	9.18
Yardlong bean, raw",	LOW	8.35
Yardlong beans, mature seeds, cooked, boiled, with salt",	LOW	21.09
Yardlong beans, mature seeds, cooked, boiled, without salt",	LOW	21.09

Food name/ Category (100 g)	Status	Carbs content in g
Yeast extract spread",	LOW	20.42
Yellow rice with seasoning, dry packet mix, unprepared",	HIGH	74.68
Yogurt parfait, lowfat, with fruit and granola",	LOW	15.86
Yogurt, chocolate, nonfat milk, fortified with vitamin D",	LOW	23.53
Yogurt, chocolate, nonfat milk",	LOW	23.53
Yogurt, frozen, flavors not chocolate, nonfat milk, with low-calorie sweetener",	LOW	19.7
Yogurt, fruit variety, nonfat, fortified with vitamin D",	LOW	19
Yogurt, fruit variety, nonfat",	LOW	19
Yogurt, fruit, low fat, 10 grams protein per 8 ounce, fortified with vitamin D",	LOW	19.05
Yogurt, fruit, low fat, 10 grams protein per 8 ounce",	LOW	19.05
Yogurt, fruit, low fat, 11 grams protein per 8 ounce",	LOW	18.6
Yogurt, fruit, low fat, 9 grams protein per 8 ounce, fortified with vitamin D",	LOW	18.64
Yogurt, fruit, low fat, 9 grams protein per 8 ounce",	LOW	18.64
Yogurt, fruit, lowfat, with low calorie sweetener, fortified with vitamin D",	LOW	18.6
Yogurt, fruit, lowfat, with low calorie sweetener",	LOW	18.6
Yogurt, Greek, nonfat, vanilla, CHOBANI",	LOW	8.09
Yogurt, Greek, plain, nonfat",	LOW	3.6
Yogurt, plain, low fat, 12 grams protein per 8 ounce",	LOW	7.04
Yogurt, plain, skim milk, 13 grams protein per 8 ounce",	LOW	7.68
Yogurt, plain, whole milk, 8 grams protein per 8 ounce",	LOW	4.66
Yogurt, vanilla flavor, lowfat milk, sweetened with low calorie sweetener",	LOW	13.8
Yogurt, vanilla or lemon flavor, nonfat milk, sweetened with low-calorie sweetener, fortified with vitamin D",	LOW	7.5
Yogurt, vanilla or lemon flavor, nonfat milk, sweetened with low-calorie sweetener",	LOW	7.5
Yogurt, vanilla, low fat, 11 grams protein per 8 ounce, fortified with vitamin D",	LOW	13.8
Yogurt, vanilla, low fat, 11 grams protein per 8 ounce",	LOW	13.8
Yogurt, vanilla, non-fat",	LOW	17.04
Yokan, prepared from adzuki beans and sugar",	HIGH	60.72
Zwieback",	HIGH	74.2

Made in the USA
Las Vegas, NV
08 June 2022